ROAD TO RECOVERY

FROM

PARKINSONS DISEASE

Natural Therapies that help people with Parkinsons reverse their symptoms

ROBERT RODGERS, Ph.D.

PARKINSONS RECOVERY

WWW.PARKINSONSRECOVERY.COM

© 2013 Parkinsons Recovery

Parkinsons Recovery provides support, information and resources to individuals who have the symptoms of Parkinson's disease. Road to Recovery from Parkinsons Disease reports discoveries from interviews and reviews of the research literature on Parkinsons Disease.

TABLE OF CONTENTS

© 2013 Parkinsons Recovery

© 2013 Parkinsons Recovery

© 2013 Parkinsons Recovery

© 2013 Parkinsons Recovery

© 2013 Parkinsons Recovery

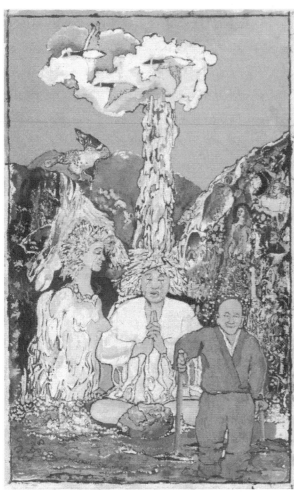

Entering the Stream (2005), Michael Sawyer

INTRODUCTION

Why do I provide support, information and resources for persons who have the symptoms of Parkinson's disease? My mother was diagnosed with Parkinson's. She suffered from several of the common symptoms including depression, mental confusion, mobility challenges and illegible handwriting.

At the end of her life she was taking a huge number of prescription medications that were causing horrible side effects. I urged her to cut back on medications she took daily, but to no avail. She died from a stroke after being kept alive on life support for 60 days.

My uncle Gordon was diagnosed with Parkinson's disease 15 years ago and died in 2009 from what was reported to be complications of the condition. He donated his body to the Harvard Medical School for research purposes. I recently learned that Harvard researchers determined that Gordon had Hepatitis C, not Parkinson's. That discovery is consistent with my research findings that as many as three-fourth of persons who have been diagnosed with Parkinson's disease actually have something else wrong.

© 2013 Parkinsons Recovery

I do not have Parkinson's myself. But if I did, I would pursue a wide variety of diagnostic protocols to assess the causes and pursue therapies that are offered by medical specialties such as Biophoton therapy, BioAcoustic therapy, quantum healing, homeopathy, craniosacral therapy, acupressure, herbs, essential oils, Bach Flower essences, aromatherapy, light therapy, hypnotherapy, vocal profiling, Emotional Freedom Technique, Alexander Technique, Healing Touch, Reiki, psychics – and this is a short list!

I would also elect to eat live food that my body needs to recover and exercise regularly. I believe in my heart that recovery from any disease is possible and have set my intention to document story after story of recovery from the symptoms of Parkinsons. I thus document the specialties that offer the possibility of relief.

Many health care providers believe that "Parkinson's Disease" is degenerative. Isn't that a horrible word - degenerative? Many people believe that it is "progressive," meaning the symptoms will continually get worse. Government publications say Parkinson's is "progressive." Most web sites with a focus on Parkinson's also declare this to be true.

Such thought forms are clearly not the foundation for launching yourself on a road to recovery. More importantly, these beliefs are blatantly false. Symptoms are signals that something is out of balance in the body itself. The body thus may be deficient in some essential building blocks, or it may be overloaded and overwhelmed with pathogens, bacteria or viruses of one form or another.

Recovery is possible as long as the body is given the support it needs to heal. Eating live foods helps. Finding ways to relieve stress helps. Eliminating toxins helps. Identifying negative thoughts that lie at the root of imbalances in the body and replacing them with positive thought forms helps. There may also be reasons for the condition that are rooted in the family system that may need to be cleared. With a little help the body can be brought back into balance.

I also believe recovery is possible now and have been experimenting with one approach or another to discover what makes that happen. It is possible to find relief from the symptoms of Parkinsons. Recovery is possible. At a minimum, relief of symptoms is a sure bet. There is no "cure" from any disease state of the body, but the body always knows how to heal itself.

You will find discussions in this book about therapies, supplements and other treatments that my research has shown help people get relief from their symptoms.

You will not find a lengthy biography of research references at the end of my book. Some of my published work includes bibliographies which are as long as the article itself! I am personally not convinced bibliographies accomplish much other than to convince people you have researched the relevant literature. After a few months, these references become quickly

© 2013 Parkinsons Recovery

outdated. Of course, science works at such a snail's pace that it does not matter if your references are outdated.

If you want back up data or information for any assertion I make in my book, please do your own research. If you question any assertion I make here, check it out. The internet is now sophisticated enough that you can find answers to virtually any question by typing the question in your search engine. Type in the full question you want to ask and see what web sites come up.

What you will find here is the wisdom about treating Parkinson's with natural methods from persons I have interviewed over the past six years. I also offer summary conclusions about the research in general which I have reviewed extensively.

When I quote a person (whether they are a health care practitioner or individual with the symptoms of Parkinsons), the quote is often taken from an interview I did with that person on my radio program. I provide a link. Click on the link to locate the interview. You can listen to the full interview of any person I have interviewed in the event you are interested in discovering more about what any person I have quoted has to say. I have extracted jewels from the interviews. You will find a huge reservoir of insight, help and wisdom by listening to the full interviews if you have not already done so.

I also want to be clear about what you will not find in my book. You will not find discussions about medications or surgeries. There are two reasons. First, there are excellent books and resources already available that can answer any question you might have about medications and treatments that are prescribed by the western medicine specialty. These books are authored by knowledgeable and highly trained medical doctors who have spent years learning about the effects of various medications, when to prescribe them and for what symptoms.

Second, I am not a medical doctor. I am not qualified to address issues you may be having with medications or surgeries. Please find answers to your questions about medications, diagnoses and treatment by consulting your medical doctor. It is imperative that you consult with your doctor and other health care providers before deciding to use any therapy, treatment or approach that is discussed in Road to Recovery.

Road to Recovery from Parkinsons Disease is all about helping you help yourself.

Robert Rodgers, Ph.D.
Parkinsons Recovery
Olympia, Washington

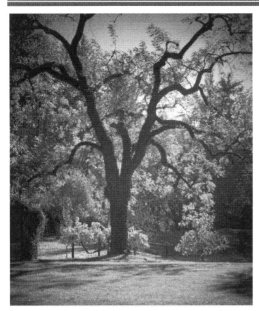

Tree of Life by Cindy Deluz[1]

RECOVERY IS POSSIBLE

Here is the simple truth. People recover from Parkinson's when they hold the belief that recovery is possible. People who believe their health will improve do improve. They take responsibility for their own health and well being and commit to a program that gives their body the support it needs to heal. They take control over their health and wellness.

Consciously or unconsciously many persons with Parkinson's hold the opposite belief. They believe recovery is impossible. They believe every year they will become more and more physically debilitated. They are convinced they have a "disease" and that their health is destined to deteriorate over time. Perhaps the deterioration will be slow, but deterioration at any pace is unavoidable. They believe that their body is broken and needs to be fixed through drugs or surgeries.

Thousands of research articles exist that evaluate the effectiveness of one treatment or another on the symptoms of persons with Parkinson's. Most of this research is funded by the pharmaceutical industry and consists of evaluating the effectiveness of one drug or another. This literature converges on the proposition that the health of persons with Parkinson's decline on average 3-4% each year.

---

[1] "I had the pleasure of greeting that beautiful tree at a ranch near the coastline in California a few months ago. Almost named the shot, "Guardian of the Grounds"...but somehow that wise old tree gave me a sense of hope, strength and endurance, so the "Tree of Life" it was." Cindy Deluz

Virtually every published source of information on Parkinson's states that it is a "progressive" disease, meaning once an individual is diagnosed with the condition, they always get worse, year after year.

When we actually examine the studies that track people who take prescription medications, there is an interesting finding that is consistent across studies. Ten percent of people with Parkinson's on average do not get worse over time. Thus, even the drug studies report that deterioration over time does not happen for 10% of people with Parkinson's symptoms.

People do recover from Parkinson's. People do feel better when they begin to take care of their body. The body is a miracle that can always heal itself when given the proper support.

EVIDENCE FOR RECOVERY

By recovery I do not mean to suggest that the condition is "cured" but that there is sustained relief from the symptoms of Parkinson's. I have a number of reasons for believing this to be true.

First, people are recovering. Relief from symptoms happens. People have done it. People are doing it. A few are symptom free. Many have found one way or another to get sustained relief from their symptoms.

I conducted an informal survey of persons with Parkinsons who subscribe to my free newsletter. The question respondents answered was: *Since Thanksgiving last year –have you been feeling better, the same or worse overall?* Thirty-six percent (36%) reported that they have been feeling better overall and thirty four percent (34%) reported they were feeling about the same. Two thirds were not worse as is presumed to occur with people who have been diagnosed with Parkinson's. The expectation that persons with Parkinson's symptoms will feel worse over time – often spoken as a condition that is "degenerative" - is an expectation that is not supported by any of the research I have done.

I interviewed Daniel Newman, MD, ND, who has a unique set of qualifications. He is a medical doctor, a naturopath doctor and is qualified in Chinese Medicine. Here is what Daniel Newman told me about his experience with Parkinson's during an interview November 13, 2009.

> *"In my experience I have seen cases where - when Parkinson's patients are diagnosed and treated fairly early - that their disease can be arrested and in some cases reversed. I don't want to be flip about it and say that is true in all cases.*
>
> *Depending on how long the case has been in force and how severe the case is, it may not be possible to reverse it beyond a certain extent… But in people who are diagnosed -*

particularly if they manage to get an integrative treatment approach in force early on in their disease process - I have seen a number of cases where it has been arrested and other cases where it has actually been reversed."

Second, my research with people who have Parkinson's has shown that relief from symptoms is possible.

PARKINSONS ENERGY PROJECT (PEP)

Zero Point Healers in collaboration with Ann Egerton conducted a study in Portland, Oregon in 2006 involving 11 individuals who had been diagnosed with Parkinson's disease. The study volunteers were all members of a support group who preferred not to take Parkinson's medications.

The study involved 6 craniosacral sessions with each participant and three group sessions over a four month period. Craniosacral therapy and energy healing is a gentle way to invite the body to release the trauma that is lodged in the tissues.

Of the 62 symptoms that were tracked, improvement from the baseline to the post-test was seen in 41, no change was seen in 5 and 16 of the symptoms got worse. This means that for 74.2% of the symptoms, study volunteers either improved or stayed the same. This startling finding is clearly contrary to the standard belief that individuals with Parkinson's experience increasing difficulty with symptoms over time.

Symptoms that did get worse over time may be a natural consequence of unwinding that occurs when trauma is released from the body. The energy work combined with the craniosacral therapy focused on helping each study volunteer release the physical, mental and emotional stress that was trapped in the tissues of their body.

When the body begins to unwind, muscle spasms, weakness in muscles, pain in joints, overall body weakness and more tremoring can be a consequence. Unwinding is a physical process. People thus often experience different and sometimes unpleasant sensations, even occasional pain, before they feel better. The unpleasant sensations are temporary.

Symptoms of weakness in the body and even pain are unpleasant to experience, yet they can be a natural consequence of the healing process. In the process of healing any condition, it is sometimes the case that a person will feel worse before they begin to feel better. The journey of recovery is clearly not pain free.

John Coleman, ND is a naturopath doctor from Australia who himself had an advanced stage of Parkinsons in 1996. He is symptom free today. I interviewed John and asked him how he came to the realization he could get better when all indications were that he would get worse. Here is his answer:

> *"I didn't know. I had no indication that I could get better. What I knew was that I had to make each day better than the last because I couldn't survive the way I was."*

> *"I set about achieving something every day. Survival was a good thing each day. Because frankly Robert, I thought I was dying, as did many people around me."*

> *"I knew it was my responsibility to make a choice to fade away or to make each day better. No one else could do it for me and there was no one else around who was willing to do it for me."*

> *"I just survived each day and did the best I could. I kept journals. Over a long period of time I started to see, reading my journals, that I was actually making improvements in my health. That gave me some hope to make each day a bit better than the last."*

The Parkinson's Energy Project study evidence confirmed John's personal experience. The road to recovery is typically riddled with potholes. Ups and downs are the norm. It helps enormously to record and track your progress.

RADIO PROGRAM GUESTS

I sponsor a weekly internet radio program – the Parkinsons Recovery Radio Network [http://www.blogtalkradio.com/parkinsons-recovery]. Different guests are interviewed each week. Some have the symptoms of Parkinsons and discuss what they are doing to reverse them. Others are health care practitioners, including medical doctors, naturopaths, homeopaths, bio-acoustic researchers, neural feedback practitioners, physical therapists, psychologists, herbalists, aroma therapists, neuro-linguistic programming (NLP) therapists, hypnotherapists, music therapists, energy healers, etc.

All Parkinsons Recovery radio programs are archived. You can download any program for free and hear for yourself what people are doing for themselves to recover by visiting http://www.blogtalkradio.com/parkinsons-recovery. The Radio Show website has 18 pages of shows. Each page of the 18 total pages contains three months of shows. Scroll down to the bottom of the first page of the Radio Show and you will find an advance arrow button where you can scroll back to previous show listings.

Alternatively, you can download any of the programs for free from http://www.itunes.com. Once you arrive on the Itunes website, search for "Parkinsons Recovery." Click on the icon for Parkinsons Recovery and the full listing of radio shows will be shown. Download any of the shows of interest.

© 2013 Parkinsons Recovery

You will hear remarkable stories on the various Parkinsons Recovery radio programs from people with the symptoms of Parkinsons who are leading vibrant, exciting and very active lives. Many of my interviewees tell me that the best years of their life began the day they were diagnosed with the symptoms of Parkinson's. You will hear this sentiment expressed in virtually all of my radio program interviews.

Pioneers of Recovery is a collection of interviews with individuals that have the symptoms of Parkinsons who found ways to reverse their symptoms. Two books have emerged – the first Pioneers of Recovery was published in 2009. The second was released in 2012. Many therapies, treatments and approaches are documented in the two books. You can listen to clips of my interviews with the 2009 pioneers that aired May 28, 2009 and to the 2012 pioneers that aired November 4, 2011.

JOHN BALL is the author of Living Well, Running Hard: Lessons Learned from Living with Parkinson's Disease. He was diagnosed with Parkinson's in June, 1983 ten years after experiencing early onset symptoms in his twenties. He has competed in 22 marathon races. Johns remains healthy, vibrant and active. Don't take my word for it. You can listen to my interview with John Ball that aired July 23, 2009.

JOHN CARLIN has recruited a medical team of ten individuals from a wide variety of specialties who provide him with the support he needs in his personal recovery program. Diagnosed in 2003, John road a tandem bike across the state of Iowa to raise money for Parkinsons Research in 2009. My initial interview with John Carlin aired on October 22, 2009. A follow-up interview aired on November 17, 2010 when he talked about his three week trip to Italy and his climb up Mount Kilimanjaro with Nan Little in the summer of 2011.

NAN LITTLE has benefited enormously from forced exercise, so much so that she is now a consultant to hospitals and health care facilities that are establishing forced exercise clinics for persons who currently experience the symptoms of Parkinson's. Nan talks about the incredible successes she has witnessed with forced exercise during my radio show that aired on November 10, 2010.

JOHN COLEMAN, ND, is a naturopathic doctor from Australia. John was diagnosed with Stage IV Parkinson's in 1995. Using a combination of natural therapies that his body needed to return to a state of health and wellness, John fully recovered in three and a half years. JOHN COLEMAN, ND attributes his recovery to a sound nutritional program, exercise, homeopathic treatments for dehydration (the Aquas), and a form of body work known as Bowen therapy which releases trauma that is trapped in the tissues of the body.

John helps many people in Australia and around the world who have Parkinson's. He tells me that a survey of 59 clients treated at his clinic for 1 to 4 years indicated that 56 showed a significant improvement in their symptoms while reducing medication usage, 2 got no worse but did not improve, while one got a little worse.

In addition, 3 clients and one colleague have completely recovered from diagnosed PD ranging from stage 1.5 to stage 4.5 on the Hoehn and Yahr scale. Those are pretty good odds for a world that believes people who have been diagnosed with Parkinson's are destined to get worse, not better. For more information about John Coleman listen to my radio show interview with him that aired July 16, 2009.

LEIF OGARD - author of I Have Parkinsons but Parkinsons Does Not Have Me - feels great, not just "good" but great. Most people without Parkinson's can't say this! He has incalculable energy. Leif owns his own business which he started after his diagnosis. By the way, his business is thriving. Leif is healthy in every respect. Don't take my word for it. You can listen to my interview with Leif that aired June 18, 2009.

WHIT DESCHNER, author of the award winning book, Travels With A Kayak talks about his experience with Parkinson's and his formula for remaining healthy, strong and active. Whit also explains the rules for the Salt Lick Contest. The contest is open for entries, though the salt licks must be sculptured by animals (not humans). You can listen to my interview with Whit Deschner that aired July 9, 2009.

LEE BENDER, eighty-three year old dairy farmer, entrepreneur and writer, has had a remarkable reversal of his symptoms using the SMART Lounge, a therapy that helps to reenergize the body-mind connection. Get a great preview of everything Lee is doing these days by visiting his website [http:www.leebender.org]. Listen to my interview with Lee on the Parkinsons Recovery radio program and you will hear a remarkable story of hope and recovery. My initial interview with Lee Bender aired August 13, 2009. Information about the vibration therapy that Lee raved can be seen by visiting: http://www.vibrationtherapy.org

In a follow-up interview that was aired on March 4, 2010 Lee reports he continues to get unbelievable results from using Vibration Therapy that is helping restore, rejuvenate and regenerate the neurological connections between his mind and his body. Lee is now helping other people with Parkinson's at his nursing home hop onto the road to recovery. The Vibration Therapy Lee raved about during both radio shows is being studied this year by Rush Medical Center researchers.

MARY PAUER shares her recent experience with Deep Brain Stimulation and with a wide variety of healing modalities, including Emotional Freedom Technique (EFT), Reiki, massage, Bowen Therapy, chiropractic care, hypnotherapy, psychic readings and the SMART lounge. Find discussions of her experiences on her blog and see her artwork. My interview with Mary Pauer aired July 30, 2009.

© 2013 Parkinsons Recovery

CAROL MEENAN, Senior Advisor with the Parkinsons Action Network, is about as active as a human being can get these days. On my radio show October 8, 2009 Carol talked in detail about her experience with Deep Brain Stimulation which has helped her to reduce the medications she takes, lift the heaviness in her chest and regain her sense of smell. Since being diagnosed, Carol has discovered her awesome gifts as a poet and songwriter. She read a number of her delightful poems on the radio program.

DANIEL LONEY is virtually symptom free today. During the initial years after his diagnosis, he struggled with his symptoms. Daniel found the answer in Tai Chi, a practice he had initially given up after being diagnosed and experiencing rapid deterioration. Daniel tells the fascinating story of his recovery during my radio program on December 3, 2009.

HOLLY HUGHES was diagnosed with early onset Parkinson's in 2009. She has discovered several fascinating therapies that are offering her incredible relief from her symptoms. Holly also raves about the SMART lounge (as does Lee Bender). She offers opportunities for anyone with Parkinson's who lives in the Chicago area to receive therapeutic sessions on the SMART lounge in her clinic offices for free. Holly is committed to helping others with Parkinson's join her on the road to recovery. To hear a smashing interview, scroll down the Parkinsons Recovery radio program page [www.blogtalkradio.com/parkinsons-recovery] to locate two radio shows that featured Holly as my guest that aired February 18, 2010 and May 18, 2011.

SANDRA from Tennessee gets unbelievable relief from her symptoms from taking a drop or two of a tincture formulated from the tops of dried fava bean plant tops. Sandra's story does not stop here. She grows her own fava beans, harvests them and makes the tincture herself. Her tincture gives her consistent relief from her symptoms. Listen to the radio program to find out how she makes her tincture. Sandra is able to get relief from her symptoms day in and day out the natural way. Her radio show aired February 4, 2010.

Sandra is getting dead serious about her fava bean project. She purchased four acres of Tennessee farm land in 2010 to grow fava beans, mucuna and other herbs that are useful for treating the symptoms of Parkinson's. If you are thinking about growing your own fava beans it would be a good idea to connect with Sandra though the Parkinsons Recovery fava bean blog at: http://www.favabeans.parkinsonsrecovery.com

KAREN has had a remarkable recovery over the past several years. She talks about therapies that have made a huge difference in providing her with relief from the symptoms of Parkinson's. Karen also talks about therapies that are absolutely free and easy to do. If you ever find yourself questioning whether recovery is possible, Karen will put all of your doubts to rest. My interview with Karen aired on Parkinsons Recovery radio program January 7, 2010.

GITA FENDELMAN**Error! Bookmark not defined.** is a certified Laughter Yoga Teacher. Diagnosed with Parkinson's disease in 2004, Gita is still laughing today. Laughter Yoga is a therapy that gifted her with a profound relief from her symptoms. Gita's web site has a wealth of great information about laughter yoga and how you can make dopamine by laughing for the health of it. The only medicine she gives herself is the natural medicine of laughter. My interview with Gita on the Parkinsons Recovery radio show aired April 8, 2010.

RICHARD LONDON was diagnosed with Parkinson's disease two years after his cancer surgery. He has his commercial pilot's license, is a third degree black belt and has practiced martial arts for over two decades. Author of A Handbook for Life: A Practical Guide to Success and Happiness, Richard is a motivational speaker and entrepreneur who just happens to currently have the symptoms of Parkinson's. His handbook for life seminars are transformational. My radio show with Richard London aired on December 1, 2010.

HEATHER MACTAVISH, diagnosed with Parkinson's in 1995, founded the New Rhythms Foundation in 1998. She uses drumming, music and song to help herself and others heal and recover from the symptoms of Parkinson's. Here is what Heather has to say about the value of drumming to her recovery on her website:

> "When she drummed, amazing things happened: the pain in her body lessened; it became easier to move her arm; her depression decreased, and while she was drumming, her hand tremor disappeared. She also found that the drug that she was taking, Sinemet, which helped the body produce Dopamine, could be reduced. After four years of drumming, she was able to half her dosage from eight to four pills per day. Heather felt that "before the Parkinson's disease was all-consuming... now it was like wearing glasses."

Heather combines creativity, science and art with spirit, acceptance and humor. Her radio show aired April 22, 2010.

MARILYN MURRAY announced she "is recovering" during my show on May 13, 2010. She is now in charge of Parkinson's rather than it being in charge of her. Marilyn exercises regularly with Chi Gong and Somantics, takes Mucuna to support her prescription medications, receives craniosacral therapy, gives and receives Healing Touch treatments and meditates daily. She underwent Deep Brain Stimulation surgery in 2012 to facilitate the effectiveness of the medications she is currently taking.

JOHN GOLD says that the therapy which helps him the most is to ride on his stationery bike for the equivalent of 10 miles a day. His positive attitude and prayer work have also made a huge difference, as have regular singing lessons that have insured that his voice is strong and vibrant which you will hear when you listen to my radio show interview with him on May 13, 2010.

ELIZABETH reported during my show on May 27, 2010 that her neurologist told her to con doing everything she was doing because she was better now than when she was first diag. 18 years ago. What does Elizabeth do? She does regular exercises through Curves, is a member of a singing group, makes picture albums for her children, participates in Parkinson's research studies, maintains a positive attitude and plans her day ahead of time to minimize stress.

DAVE believes it is important to be open to the expression of symptoms, however, that might be revealed. He recounts a 9 day hike he took across the Olympic Mountains in Washington state during the show on May 27, 2010 and offered advice for medical doctors who treat Parkinson's. If he were a medical doctor who treats Parkinson's, the first thing Dave would do for his patients is to write out a prescription for walking.

SUE RICHARDS has developed her own recovery program since being diagnosed in November, 2007. She has gone from using a wheelchair and walker to being able to walk without any aid whatsoever. Sue discusses the therapies that have helped her recover during my radio show on September 16, 2010. One of the therapies in particular that has been helpful for her is Forceless Spontaneous Release, a form of Chinese Acupressure known as Yin Tui Na.

Sue maintains a post menopausal blog [http://www.mymenopauseblog.com] and contributes photographs to a superb photographic blog: http://www.blogguelph.com. If you need to have an uplift of your mood visit her photographic blogs. The pictures are stunning.

In the early stages of her recovery program a few of Sue's friends designed a website which made it possible for her friends to support her recovery program through a single donation or automatic monthly donations of $10 or $20 through the Paypal secure online payment system. By way of example, here is the link to her website: http://www.helpingfriends.ca/supportsue Sue suggests that anyone currently in need of assistance consider using this approach as a useful mechanism to raise funds to support a recovery program. Obviously, the support Sue has received has helped her enormously. She has also had to learn how to be more open and willing to receive help in the form of monetary donations. Sue says that her decision to accept help from her friends in itself has made a huge difference to her recovery.

PAMELA QUINN danced professionally for 20 years with ODC/San Francisco and with actor/writer Michael O'Connor before being diagnosed with Parkinson's disease at age 42. She made a video entitled 'Welcome to our World' which shared first prize at the 2010 World Parkinson's Congress. Pamela discusses an amazing range of creative movements, exercises and dances on my show September 30, 2010 that have helped her and many other people cope with the symptoms of Parkinson's Disease.

ANGELA WENSLEY discusses on October 29, 2010 a variety of natural and safe therapies that have made a huge difference to her recovery including Myofascial Release (MFR), tennis, kick

© 2013 Parkinsons Recovery

boxing, exercise, nutrition, cranial electro-stimulation, Hakomi and intramuscular stimulation (IMS).

CHERYL shares her excitement on October 21, 2010 about a dental appliance she is using to correct for Temporomandibular Disorders (TMD or misalignments in the jaw bone). She has been getting profound relief from her symptoms which she discusses in the December 2010 issue of the Parkinsons Recovery Magazine.

JOHN BAUMANN, Adjunct Law Professor at the University of Louisville and widely known as the Inspiring Esquire, knows just about everything there is to know about living well with Parkinson's and the power of the positive. He offered an inspiring explanation of the 12 critical steps to success during my radio show that aired November 3, 2010. The steps apply to any goal, including recovery from the symptoms of Parkinsons which he has applied personally with remarkable success. John married Bernadette Baumann in 2011 and both he and Bernadette were guests on my show November 14, 2012. His progress on the road to recovery has been nothing short of miraculous thanks in large part to Bernadette's support and guidance in the all important areas of supporting his nutritional intake and motivating him to exercise regularly.

GORD SUMMER, former owner and operator of hotels, traces his symptoms back to 1999. Martial arts instructor and master scuba diver, Gord is more active today than ever. He considers Parkinson's a new lease on life.

Gord reported during my radio show on December 29, 2010 that martial arts had been the most powerful tool for harnessing his symptoms. He uses his martial arts skills to move energy from one part of his body to another for the purpose of revitalizing and regenerating the weak side of his body that happens to be on a temporary vacation – whether it is a finger, hand, arm or foot. For example, if he happens to be having difficulty using his fork with his right hand at the dinner table, Gord uses his breath and intention to transfer energy from his good side (the left) to his lazy right side. Presto – his right hand begins functioning normally again. It is quite magical and works every time. Gord explains precisely how to make this happen during the radio show.

Gord has also found that maintaining a state of calmness, sustaining a positive attitude, practicing tai chi and pushing his body to the point of exhaustion are factors that, taken together, contribute to his excellent health today. What advice does he offer?

> *"Don't mothball yourself in a glass cabinet. Parkinsons is a new lease on life if you stay active, defiant and stubborn"*

RICHARD SECKLIN, author of Parkinson's Disease – Looking Down the Barrel, was once the national gold classic bodybuilding champion, a health club owner and a career Texas law

enforcement officer. He quit his career as a law enforcement officer and found himself
down the barrel of a gun contemplating suicide. Rick is a true survivor living with Parkin
He offers specific suggestions on how to find the best doctors for your medical team on ...,
show that aired December 22, 2010.

HOWARD SHIFKE was diagnosed in November of 2009 with a full complement of the symptoms
neurologists use to diagnose and treat Parkinson's. Howard decided to use a holistic approach
to address his symptoms. Instead of numbing his symptoms with medications, he listened to
them. He found that the issue in his body was electrical, not chemical and took positive steps to
address the full range of neurological challenges he faced. For a play by play description of his
program of recovery, listen to both radio shows with Howard as my guest on March 15, 2011
and March 30, 2011.

BIANCA MOLLE found answers to her challenges through a regular practice of GiGong. Fully
recovered today, Bianca offers coaching services to persons with Parkinsons symptoms who are
interested in connecting with someone who has traveled down the road to recovery. Bianca
writes an awesome blog. Her writing and insights are spectacular. Bianca's radio show aired
June 15, 2011.

Songwriter Singer Arlon Bennett's music has won a number of music awards over the years. He
played to the first time his song, Consider the Possibilities, at the 2012 Parkinsons Recovery
Summit in Cincinnati. Arlon plays a number of his amazing songs from this album on my radio
show December 5, 2012.

LIDIA EPP is a molecular biologist who is proficient in biochemistry and clinical molecular
diagnostics. Her former husband had been diagnosed with Parkinsons Disease several years
before she developed symptoms of Parkinson's. She found this connection curious. After her
new husband began to experience Parkinson's symptoms, Lidia concluded the root cause was a
Candida infection that the three of them had in common. This speculation motivated her to get
serious about doing a Candida cleanse. After she and her new husband did a cleanse for the
excessive Candida in their bodies, all of their Parkinson's symptoms vanished. Lidia Epp
subsequently published an article that offers a scientific explanation of the connection between
Candida and dopamine depletion. She offers a lucid explanation of the scientific basis of her
discovery during my March 23, 2011 radio show.

JIM, a former competitive cyclist from Florida was initially devastated by severe symptoms
associated with his diagnosis of Parkinson's disease. Determined to ride again, he spent hours
working out at the Cypress Palms assisted living facility with unbelievable results. The people
responsible for coaching Jim joined with him on my radio show March 14, 2012 to tell his most
amazing story of recovery. Jim's symptoms vanish when he rides his recliner bike.

KARL ROBB, diagnosed with early onset Parkinson's disease at the age of 23, has experienced the symptoms for over 20 years. One therapy in particular that has had a profound impact on Karl's recovery is Reiki, a form of "hands on" energy healing which has become popular over the past decade. Karl is now a Reiki master himself and offers treatments to others. He continues to administer Reiki treatments to himself and writes a stunning blog about his experience with Parkinson's. Karl was a guest on my radio show March 20, 2012.

JYDITH LYNNE has been recognized in Hawaii as "La'au Kahea," a rare healing form where she utilizes the alchemy of her 5 octave voice to catalyze harmonic alignment for people and places. Diagnosed with Parkinson's in 2009, Judith has included her own work in her healing protocol and is very excited about the noticeable improvement of her health, believing that her regular meditation practice of Vocal Toning is accelerating her recovery.

Her profound understanding of the physical-psycho-spiritual power of the voice led to her development of Vocal Energetics™ and Harmonic Healing™. Both methods are grounded in the understanding that everything in the manifest world is frequency and that the Voice is our most powerful and accessible tool for achieving multi-leveled harmonic health and spiritual fulfillment. Judith was a guest on the Parkinsons Recovery Radio Show March 28, 2012.

PHYLLIS ROGERS was diagnosed with Parkinson's disease in 2007. Today she is virtually symptom free. After doing her own research, Phyllis figured out what really matters when it comes to therapies that make a difference for her. She had a serious conversation with God and they agreed that she did not need to have Parkinson's. Among other incredible contributions to the Parkinson's community, Phyllis works with adults to help them become physically fit. The author of Over 40 and Gettin' Stronger, Phyllis Rogers was a guest on my radio show April 11, 2012.

I continue to air weekly radio programs with guests who tell their stories of recovery. Tune into any of the programs [www.blogtalkradio.com/parkinsons-recovery] as they are aired live Wednesdays at 3:00 pm Pacific time. Call toll free (877) 590-0733 if you live in the United States. If you live in other countries, connect to any live radio show through your computer using Skype when connected to the radio show website. All of my radio shows are archived.

If you find yourself down in the dumps and depressed, listen to either a live show or an archived show. The radio shows are uplifting and informative. It also helps to hear the stories of other people who are on the road to recovery or who have fully recovered.

WHO RECOVERS?

Some people follow a gentle path of steady improvement with increasing evidence of symptom relief. A few people are now symptom free. Most people on the road to recovery say that their symptoms are tightly correlated with stress. When they not under stress their symptoms are either not present or inconsequential in character. When they are stressed, symptoms smack them in the face. Fluctuation in symptoms can be dramatic moment to moment.

Others experience a graduate decline in their health which is text book in character. The textbooks after all say that if you have Parkinson's you are supposed to get worse over time.

What distinguishes those who get better and those who do not? From my research and observations, two factors make the difference.

First, if you believe in your heart that you can recover you will recover. You will treat your body well and give it what it needs to heal. I have written an entire book on the subject entitled Five Steps to Recovery [www.fivestepstorecovery.com] to help people transform their beliefs and thought processes. I discuss the five steps in some detail and play several meditations from the book during my radio May 7, 2009.

Second, people who see a relief of symptoms believe that their healing comes from a place deep inside themselves. That is to say, healing comes from within, not without. People who experience a gradual deterioration in their health tend to hold the belief that their healing must inevitably come from a source outside themselves.

The source depends on the person of course. Some wait for a miracle cure. Some believe medications will be discovered tomorrow that will fix the problem. Some hope for relief that might come from surgery. Some travel to one shaman after another with the hope they will fix them. Others scan the internet everyday for a tip on a supplement that will "cure" them.

Still others identify with their disease. This is how John Briggs, ND, explains the consequence of identifying with a disease like Parkinson's.

> *"We need to adopt the philosophy of being healed and not of being sick. So many times we identify with some disease. It becomes part of our identity. I have had people who are very difficult to help because they have so identified with their disease. If they were to get rid of the disease they would lose their identity."*

Wouldn't it be wonderful if there were a simple solution to the pain and agony of Parkinson's? Isn't there something or someone out there that will fix the problem? I personally identify with this attitude myself. Just fix me. Fix me now.

Waiting for something or someone to fix us is like waiting for Godot. Recall Godot never shows up. As we wait, we ignore valuable signals our body gives to us. Our body will tell us what we need to know. We just have to listen carefully.

© 2013 Parkinsons Recovery

n't listen, guess what? We gradually get worse.

ole who get better acknowledge to themselves that sustained healing does not come from a source outside of us. Rather, healing comes from a magical place deep inside ourselves as we listen to the messages our body sends. Of course the outside therapies will help and can be very beneficial, but true healing comes from a place deep within.

The route to health is to disengage from being suspended in a persistent state of stress, fear and anxiety. Allow the pulse of life to move in and out of your body with its natural cycle of expansion and contraction. Hormonal balance and harmony will return in its own time and place. My hope and intention is for this to happen for everyone now.

FIX ME NOW

Everyone encounters days when they feel lousy. Some people encounter a depressing day when they are told by a medical doctor they have a disease. Perhaps the disease is Parkinson's or diabetes or high blood pressure. Whatever.

I'd like to speak for myself here. When I am not feeling well or when my doctor tells me I have a disease, my immediate reaction is to ask:

> *"Isn't there someone out there who can fix me?*
>
> *Isn't there a pill?*
>
> *Isn't there a shot?*
>
> *Perhaps surgery can make me well again?"*

The motivation for a cure that comes from a place deep inside me is compelling. Take the problem away - now. I want to feel good again - now. I launch a search to find a cure, a quick fix. I am frantic to find ways to fix my problem.

> *I talk with friends.*
>
> *I search the internet. It is always possible to find cures on the internet.*
>
> *I visit the library.*
>
> *I ask medical doctors or naturopaths or whoever might know about a cure.*
>
> *I consider traveling to Mexico to get experimental gene therapy.*

© 2013 Parkinsons Recovery

There is an ending to my quest. It is always the same. I have gone through this process before. I find a treatment that cuts away at the edges of my problem. I decide to try it. The symptom is relieved temporarily. If I am lucky I find relief for a few months or longer.

Then when I least expect it – just when I had convinced myself that the problem was solved – a pain or discomfort in a different part of my body starts screaming at me.

Yesterday my left foot hurts. I take a pill. Today my left shoulder hurts. The pill I took yesterday does not relieve the shoulder pain. The pain is sneaky. It just traveled to another place in my body. I am nagged no matter what I do to fix the pain.

Here is the truth of the matter. The chance there will be a "cure" for Parkinson's - a quick fix - is as good as hitching a ride to Mars. You are probably thinking to yourself - but medical science has "cured" other diseases. Really? Just consider our modern experience with other diseases.

Polio was never "cured" with the polio vaccine. People who had polio as children often see the symptoms of polio come out of hibernation 25 years later.

Infections were never "cured" by antibiotics. Even if we feel "well" after taking a 3 week prescription of antibiotics, there are always vestiges of the infectious bacteria that remain locked in the cells. More and more people are dying from the ravaging effects of infections that are unresponsive to antibiotics. You get the point.

Many people do hope for a Parkinson's "cure." Wouldn't that be awesome? The frustration of waiting for a "cure" is the limitation of time.

How long do you have to wait for a cure? One hundred years? Perhaps two hundred? I have been a research scientist for many years, so I am very familiar with the snail's pace of scientific "progress".

Science works in tiny, incremental steps. Consider the hope there might is a drug that will potentially bring symptom relief. Consider what happens now.

The drug is first evaluated on animals.

Results are gathered and evaluated.

Results look promising.

The study is written and submitted to an academic journal for review.

The journal editor sends the study out for review.

The editor evaluates the reviews and asks the authors to revise and resubmit.

© 2013 Parkinsons Recovery

The authors revise and resubmit the study to the journal editor.

The editor sends the revision out to the same reviewers for further evaluation.

The editor winds up rejecting the paper.

The study is submitted to a second journal for review.

The same process above is repeated.

And if rejected, the study is submitted to a third journal.

And so forth.

Years pass. We all get older.

Finally the study is published. Other studies on animals are done to see if the results replicate. The process above is repeated.

Years Pass. We all get older.

Approval from the FDA is obtained to evaluate the drug on humans. The process above is repeated.

Years pass. We all get older.

The drug is finally approved for use by humans. Now the true challenge emerges. Virtually all prescription drugs have a positive effect on a small, selective set of symptoms. How many of the symptoms you experience today can be relieved by taking this newly approved drug for use by humans? One out of ten? Two out of ten? And, what are you going to do about finding relief for the other symptoms this drug does not treat?

Oh, and there is one other tiny complication I should remember to mention. Virtually all drugs have side effects – some of them quite serious. That is why the FDA (or other government monitoring agencies) become involved. My mother was diagnosed with Parkinson's. She wound up taking an array of 10 different medications. I am convinced she died from taking too many prescribed medications at the same time.

Healers have a very different perspective on disease. When we are in pain and our bodies are screaming at us to pay attention, the response is to say:

> *"I have good news to report to myself today. My body is giving me important information. Something is not quite in balance here."'*

"Why don't I take a break from my daily routine and simply listen to my body? What is my body actually telling me? Obviously I need to be doing something different. I just need to figure out what and then do it."

- *Perhaps I am eating the wrong food.*

- *Perhaps I need more exercise.*

- *Perhaps a friend is toxic.*

- *Perhaps I am drinking water from plastic bottles and I am poisoning my body.*

- *Perhaps I am cleaning my bathtub with a toxic chemical that is poisoning me.*

- *Perhaps I am using make up or soap or deodorant that is poison to my cells.*

- *Perhaps the meat I am eating or the water I am drinking has toxins.*

The point is that old habits must be changed in some way. Listen to your body. Make some changes. Wait. See if you feel better.

Make more changes. Wait. See if you feel better. Create your own personal experiment. Your body knows the answers. All you have to do is listen to your body and act accordingly.

Hoping for a cure? Here is <u>John Coleman's</u> perspective on a cure.

> *"You are healthy today. You are precisely where you need to be now regardless of any symptoms that may be present.*
>
> *The body is always giving us signals of what it needs. We just need to listen.*
>
> *People say they want to be cured. From what? Bacon is cured. Concrete is cured. Why in the world would anyone want to cure people? Disease is simply a manifestation that something is wrong with how we treat our body."*

Consider the various meanings of cure. We cure bacon. Do you want to be cured like bacon? I certainly don't. We cure concrete. Do you want to be cured like concrete? I certainly don't.

The underlying message behind the hope of a "cure" is to isolate and identify a single cause. Treatment of symptoms alone in the long run does us little good. So let's all celebrate the challenge to find the "cause" so that it can be "cured."

But wait. There is not just one "cause." Factors that cause neurological problems are complex and multifaceted. When one source of a symptom is isolated, there is a welcome opportunity to find a solution. But that is only the start of the road to recovery. For most people, there are a cluster of causes.

Neurological challenges will linger until all of the causal factors that are causing the imbalance have been identified. Once each of the causal factors is isolated, a treatment can be found.

The idea of finding a cure connotes a fixed condition. Suppose one cause of hormonal imbalances is identified and addressed - whether through surgery or medications. That is certainly something to be celebrated. I assure you, however, that a multitude of other influences will remain that have the potential to cause hormonal imbalances. Such factors include stress, negative thinking and unresolved trauma.

The body is never in a fixed state. It is changing from moment to moment. If systems in the body were fixed, we would be dead.

Personally speaking, wishing for a cure of any disease is not my cup of tea. I would much rather opt for the thrill of the journey as I return back home to myself. The presence of troubling symptoms means that for one reason or another I have lost contact with my body. I have deserted it.

You can wait for a cure if you wish, but do not keep your fingers crossed. I believe the better bet is to figure out ways to heal using a variety of safe, nonintrusive approaches. Healing was actually a lot more sophisticated hundreds of years ago. We are just now relearning the wisdom of our ancestors.

Disease, pain, discomfort, despair and depression are all gifts in disguise. It is the body's way of giving us early warning signals that something is wrong. Action and attention are necessary if you want to feel better. Take it now. Be surprised with the results. The answers lie within you and no one else.

RECOVERY CAN HAPPEN NOW. MAKE IT SO

What constitutes recovery? Is recovery a matter of returning to the state which existed prior to the illness? If so, when was that?

Bodies are in a perpetual state of change. It is a rare day when everything is balanced. It is abnormal when all systems are fully functional.

What day in your life do you want to "recover?" There are days of tears, days of agony and days of frustration. There are also days of joy, exhilaration and unqualified happiness. Again I ask, what day of your life do you want to "recover"?

Parkinsons Recovery has little to do with returning to a moment of the past which has vanished as is the custom with each and every moment of our lives. Rather, Parkinsons Recovery is all about:

- *Recovering our unlimited and unqualified life force.*

- *Claiming our full power to become whole and complete.*

- *Nurturing our creativity whenever and wherever we are inspired.*

If a symptom is a barrier to becoming all that you are, may that symptom be addressed, resolved and healed now. If a critical and deprecating thought is pulling you down into the bottomless hole of depression and despair, may that thought be ejected, removed, released and dissolved now.

Why suffer from debilitating symptoms for the rest of your life? Make recovery happen for yourself today. Now. Eject the thoughts that are dragging your life force down into the gutter.

Honor your unfulfilled dreams today.

Embrace the thoughts of a new way of being in the world with your family and yourself.

Acknowledge the pulse of your soul, your body and your heart now.

It is beating. Listen. It is calling out to you now.

"I am alive. I am all that I ever needed to be."

Hear the gentle whisper of these words in your heart and your body will return to that sacred place of balance and harmony instantly. Healing happens now if you declare it to be so.

© 2013 Parkinsons Recovery

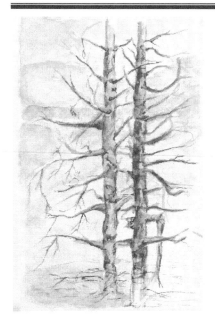

Pioneer Trees by <u>Mary Pauer</u>

THE FALSE BELIEF TEMPLATE MOST PEOPLE BELIEVE IS TRUE

My mission at Parkinsons Recovery is to offer hope to people who have been diagnosed with Parkinson's. People with Parkinson's do recover. People with Parkinson's do find ways to get relief from their symptoms.

Parkinsons Recovery is all about bringing to center stage stories of hope. "Progressive" and "Degenerative" may be the accurate experience for some people - perhaps even many - but it does not have to be the experience for you.

My work with persons who have been diagnosed with Parkinson's reveals that health care providers are entirely pessimistic about any prospects for recovery. The following questions are never asked:

- *How long will it take for me to begin feeling better?*

- *How long will it take for me to fully recover?*

- *How much better will I feel next year at this time?*

- *When will I feel strong enough to ski again - or run - or play baseball?*

Rather, the questions on the dinner table for people who have just learned they have been diagnosed with Parkinson's are:

- *How fast will I deteriorate?*

    ○   *How much worse will I feel next year at this time?*

    ○   *How long will it be before I am in a wheel chair?*

    ○   *When will I fall and break my hip?*

I have a simple point to make which I want to make simply. When people are first diagnosed with Parkinson's, the news they hear about their future is depressingly pessimistic.

The following are quotes from individuals who participated in the Parkinsons Energy Project in Portland, Oregon. Our research project evaluated the effects of energy healing on the symptoms of persons with Parkinsons. Before the project began each participant answered the following question:

What has your doctor told you about Parkinson's?

"I guess the symptoms increase to the point that you are disabled. I understand that one doesn't die of Parkinson's but you get so weakened that you can't fight it off."

"He told me be sure to have prescription drug coverage - that I was going to need it. He said I would live probably another 20 years. They just try to reassure me that I do not have a terminal illness. He said that I wouldn't die of Parkinson's. He said I probably had it at least 5 years before my symptoms showed up."

"I will use a walker and wheelchair at some point. It is going to be hard for me to keep my balance. I have already noticed bobbing now and then. I haven't fallen. Everything I have heard about people is that it is going to be horrible. So, I do not have any reason that it is not - nobody has ever said that it is going to stop progressing and it is not going to get worse. I have never heard anything positive to make me feel hopeful."

"I had done some research and I said (to the doctor) so, what we can expect is steadily deteriorating in condition, but Parkinson's will not kill her, is that right?"

 He said, "Yes, that is correct."

"It is a progressive disease but different people progress at different rates. I can remember sitting in his office and saying to him that some people never progress beyond the initial stages and he said yes, some people don't. Most people do. I do not think he said a lot about long term. But I have read enough to be scared about that. One thing he did say was that the medications did not stop the progression so I connected A and B and said why take medications if you do not need it."

"It is a progressive disease. How fast it progresses and how far it progresses could be individual. There is no way of determining that beforehand at the present time and there is no way of absolutely assuring that it is Parkinsons - the only definitive diagnosis is post mortem. And that seems a little radical."

"Besides the original diagnosis more or less my neurologist said that this is a progressive disease. Here is a box of pills. Go take them and have a good life."

"The neurologist tells us more than anybody ... he hasn't told us that much other than he has this medicine."

"The doctor just says it is degenerative. Come back in 6 months. We will treat the symptoms the best we can."

"He actually did not tell us a lot. When he told us that my husband had Parkinson's Plus, my husband just said 'That sounds like a death sentence.' And the doctor was very unresponsive."

"He just said I could expect to have more and more symptoms over the years."

*"Not a great deal. He talks about what a chronic disease***Error! Bookmark not defined.** *means and it is not treatable other than reducing the symptoms. It was a very brief conversation and I have not seen that neurologist since."*

"Standard answer was that it was a degenerative disease that cannot be stopped and so my husband's symptoms will progress and get worse. Now they don't identify which symptoms but they just say he will get worse. No time table. No definitive answers. Just a general answer."

"We had a short conversation - the worst case scenario is total paralysis. You aren't going to die."

Not one person we interviewed was given a shred hope by their doctors that they could get relief from their symptoms or that they could actually feel better. We steadfastly challenge this belief template at Parkinsons Recovery. Evidence proves it is simply not true.

We are assembling stories of people who have recovered fully or who have found relief from their symptoms. We are analyzing research that evaluates the impact of natural therapies on the symptoms of Parkinson's which offer a promise of hope. We are assembling a compelling body of evidence that demonstrates relief from symptoms happens to people every day. Recovery can happen for you.

Our purpose is to acknowledge and honor the healthy belief template that recovery is possible. There can be "progression," but the progression is toward health and wellness and not toward a wheelchair. When hope is held close to the chest, a journey of recovery unfolds.

- *It is possible to feel better.*

- *It is possible to find relief from symptoms.*

- *Some people have even proven it is possible to recover.*

THE TRUE BELIEF TEMPLATE THAT MAKES RECOVERY POSSIBLE

Even if you are enthusiastic and optimistic about getting well today, most people with Parkinson's eventually revert back to the belief that Parkinson's is a "progressively degenerative disease." Since this belief is held by many people, it is easy to be convinced it is true.

It is difficult to sustain a belief that differs from what knowledgeable authorities say is true. When a bad day creeps up on you, the normal reaction is to say to yourself:

> *"Oh, right. The evidence is staring me in the face. I am feeling worse today than yesterday. This means I must be getting worse, just as 'they' said would happen."*

We feel good some days and lousy other days. Note that I say "we." By "we" I mean everyone - people who are healthy and those who are not. The difference is that people who are healthy say to themselves:

> *"I will be better soon."*

People with Parkinson's say to themselves:

> *"Oh God. Here it is."*

The recovery process involves good days and bad days that come in strange and unpredictable patterns. When the body makes adjustments in its journey to return to a state of balance the aftermath can sometimes be pain and discomfort.

My research shows that as symptoms improve, people may report slightly more pain in the short run. Why is this so? They are paying attention for the first time in their lives to the messages their bodies are giving them.

Ever had an entire day of being virtually symptom free? It is so wonderful when this happens. Then, a bad day comes out of nowhere. Symptoms smack you in the face. It is challenge to get out of bed. Brushing your teeth is more difficult than yesterday.

© 2013 Parkinsons Recovery

On a bad day it is tough to dispute the belief that you are deteriorating. After all, you feel lousy. Those who love you probably hold the same belief that most other people hold. What is this belief? Your ill health today means you are deteriorating.

The path to recovery is not a gentle slope in an upward direction. Our observation from working with clients with Parkinson's reveals that recovery zigzags all over the place. Recovery is difficult to track for this reason, especially when you happen to be the one who is experiencing the unpleasant symptoms.

The last ditch hope is always for a quick fix. A miracle would be nice. Surely there is a supplement, a drug or some therapy that will cure Parkinson's? Isn't a cure just around the corner?

Wouldn't it be wonderful if a cure were just around the corner? Waiting for a cure is just a lame excuse not to give your body what it needs to recover.

The problem in a nutshell is this. If you believe you are getting worse, you will get worse. If you sustain the belief that you are in recovery, you will recover.

The belief in recovery will be absorbed by each and every cell in your body.

> *Your cells will exude hope.*
>
> *Hope is infectious.*
>
> *Hope heals.*

THE BODY IS NOT BROKEN. IT IS WORKING PERFECTLY

The natural condition for the body is to be well, not to be sick. When the body has the support it needs to return to a state of balance and harmony, recovery happens. When hormones are balanced you feel good. When they are out of balance you feel lousy

Symptoms of Parkinsons are not pleasant for anyone, but they do offer valuable information about the type of support that is needed for the body to heal.

The body of the person with Parkinsons is actually working perfectly, just as it was designed to work. There are a myriad of cells which are specifically configured to help the body heal illness. Neutrophils rush to the site of an infection. Monocytes devour dead tissues and help control inflammation in the body. Osteoblasts knit the rough edges of broken bones. An army of other microscopic cells work individually and in teams to reverse cell damage that is caused by illness.

Some cells are so specialized they do not even have names. They have not yet been seen or detected by scientific research. It is all so cool really.

I do not think of Parkinsons as a "disease." Nutritional Counselor and author Dorit summarizes the issues with identifying with a diagnosis of Parkinsons beautifully.

> *"We are not Parkinsons. We are not the ramifications or the manifestations of the tremors or the tightness and the stiffness. That is not who we are. Who we are is so beyond that. It is just an experience that is just taking us to another, higher level."*

Heather MacTavish expresses this sentiment beautifully:

> *"I am not a 'wheelchair' or a 'Parkinsonian.' I am an individual."*

The body is not broken. It is not diseased. It is simply out of balance. The key to getting well is to acknowledge the meaning of the messages that our bodies give us each day.

Any cover up of symptoms undermines the body's natural ability to heal. Cover ups, regardless of what form they take, make the messages our bodies give us terribly difficult to interpret.

The foundation for recovery from Parkinsons is thus founded on a powerful truth. Acknowledge the meaning of what our body communicates to us from one moment to the next. Then answer the call. Give your body what it needs.

Recovery then unfolds effortlessly. Be sure to add a little patience to the recipe too.

Our bodies are well equipped to heal whatever imbalances that may be present. They just need a gentle nudge remembering how sometimes.

OUR BODY ALWAYS KNOWS HOW TO HEAL

I asked John Briggs, ND, whether he believed it was possible for a person with Parkinsons to become symptom free. Here was his answer:

> *"I truly believe that with all my heart. The body knows how to heal itself. If you cut yourself, what happens? Do you have to try and think about making your body heal? It heals on its own.*
>
> *As long as your body has the nutrition that it needs to be able to function normally, then we really shouldn't have to worry about it healing itself. Normally, why we don't see healing is because we are lacking specific nutrition that the body needs for different tissues.*

© 2013 Parkinsons Recovery

I was in an explosion in 1976 that gutted me. I was rather severely wounded. I had my intestines in my hands. For the longest time I had areas in my abdomen that were very numb and felt like rubber because there was no feeling there. Gradually, as time went by, the nerves re- grew into those areas.

Can nerves grow? Absolutely.

Can nerves be healed? Absolutely.

Does your body know how to heal itself? Absolutely.

Just have to give it what it needs and remove what it doesn't need. It can heal."

Our bodies do know how to heal themselves. They just need a little help remembering how sometimes.

The body is a complicated network of inter-related systems. The intricacies are mind boggling. And, the truth is that scientists have not really figured out how the various systems in the body relate to one another.

Medical researchers continually research various interventions in the form of drugs and surgeries that can relieve pain and heal disease. We are thankful to their work because it saves lives.

There is one difficulty with any such intervention however. Cells in the body have a consciousness in their own right. They stop suddenly and say to themselves:

"Hey...What's going on here? What's happening? I thought that was my job!"

After getting out the resentment, the cells in the body conclude

"Ok, fine."

Think about it. This is the same response we are likely to have when someone volunteers to do something for us. We usually are happy for them to do it because it frees us up to spend our time doing other things.

The cells in the body respond in the same way. The cells conclude:

"Ok, I'll simply turn off that system. If someone else is going to do it for me, I'll pay attention to the other important matters at hand."

Notice what happens. The body deliberately turns off an intricate control mechanism that makes it possible for it to function so beautifully day in and day out.

In what circumstances does the body respond this way? If we are giving our bodies wha[t] need to function in the form of nutrition, vitamins and minerals, the cells are thankful f[or] nourishment. But any synthetic medication or surgery that offers more than nourishm[ent] trigger a knee jerk reaction from the affected cells in the body.

When we ingest synthetic medications, the systems that are naturally used by the body to regulate hormones are disabled. The body instinctively switches off the complex mechanisms it uses to regulate hormones, functions and regulatory systems.

We disable control systems in the body because we decide our bodies can no longer perform that particular function. More simply put, we do not trust our body to perform its job any longer. This decision disrupts the body's natural ability and wisdom to maintain health. Each cell has a consciousness in its own right which is profoundly disturbed.

The reality is that when we intervene into the natural functions of the body whether through surgery or drugs, the systems in the body are jolted. Most interventions are rather crude. They affect a very specific subsystem of the body and thus wind up shutting off other systems that the body uses to keep us healthy.

I believe that natural remedies should be the preferred choice initially. By natural remedies, I mean any support we can give to our body so that it is able to perform the job it knows how to perform perfectly. This includes, among other options, eating fresh, organic food and exercising regularly. After all, a supplement is simply nutrition in the form of a pill.

It is important to consult with your doctor and consider all the options, including taking drugs or having surgeries performed. Clearly, drugs and surgeries can and do save lives.

My suggestion is quite simple. Give your body a chance to heal itself. It takes time for the body to heal. It takes patience. The body knows how to heal itself. I am acknowledging here what people have known for thousands of years. We simply forgot the truth of who we really are. It is high time to reclaim the wisdom of our ancestors.

If your body is out of balance for any reason, review all the options. There are a multitude of natural remedies that will support your body's natural ability to heal. When given the proper support, it is easy and natural for your body to do what it knows how to do best: return to its preferred state of health and wellness

WHY IS IT SO HARD FOR THE BODY TO MAINTAIN A BALANCE OF THE 40 OR SO HORMONES?

So what is the big deal anyway? Everyone knows that there are hormones that heighten the level of excitement in our bodies and there are other hormones that calm us down. The calming ones (like dopamine) make us feel good inside. Who doesn't want to feel good inside?

Good enough. So the answer must be simple. Spend a little time every day doing exciting things and a little time doing relaxing things. When you divide up the day like this your hormonal scorecard should be just about balanced. Shouldn't it?

Unfortunately not. Let me explain why.

Have you ever noticed that when you are frightened unexpectedly it takes a long time to come down from the excitement? Perhaps you cannot stop talking about what happened or you can't sleep or you keep worrying that the same scary thing will happen again.

The effects of stress hormones linger in the body for - get this - as long as 48 hours. One frightening moment that lasts a fraction of a second can have a continuing impact for two days.

OK, now consider the opposite situation. You are doing your meditation for the day. You are calm. You are collected. You are enjoying just being with yourself. No worries. No fears. No bothers.

Until the phone rings and a dear friend has an emergency. They were in an accident on the interstate minutes ago. How long does it take you to shift from your state of full meditative relaxation to that familiar place of alertness and concern? If you are like most people, the shift happens instantly.

The physical staying power of dopamine last a few minutes. The effects of adrenaline last for 2 days. Is it any wonder then why it is so tricky to maintain a balance of hormones in the body? The difference in "staying power" of the two types of hormones is huge.

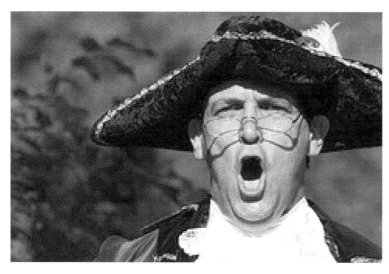

Photo by Peter Thompson

SHOULD I FIGHT OR SURRENDER?

I know what you are thinking. The answer is obvious. Of course you fight, right? This will not be my answer. Since there are only two choices, you now know my answer. Read on.

One of my favorite past times is reading obituaries. OK. I agree this is weird, perhaps even demented, but give me credit for a little self-disclosure here.

What do people say about their loved ones in obituaries when they die of cancer?

> *"She fought a courageous battle."*

It goes without saying (although I am now saying it) the obituary never points out that the battle was lost. For all of the thousands of obituaries I have read, no one - I repeat no one - won the battle. These odds are not encouraging.

This is my twisted way of alerting you to what you are not expecting. I will argue that a healthy way to heal the symptoms of Parkinsons is to embrace the meaning and information the symptoms are giving us.

My explanation starts with a story about horse racing. How in the world is horse racing related to Parkinsons? Ah, is impatience an issue for you? It is for me. Let's each tolerate our impatience as I write and you read the next section.

HORSE RACING AND PARKINSONS

One of my pleasures in life has been to live at one time in the beautiful city of Lexington, Kentucky which is home to some of the fastest and most famous thoroughbred racing horses in the world. Part of the Lexington folklore revolves around Patrick Henry, a horse that won over 6 million in purses.

© 2013 Parkinsons Recovery

In his retirement years Patrick Henry lived on a horse farm near the famous racing track known as Keeneland. His handlers told me that the most dangerous time to be inside Patrick Henry's horse stall was when the racing horn at nearby Keeneland signaled the time for a race to begin.

Patrick Henry knew he was not at the starting gate. He knew he was not racing. He knew he had been "put out to pasture." He did not like it one bit.

Patrick Henry would become angry, even violent. His entire body would shake, rattle and roll. He tore up anything in his way - his hay rack, the walls to his stall and even his handlers if they were inside the stall with him. It was dangerous business for his handlers on racing day.

Patrick Henry was determined to race. He had no interest sitting on the sidelines. He got no pleasure from hearing the shouts of the crowd nearby.

His handlers quickly learned that you could not confront Patrick Henry during such occasions. His fury would be ignited. He temper would intensify. His frantic behavior would become measurably worse.

His handlers explained to me that the only response was to allow Patrick Henry to have his pout, shake like a mad horse and scream out his anger from the bowels of his life force. The only response possible was to allow the energy to be expressed.

Once he was able to fully and completely express his feelings they would pass. The shaking would stop. The fury would pass.

Patrick Henry was processing his own feelings of inadequacy. His handlers and owners decided he was too old to race. Part of him certainly knew that he was too old to race.

But this was all too much to stomach for this proud horse. Patrick Henry needed to release his own feelings of inadequacy in his own way.

Let me now explain the connection between Patrick Henry's frustration and Parkinsons. Having interviewed many persons who currently have the symptoms of Parkinsons, I have observed that there is an underlying intensity that is typically present. The intensity is coupled with a genuine sense of power and focus, two remarkable traits that help people succeed in life.

The intensity and focus is a good thing. It is a precursor to success in life. It is the reason why so many people with Parkinsons have a long record of amazing accomplishments. No one, however, can sustain this intense level of intensity without paying the price of serious harm to their neurological system.

Patrick Henry's handlers relocated him 20 miles away from the race track. Had he remained near the race track he would have destroyed his body and departed this earth at a young age.

© 2013 Parkinsons Recovery

If persons with Parkinsons insist on leading a lifestyle that is characterized by unrelenting intensity, neurological integrity will most assuredly suffer.

The solution for Patrick Henry and for anyone who is challenged with neurological symptoms is to find that magical place of balance – not too much in the way of intensity and not too much in the way of moderation.

PLACE OF BALANCE

When the symptoms of Parkinsons present themselves what is the typical response for anyone? For most people (myself included) the typical response is to fight the symptoms, to engage an internal war against them.

This response works beautifully for some people, but I want to offer a companion response for you to consider. Consider the possibility that our body will find a place of balance no matter what circumstances you confront or how you respond.

If you operate in high gear day in and day out - running marathons, accomplishing miracles, running a business, setting high goals, handling the traumas of everyday living - your body will find a way, anyway, to find balance in your life.

You cannot stop this process no matter how hard you try. You have no control over it.

YIN VERSUS YANG

We need both yin and yang. Aggression needs to be balanced with receiving the pleasures of life. The war inside us needs to be balanced with making peace within us.

If it suddenly becomes more difficult to move, your body may simply be finding a way to slow you down. If it is more difficult to talk, maybe your body is telling you it is time to listen more often. If your body wants to shake uncontrollably, perhaps there is tension in the tissues that needs to be released.

In other words, any symptom you experience is valuable information. All you need to do is to listen to your body. Give in to the pain, discomfort and frustration. Set your intention to learn more about its underlying meaning. The symptoms -however unpleasant they may be -are gifts in disguise.

The best analogy here is to think of what happens in martial arts when you absorb the blows of your opponent rather than counteracting with equal force. There is limitless power when you flow with the energy of the moment - absorbing the blows rather than fighting them.

If you counteract the blows of your opponent you will ultimately lose the fight. In the end the route to victory is "giving in" and yielding.

© 2013 Parkinsons Recovery

BALANCE YOUR HORMONES USING ENTRAINMENT

What does it take to maintain a perfect balance of hormones in the human body? I have a video that I would like everyone to see. This is the most amazing video of a man who is doing a 5 minute juggling routine at the conclusion of his comedy routine before a live audience.

What does jugging have to do with Parkinsons? Nothing actually. It is the presence of Chris Bliss that is remarkable to experience. His body is balanced, centered and in perfect harmony. He is in a space where every movement is effortless. It is a place of no thoughts, no forcing and no time.

When you invite yourself into this place, you will also connect with a place for yourself that is familiar. It is the place you were also in when you accomplished similar feats in your life, accomplishments that for you were also effortless.

Hormones get out of whack when we force ourselves to do something that is not right for us. Hormones get out of whack when we try too hard, work too hard and forget about what is really important in life.

As you watch his routine, connect with the same space he is in. Invite your own body to remember this place of solidarity, assurance, confidence and balance. It is a sweet place that allows you to accomplish anything without angst or agony or anger or frustration. Everything is possible when you slip into this place of harmony.

The video lasts 5 minutes. Allow your own groundedness and centeredness to be entrapped by Bliss' unbelievable juggling act. Allow your body to become entrained to Chris' blissful state of balance and harmony (no pun intended).

Get into his space of balance and harmony. As you do, watch your hormones (and your life) come back into perfect balance. Click on the link below to watch Chris Bliss' amazing juggling routine

http://www.youtube.com/watch?v=5uaBBl3gXRs

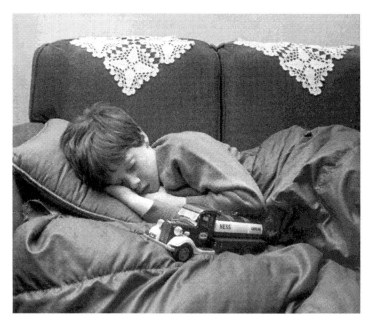

Dreams by John Fasulo

"If our lives are indeed the sum total of the choices we've made, then we cannot change who we are. But with every new choice we're given, we can change who we're going to be." The Outer Limits Television Series

There are two ways people respond to the symptoms of Parkinsons. The first is to ask other people to treat the disease. The second is to become an advocate for your own recovery. I am a steadfast advocate of the second approach. Let me explain the difference by reporting my response to a question I received recently about treating Parkinsons Plus.

Question:

> *"I was diagnosed with Parkinsons in 2002. In 2006 I was told that I probably had Parkinsons+ or CBD. Since then neurologists have no suggestions for help with CBD".*

> *"I am wondering if you knew of anything being used for Parkinsons+".*

My Response: Your question is the perfect question for a medical doctor who is trained in a two step process for treating disease. First, the condition is given a diagnosis. Second, the diagnosis informs a treatment (though in this case the neurologists do not have anything to follow-up with).

Medical doctors have to be very concerned about following this protocol or else they could be sued if something goes wrong. I am not a medical doctor. I am a researcher. I have the flexibility of approaching the challenge of healing illness differently.

ACKNOWLEDGE YOUR POWER

At Parkinsons Recovery I propose a different model to follow, a model of wellness. The argument that underpins everything I am writing about and everything I am discovering in my research is that the body has an inherent wisdom to heal.

The body is simply giving us valuable information about an imbalance if there are symptoms: Perhaps too much stress in your life; Perhaps too much trauma; Perhaps too many toxins. Something is out of balance or overtaxed.

Some people choose to respond to troubling symptoms by covering them up, numbing them or otherwise killing them in some fashion or another.

I say – allow symptoms to be expressed. They are giving us valuable information about what is up.

With my approach, there is no emphasis on the disease state. The name is inconsequential - Parkinsons, Parkinsons +, MSA - it is of no consequence. Rather, the focus is on giving the body what it needs to become healthy. I propose a positive mind set rather than a negative mind set.

PAY OTHERS TO TREAT THE DISEASE

If you follow down the path where the "disease" is treated, here is what happens:

(1) You receive a diagnosis (and I certainly have no doubt in your case but that the diagnosis is sound)

(2) You discover little or nothing can be done for this particular "disease."

(3) You get depressed, crawl into a hole and wait to feel worse.

When you operate on the basis that the body knows how to heal itself, the sequence is dramatically different:

BECOME AN ADVOCATE FOR YOUR OWN RECOVERY

(1) You receive information from your body that something is out of balance. Perhaps there is a nutritional deficiency. Perhaps stress hormones are overpowering everything in your body. Perhaps your elimination organs cannot handle the heavy traffic of toxins.

(2) You discover through your own research that there are hundreds of options for addressing the problem.

(3) You start experimenting with one approach or another and determine what works for you.

(4) You become hopeful, launch out into the world and begin feeling better.

I prefer the second approach, but I am a little biased. Control is a fundamental issue that is reported to me by many people with the symptoms of Parkinsons. It feels as though there are many circumstances that defy order and control. It feels like chaos reigns every day.

What better way to address the fear of losing control than to take control over your own health. Let no one else decide what is right for you and your body. Assert your authority. Claim your power. Maintain full control over decisions that affect your health. Allow others to assert their authority over you and you lose all control.

Where do you start? Where do you find out about the hundreds of options? One place is Parkinsons Recovery. I interview people every week who have the most interesting and helpful suggestions for treatments. I have been amazed at the number of therapies and approaches people have tried that are helping. More interestingly, each person's list is different!

The fun part is to review the options and determine which ones you want to try on for size. Keep experimenting and you will find therapies that will help give relief from symptoms. That is the one solid conclusion I have drawn from my research.

THE VALUE OF EXPERIMENTATION

Steven Fowkes from the Cognitive Enhancement Research Institute says that people who experiment live significantly longer than those who give their power of choice over to others.

> *"If you grab an animal, like a rat or mouse, the animal freaks out and wants to get away. It struggles. If you release the animal when it is still struggling, it is left with the message that struggle leads to a solution. That is hopefulness.*
>
> *If you hold on to the animal until it stops struggling and then let it go, the message is: Struggle is useless. There is nothing they can do to escape the capture, the torment, whatever it is that the grabbing constitutes.*
>
> *If you look at those two animals, the animal that you let go before it stopped struggling, that animal lives an almost normal lifespan. The animal that you grab and hold onto until it is helpless and stops struggling dies very young.*
>
> *That message is about the belief that your action is actually going to make a difference. Doing something is better than doing nothing. Being proactive is better than being passive.*

© 2013 Parkinsons Recovery

I also have seen this in clients during my HIV-positive volunteer days. The people who lived much longer that were developing AIDS (advancing from HIV positive to full-blown AIDS) went off to seek the cure of the month, such as…

- *cucumber extracts or*

- *BHT or*

- *acupuncture or*

- *selenium supplement or*

- *antifungal drugs*

They would go off, look at the literature and then go after it. Those people lived for years. The people who just accepted the doctor's advice, took the nucleoside drugs and passively cooperated with the system died young.

That told me that attitude was a key issue. It wasn't the specific therapy that was chosen. It could be anything. It could be at the top of my "flaky" meter and still seem to significantly extend their survival, even double it or triple it. That taught me you need to believe in what you are doing."

Steven Fowkes, CERI

I interview many people who are hesitant to take action. They want to gather the evidence and the facts about a particular therapy or treatment. They conduct research (as do I). They ask questions in chat rooms. They conduct research on the internet. They call me on the phone and ask if I have heard of the therapy or treatment. They conduct research at university libraries. They ask health care specialists for their advice and counsel.

Weeks pass. Months pass. Years pass. No action is taken because the full evidence is not yet in or because the feedback is mixed. Some people say go for it. Others say it is a waste of time and money. Still others may tell you it will harm you.

But wait. Doctor Smart Mouth, Ph.D. from University Big Wig in Smarty Pantsville is currently doing a smancy fancy study to evaluate the therapy you are considering. It has all the publishable criteria: double blind, large sample, well controlled and quantitative.

Smart mouth will be able to tell us all whether it is worth trying in several years. Of course his study will recommend follow-up studies, so the jury will be out for another 30 years.

Symptoms get worse. The person loses the motivation to continue their investigation. The person gives up. The person dies at a young age. End of story.

I say this. Ask yourself - what therapies do I want to try? What does my own intuition tell me? Make sure the therapy is safe of course. It is certainly best if the therapy is noninvasive. Sure it is a good idea to make some preliminary checks on the internet, with your doctor, with your friends, with specialists.

Beyond these basic checks, take action if your intuition tells you to go for it. Try out whatever therapy you are drawn to.

You cannot go wrong if you take action. Why? Even if it is not the right therapy for you and your body, you will get valuable information that will guide the choice about the next therapy to pursue (whether it is a supplement or exercise program or nutritional program or …). Steve Fowkes explains the value of taking action by way of this example:

> *"Some people with Parkinsons disease are going to have a blood coagulation problem that goes along with it. When they take nattokinase, all their symptoms are going to ease significantly. Until you try it, you do not know that."*

The people I interview who are getting remarkable improvements in their symptoms do not focus on one treatment or therapy. They use multiple treatments and therapies. They keep searching. They continue to experiment. They keep taking action. They keep getting better and better.

Steve Fowkes recommends a draconian rule that works beautifully:

> *If I don't get better, I don't spend my money on it and I don't spend my time on it. It actually comes down to a fairly simple program.*

Please note that I have not said what action to take. I do not need to. If you access your own intuition, you will be able to figure out a starting point for your own recovery program. Dr. Smart Mouth does not know what you need. I certainly do not know what you need. You do. Check in with yourself.

Or wait. Perhaps you do not have the "money"? That is a silly excuse. There are many therapies that have yielded huge benefits for people that cost nothing. Take one small step forward. Monitor the result. The chances are good you will be feeling better. This will give you the energy and motivation to take the next step on your Road to Recovery.

If you are getting good results from the therapies you are using and the medications and supplements you currently take, be happy about it. Stick with what you are doing. If you are not getting good results, try something else.

© 2013 Parkinsons Recovery

THE SPECTRUM OF MEDICAL SPECIALTIES

There are many specialties to consider when searching for therapies and treatments. I will preview several by way of opening up ideas for widening your search to find relief from the symptoms your currently experience.

One of the places familiar to most people is western medicine, a specialty among many other possible specialties that can be considered. Western medicine treats symptoms with prescription drugs and surgery. This approach for treating illness has become a commonly accepted method of treating disease for about 100 years now.

It is losing some of its popularity because of the side effects of the medicines and the consequences of surgeries. It is important to remember, however, that the mainstream medication specialty is precisely what some people need to jump start their recovery program.

Thank goodness the western medicine specialty is stringently regulated. Prescription medicines make molecular changes to the cellular structure of the body. Most prescription medicines have significant side effects. This is why Federal Drug Administration (or a similar agency in other countries) legally regulates the availability and sale of all prescription drugs. Stringent certifications are required for the medical doctors who prescribe the medications and for the pharmacists who sell them.

The standard treatment approach in western medicine is to perform diagnostic tests to determine the cause of the symptom. Unfortunately administration of the tests can of course take months and require considerable expense. Unfortunately, the diagnostic tests sometimes cause illnesses in their own right.

After determining a diagnosis, the standard approach is to prescribe medications or surgery. If the medications and/or surgery succeed in alleviating the symptoms, the treatment is declared a success. If it is unsuccessful the treatment is suspended in search of alternative drugs or surgeries that are hoped will provide relief. Sometimes medical doctors have to go back to the drawing board to consider other possible diagnoses. Some people have a long list of diagnoses for a variety of symptom sets.

The western approach to medicine works beautifully for some people and some symptoms. For other people and other symptoms, such treatments can be disappointing. Many people prefer this specialty over other alternatives. Others use both.

There are also a wide variety of other specialties that offer the potential to provide relief which rely on natural methods to heal the body. An advantage of such specialties is that they have been practiced for many thousands of years with great success. The worst side effect you are likely to experience when using natural therapies is improved health on some level.

The number of specialties other than western medicine is extensive: homeopathy, acupuncture, herbs, meditation, energy healing, physical therapy, tai chi, Chi Gong, naturopathy, exercise, hypnosis, counseling therapy, nutrition, body work - you name it.

This is the short list. Most of these specialties have been practiced for thousands and thousands of years. The standard approach to illness in the United States was to use homeopathic remedies until the beginning of the 20th century, a time when most of us alive today were not living.

Many people get a huge advantage when they use a combination of specialties. Why? When used in combination, the benefits from using the treatments from more than one specialty are usually synergistic.

In the countless interviews I do with individuals who have the symptoms of Parkinsons I am overwhelmed with what people do that helps - not just a little - but a lot.

Open the door to consider what all specialties have to offer. That is what I have been doing with my own research strategy. I am unearthing exciting discoveries. You can pursue the same path of discovery with the same dazzling results.

Join me with investigating other specialties that have the potential to help you feel a lot better. The people who are getting great relief from their symptoms are willing to experiment with many different specialties. The sky is the limit. The potential for healing is limitless.

CRITICISM FROM FAMILY AND FRIENDS

There is usually one black sheep in any family. Black sheep insist on doing things differently. Their family believes their way is weird, unsafe, unsound and just plain stupid.

I am the black sheep of my family. I am always trying out new therapies of one type or another. My current mission is to reverse the color of my graying hair back to black.

New therapies are continuously being introduced. Is it likely that some of them will help? I figure, why not give them a try. They are natural, noninvasive and safe to try. What is there to lose? I have only one life to live and the life I get to live does not last forever.

Reactions I get are blank stares and questions.

1. *Is there any research to indicate this will help?*

2. *Why do you want to pursue a therapy that your doctor does not even know about?*

In short, there is usually significant criticism from family members when the black sheep decides to branch out and try out treatments or therapies other than prescription drugs and/or surgeries.

Are you the black sheep of your family? If so, I need to clue you in to the reactions you can expect from your family when you announce you are pursuing therapies that are not familiar to medical doctors or approved by the FDA.

> *You have to be kidding me. You are going to try tai chi? Isn't that what backward Chinese people do?*

> *You want to eat differently? What is this? You don't like southern cooking? You don't like barbecue? What is wrong with you?*

> *You really shouldn't exercise. You may hurt yourself.*

> *You shouldn't try to improve your driving skills. You are bound to have an accident.*

> *What? You are going to see an energy healer? Did they graduate from medical school?*

> *You are going to take a supplement that has not been proven by research to help Parkinsons? That is pouring your money down the drain.*

Do any of these sound familiar?

From my extensive interviews with persons who have the symptoms of Parkinsons, a family drama often unfolds when the black sheep announces they are branching out of the family mold to try natural therapies.

Why do family members get so upset with the black sheep of the family in such cases, especially when treatments they have been using are not working? My answer to this curious question is that they are threatened. You are challenging sacred beliefs about illness and recovery that are limiting their ability to maintain their own health.

Family members may very well have bothersome symptoms of their own. They hopefully have taken the smart step by seeking the advice from the specialty of western medicine. If they are not considering other specialties that have the potential to provide relief however, they have given up their power of control over their own destiny. They have resigned themselves to being told what to do.

It is frightening for anyone to acknowledge they have given up the power of choice, especially when it comes to their own health and well being. Learning that someone else in the family is

© 2013 Parkinsons Recovery

stepping up to the plate and taking responsibility for their own health elicits deep questions about the decisions they have made regarding their own health care.

It is tough for all of us to face the truth of our actions. Denial runs deep in everyone (can you see my hand raised now?) Of course there will be emotional reactions when a black sheep of the family branches out of the grip of "mainstream" medical care and to take control over their own health. They are not discarding the value of western medicine. They are simply considering other options for themselves. The decision to broaden a decision context triggers unexpressed doubts about the power of choice everyone else has given up with regard to their own health care.

No one likes to see denial unwrapped and confront the harsh reality they have given up all their power to decide what is in their best interest. After all, it is their body and their life. Viewed in this context, it makes perfect sense that many people in your family will try and convince you to limit your choices because that is what they have done. Everyone likes to have company in the sewer of their own limiting beliefs.

Incidentally, the color is my hair is turning back to its natural color of black from gray. I am doing it naturally - no dyes involved. Isn't that cool? I suppose I could turn it back to black with hair dyes, but then I would be giving up my power to choose an alternative method.

Do you want to know how I am doing it? You will have to make the explicit decision to consider another alternative besides using hair dye. If you want to know the secret, join us for one of our Jump Start to Wellness Program which is where I give away the big secret to reversing hair color naturally. I have had to update my picture on the cover of this book. I look younger now because my hair color is much darker.

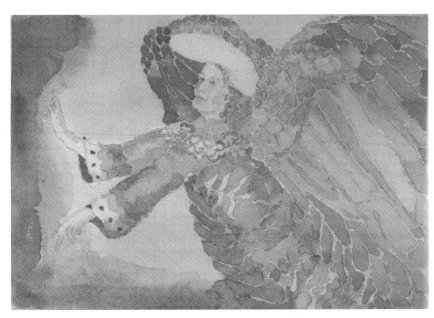

Photo by Anne Davis[2]

Thoughts create our reality. If we hold the thought (either consciously or unconsciously) that we have a disease that is destined to become worse over time, this is precisely what will happen. We will feel progressively worse over time.

Alternatively, if we believe that we can heal from disease we will heal. We will eventually feel better. Or, we interpret our symptoms from a very different perspective.

THOUGHTS ARE THE
MOST POWERFUL
INFLUENCE ON
RECOVERY

---

[2] "I have asked myself what the painting has to do with PD. After all, I might have started this without PD, right? I can't know this for sure, of course, but I think that Parkinson's is essentially a stress related situation. Drawing and painting in my case are the exact opposite of stress. There can be no rush, because time as linear just doesn't exist when one is engaged in 'seeing.' The attention called upon is high powered, but also gentle, just the kind of attention my body needs to counteract the stress response. And the state I get in is essentially joyful, just the state of a sort of living prayer; also needed by my faithful body. People are relieved to have me doing something interesting, as they are slightly scared by my PD, I think. I have something to offer, and have given away lots of paintings, and sold a few too. I am immensely grateful to have a new way to express myself and so I don't miss the children and the classroom as I did at first.

I then started to see angels and paint them. This was a total surprise, and I have no idea what to make of it. However, it is crystal clear to me that not complaining, demanding much of myself, the lovely act of self-forgiveness, the generosity required to accept help from others, patience, solitude and all activities of the spirit are directly called for by Parkinson's. My daily life, it's small moments, is like a sensitive geiger counter... shaking or not... walking or not, all tied up with how sensitively I live. Each year I paint an angel and have him/her made into a card. Like the lady on your resources page, I paint for the state it engenders in me. Sometimes I shake, sometimes I don't. Parkinson's gave me the gift of time and so is the mother of my creativity." Anne Davis

Michael Soyer was an artist and Zen Monk whose paintings are masterful. He was physically challenged over the last five years of his life. During an interview a year before he died, Michael said the happiest years of his life had been the last five. Why? He was able to devote all of his time to the love of his life – painting. Three of his remarkable paintings are featured in *Road to Recovery from Parkinsons Disease*.

Thoughts are so fundamental to the recovery process that I have written a book and recorded a series of meditations that explains the five steps that are necessary to transform your thoughts and get sustained relief from the symptoms of Parkinsons. The book is titled The Five Steps to Recovery.

The process for Parkinsons takes a familiar course. Eventually there is a spell of feeling worse. Fear rears its ugly head. The following thought emerges:

> *"I will never heal from this disease. Everyone says that my condition will get progressively worse. Look what is happening to me today. I must finally accept the reality that I am getting progressively worse."*

What we know from quantum physics is that this belief will eventually be confirmed. The truth of the matter is that this belief is not - I repeat not - true.

It is possible to heal from any condition or disease. Hold in your consciousness the belief that your body knows how to heal itself.

- *Wait.*

- *Listen to your body.*

- *Give it what it needs.*

- *Give it time.*

- *Watch what happens.*

- *You will be delighted.*

QUEST FOR A CURE

Many people I interview have a passion to become "symptom free." They identify with this goal. Thoughts about becoming "symptom free" dominate their day. Some people have asked me to count the number of people who have in fact had a diagnosis of Parkinsons and subsequently become "symptom free." If it is possible to recover fully and completely, then let's see the proof, eh?

I have sponsored guests on my radio show and included interviews in Pioneers of Recovery of people that are symptom free today: John Coleman, ND, Howard Shifke, Lidia Epp and Nathan Zakheim. Many other guests are close to being symptom free. You will discover other inspiring reports of recovery at [http://www.blog.parkinsonsrecovery.com], the Parkinsons Recovery blog. Generally speaking, most people report that their symptoms fluctuate widely. Symptom free weeks are interspersed with weeks when symptoms flare. Difficult weeks are usually triggered by stressful circumstances.

When I launched Parkinsons Recovery several years ago my plan was to maintain a count of people who are symptom free and those whose symptoms are improving. My research skills are primarily quantitative, so this was just my cup of tea.

Early on, I encountered some obstacles. I talk with many people who are feeling much better, but I often do not get their permission to tell their stories or even add them to the count. I hear many reports from people who know others that have fully recovered. The only stories I can report during the radio program, the e mails and the blog are about people who give me permission to post them. I only post first names.

Several years into my research I decided not to construct a "count" on the basis of symptoms as a function of whether they fully or partially resolved. A "count" places the emphasis on the wrong side of the coin - on the goal of becoming symptom free. What is the problem with this emphasis? You are most likely thinking,

> *"Isn't that the whole point of recovery?"*

Any successful recovery programs hinge on maintaining a healthy inventory of positive thoughts. The challenge for all of us is that our egos entangle us in a nightmare of negative thoughts throughout the day which traps us into a valley of despair. Worries that focus on symptoms actually wind up provoking existing symptoms and even creating new ones.

We get angry:

> *Why am I not feeling better today?*

We get frustrated:

> Why *did a new symptom flare up today? I have suffered long enough.*

We get impatient:

> *Why do I have nothing to show from my hard work?*

We get fearful:

© **2013 Parkinsons Recovery**

Why does my family believe I will get worse and worse. Is it true Parkinsons is "progressive"?

We get depressed:

Why should I bother trying anything new? Nothing is working out.

We get mental:

Where is the evidence for recovery? I want to see a count.

I could continue with 100 pages of questions inspired by our clever egos, but you get the point from the short list above. Our egos keep us stuck in the mud. It happens to all of us. No one in a body escapes.

Here is the rub. When our thoughts throughout the day are intent on eliminating symptoms or becoming "symptom free" we give energy to what we do not wish to manifest. If we agonize about becoming symptom free, any hope of recovery will inevitably backfire. We get the opposite of what we want. We give energy to what we do not want. If a majority of thoughts during the day focus on becoming symptom free, we nurture the symptoms, guaranteeing they will continue to pester us.

I admit this sounds counter intuitive, so let me explain. Focusing on becoming "symptom free" suspends you in a space of negative thinking that hangs out in collective consciousness. Every thought has a frequency. Those that congregate around "eliminating symptoms" are low frequency thoughts that can never manifest health and wellness. Rather, such thoughts sustain disease and illness. Consider the thought:

"I want to be symptom free."

The focus here is on what you do not want rather than on what you do want to manifest.

A key to recovery is to take control over our thoughts moment to moment. As I wrote Five Steps to Recovery (which is all about transforming our thoughts), I monitored my own thoughts each day.

Geez. I could not believe what I discovered. I roll the same negative thoughts around my head every day. The number of new thoughts was unbelievably tiny when compared to the thousands of negative thoughts I recycled every day. It was as if I was living the same day over and over as I listened to the same record of depressing songs.

Have you ever seen the movie *Groundhog Day* where Bill Murray re-lives the same day every frickin' day? The trap of negative thinking is just like the nightmare Bill Murray faced every day. You might as well read the same book every day of your life, year after year. The first day the book is interesting. After several months (much less decades) the book gets pretty darn boring. The juices of life get drained very quickly.

When I keep recycling the same negative thoughts, I have no prayer of changing any circumstance in my life. I certainly have no hope of reversing a chronic set of symptoms.

Among those who occupy a body, who is "symptom free"? I suggest that the honest answer is no one. Not me. Not you. Not anyone who occupies a human body. Everyone experiences symptoms most days: perhaps a new ache, perhaps a familiar digestive challenge, perhaps depression, perhaps low energy, perhaps a sprain, perhaps anxiety.

WHAT IS THE COUNT OF YOUR SYMPTOMS?

When I preview the list of symptoms that are associated with people who have the diagnosis of Parkinson's disease, they include just about everything wrong that can happen to a person. Perhaps this sounds outrageous, but it is true.

What follows is a streamlined list of symptoms reported by persons who have a diagnosis of Parkinson's disease. A "streamlined list" means I have not included every symptom that people with Parkinson's tell me they have experienced. As you read down the list, make a mental count of which ones you have experienced at some point in your life time.

I do not know what your count is, but I have personally experienced all of the symptoms in the list at one point or another in my lifetime. I do not have the diagnosis of Parkinsons.

* Stiffness	* Dizziness	* Frequent urination
* Numbness	* Excessive sweating	* Circulation issues
* Cramps	* Daytime sleepiness	* Haggard look
* Balance	* Insomnia	* Headaches
* Depression	* Memory loss	* Arm/leg heaviness
* Repeating yourself	* Weight loss	* Muscle spasms
* Anxiety	* Skin rashes	* Full body weakness
* Apathy	* Restlessness	* Pain
* Swallowing	* Memory challenges	* Difficulty breathing
* Walking difficulties	* Rigid muscles	* Red rash
* Standing up straight	* Muscle spasms	* Arm/leg rigidity
* Constipation	* Joint pain	* Social smiling
* Fatigue	* Nightmares	* Swollen ankles
* Diarrhea	* Hallucinations	* Chest tightness
* Urinating	* Bruising	* Tingling
* Tremors	* Changes in sleep patterns	* Tremors
* Drooling	* Speech/voice changes	* Warmth in body parts
* Faintness on rising	* Difficulty with stairs	* Weak muscles

How about now - in this very moment as I write these words? What symptoms am I experiencing in this moment?

1. I have incredible stiffness in my shoulders which always happens when I write every day.

2. I have ringing in my ears which I have learned to ignore.

© 2013 Parkinsons Recovery

3. I have an ache in the middle of my spine (T4-T5).

4. My throat is restricted.

5. I had memory loss a few minutes ago when I could not remember how to spell a word.

6. I had a tinge of tingling in my left little finger a few moments ago.

My list of symptoms above pertains only to this single moment. I will not bore you with a list of my personal symptoms from this morning or yesterday, but I can assure you my list of symptoms differs from day to day.

This is normal for most people unless you are superman or superwoman. (I do not have any research evidence on Batman or Bat Woman).

The body gives us a continuous feed of information. When we listen to the moment to moment information our bodies send us, we are in a much better position to make the adjustments that are needed for our body to come back into balance. Instead of wishing I want to be "symptom free", the better wish in my book of wishes is to be "symptom rich".

If I were "symptom free" for one day, the likelihood my body would be out of balance is reasonably high. If I were symptom free for two days the likelihood my body would be out of balance is extremely high. If I were symptom free for a week, I dare say the probability my body would be out of balance is guaranteed. My personal mantra is thus:

> *"Bring the symptoms on."*

Don't get me wrong here. I do not like symptoms one bit. I also do not know what I would do without them. I need the information they give me to hang around the earth for a little longer.

If all of my thoughts zero in on the goal of becoming "symptom free," there is no time or energy left to think about what I want to create in my life. I really do want to figure out what my soul needs to do in my life before my time is up. But if I choose to spend the rest of my day today worrying about just one of my symptoms - say not being able to spell a word this morning - there will be no time in my day to ask my soul what it needs for nourishment.

I am choosing to spend my time luxuriating in "Worry Land" which I visit frequently. Of course the process is repeated tomorrow as I worry about not being able to remember what I was worrying about the day before. And so the process unfolds day after day as my enthusiasm for life diminishes.

If I focus my thoughts on becoming "symptom free,"

* I am not listening to my body.

* I am detached from my body.

* I am not connecting with the essence of who I am.

Because I am disconnected with my body, my symptoms in the moment will be sure to fester as other symptoms surface.

As I write this paragraph, I am not even aware of any of the symptoms that I listed a few minutes ago that were pestering me. I am not aware of them because my attention is focused in the moment on writing which is a true love of my life. Focus on writing and my energy soars. Focus on getting rid of my symptoms and my energy slides into the sewer.

How to Shift Thinking

Bodies get out of balance. It happens. It happens to everyone. The body always strives to return to balance. The natural state for the body is health and wellness, not disease and illness. How do I shift my hamster wheel of negative thinking which I have been riding on since childhood?

First, I recognize I can choose the thoughts I wish to think. I am the master of my own thoughts. I can spend my day fighting against the symptoms of the day because I am determined to be "symptom free."

Or, I can nourish my body with positive thoughts that will nourish my life force. I can write. I can dream. I can forward plan my life so that I am living the life I choose to live.

Second, I can change my thinking habits. I can forward plan my day as the first activity of my day. It is 7:30 am. I have just woken up.

* How do I want to spend my time today?

* What do I want to accomplish?

* What do I want to see happen?

* What do I want to see happen in my life today?

* What do I want to see happen in my life this month?

* What do I want to see happen in my life this year and next year?

The more I can detail out what I want my future to look like, the more I can -

*sense it   *feel it   *taste it   *hear it   *see it*

This process infuses energy to the dream and provides the foundation for the dream to manifest effortlessly. If I spend my day contemplating what I do not want to experience (like symptoms), my thoughts lack focus. They dissipate my energy. My life force is diminished. My body is filled with dead energy. I nourish the entrapment of my own ego which fuels my symptoms.

If I tally the number of people who are "symptom free", I will oil everyone's hamster wheel of negative thinking. When suspended in a space of negative thought forms, no one is in a position to manifest balance and harmony in their life.

I get energy from forward planning my life. I lose energy from addicting myself to negative, depressing thoughts that drag me down into the pit of depression. This place familiar to many is yucky. My ego is always inviting me into the "mind sewer" of negative thinking.

I have decided it is in my best interest to refuse the invitations of my very clever ego. Mind sewers smell bad. Mind sewers are stagnant. Mind sewers breed disease. Mind sewers promote illness. They are not good places to live.

I choose to whisk away all the negativity in my thoughts. I do not have any control over ending wars in the Middle East or curbing drug related deaths in New York City. I can control what I choose to think.

When I choose to focus my thoughts during the day on what I want to accomplish during my lifetime, I feel lighter, more alive, more energetic and more powerful. When my mind becomes a fertile garden of positive thoughts, miracles do happen. Often.

"I have the power to heal myself.
You have the power to heal yourself.
Together we have the power to heal the world."
Zhi Gang Sha

THE GIFT OF SYMPTOMS

What thoughts are triggered by the symptoms? Does fear rear its ugly head? Do you want the symptoms to vanish instantly? Of course! But if the underlying thought is that the symptoms mean your body is not working properly, you will find yourself in a negative frame of mind that carries little of the energy that is necessary to heal.

Two examples follow that illustrate two possible thoughts that you can carry about two symptoms that are prevalent for Parkinsons: pain and tremors. The theme for each is that the body is giving you useful information about imbalances, deficiencies or system weaknesses that need to be corrected.

THE UNDERLYING MEANING OF PAIN

It is entirely understandable why we become angry at our bodies when they do not function well. We want to disassociate ourselves from the places that hurt and that do not function as we need them to function.

The body is continuously sending us signals. Sometimes these signals convey pain and discomfort. Pain is the body's way of telling us to pay attention. Something that is unknown to you needs to be brought to your attention for healing.

However unpleasant it may be, pain is spiritual guidance for us. When we learn how to listen to our bodies, we are in a position to take the action needed to heal the deep pain that resides within us. Your body is not broken. It works perfectly.

How do you release the trauma and stress that is trapped deep inside you? Connect with the consciousness of your body. What is screaming at you in the moment?

What part of your body is calling out for your attention now? Is it your left hip or your right leg or ....? Listen. Connect with that place. Ask:

> *"What is here now? What do you need? What are you trying to tell me? I am here for you now. I am ready to listen."*

When we listen to the signals that our bodies are sending us we will have a good idea how to heal ourselves. Although our body may be in deep pain, our bodies do know how to heal themselves.

> *Just listen.*

THE UNDERLYING MEANING OF TREMORS

There are many Parkinsons symptoms, so let me consider one by way of illustrating what it means to listen to your body. Consider the nettlesome problem of tremors. Do you have tremors in your arms or legs or hands?

If you are like most people, your reaction to tremors is to shout:

> *"Stop it. Stop it now"*

© 2013 Parkinsons Recovery

Consider an alternative reaction when tremors happen to riddle through your body. The alternative reaction we recommend is to say:

"If you need to shake, then shake away."

Why? Shaking is a natural way for the body to release trauma that is trapped at the cellular level.

Have you ever watched an animal who becomes frightened? Animals freeze when danger is present. It is a natural reaction to stress that the body uses when danger looms. After the danger passes the animal shakes for a few seconds or even minutes until the trauma is released. The animal then goes about its business without holding the fear in their body.

When you listen to your body, what is the meaning behind your tremors? Our work with persons who have Parkinsons reveals that the answers can vary from extreme stress to memories of one trauma or another in childhood.

If the trigger for the tremor is stress, the ideal response is to figure out how to release the stress. If the trigger for the tremor is trauma there are a variety of therapies that can help your body release the trauma that is trapped in the tissues. Most trauma that has lingered for years does not release without a little help and support from others.

Once you figure out the message your body gives you and once you respond accordingly, do not expect a quick fix. The body requires time to heal. Recovery of persons with Parkinsons takes time and patience.

The good news is that people do experience a welcome relief of symptoms when they listen to their bodies.

Your body will tell you what it needs.

Just listen.

It is not broken.

It really works perfectly.

© 2013 Parkinsons Recovery

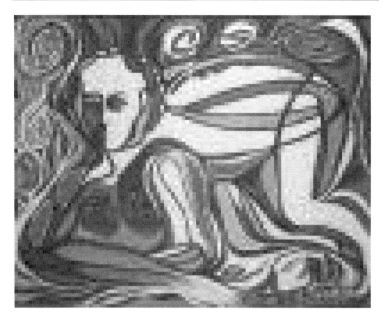

Nude with Parkinsons by Carol McLeod

DIAGNOSIS OF PARKINSONS

PARKINSONS IS A GARBAGE CAN DIAGNOSIS

I want to begin this "thinking exchange" with you by making a simple statement. Parkinsons is a "garbage can" diagnosis.

What does this mean exactly? It means that doctors have evaluated other possible causes for your symptoms by administering a myriad of specialized (and often very expensive) medical tests.

When a possible cause is ruled out, it is eliminated from the list of possibilities. The diagnostic candidate is discarded and thrown into the garbage. Many causes can be evaluated, one by one. As they are ruled out they too are pitched into the garbage can. To their credit, doctors are usually very meticulous and will evaluate a long list of possible causes.

At some point the list of probable causes is exhausted. No other condition is found through testing to be a probable cause. The doctor is finally confident in drawing the only logical conclusion that remains: Parkinsons.

Notice that the diagnosis is derived through elimination. There is no positive way of actually knowing whether or not you have Parkinsons. There is no blood test. There is no definitive DNA marker. There is no MRI that gives the information needed.

Oh, there is one possibility: Biopsies of brain tissues give the definitive diagnosis. Such tests however are only possible on people who are dead.

© 2013 Parkinsons Recovery

What does all of this mean to you? It means that the factors that contribute to your symptoms are unique to you.

What does this mean from a research perspective? It means that the variation in response to treatments is huge. For any given treatment, some people are greatly benefited while other people actually get worse.

Many people we work with are curious to discover what therapies or supplements or herbs or body work are a sure bet for helping them to feel better. There are no sure bets for any treatment.

Take John for example. John gets totally jazzed because when another member of his Parkinsons support group used supplement "x" she experienced instant relief of her symptoms.

John does exactly what I would do. He rushes out and purchases supplement "x." He takes his first dose. No change. He takes his second dose the second day. No change. And so forth, day after day. Is the supplement John purchased a sugar pill or what?

His frustration is explained by a simple truth: There are many complicated factors that can contribute to the symptoms of Parkinsons. What did John discover through his own personal experiment?

The factors that are contributing to his own symptoms are not the same factors that are contributing to the symptoms of his support group friend. His friend's body was deficient in supplement "x". John's body is not deficient. End of story.

The bottom line is that the factors that cause each person's symptoms are unique to them. We know from our own experience in working with people who have Parkinsons that the primary causes are stress, trauma, toxins and physical injuries. But how this translates for each person is very individualized. The routes to recovery are inevitably unique.

THE PROBLEM IS NOT A DOPAMINE DEFICIENCY

Most people who have been diagnosed with Parkinsons are told that their bodies do not produce enough dopamine. The implication of this belief of course is that their bodies are not working correctly.

We believe dopamine deficiency is not the real problem. Surprised? There clearly is a hormonal imbalance. But who is the real culprit here - dopamine or adrenaline?

We believe the true cause of the hormonal imbalance in Parkinsons lies with an overabundance of stress hormones: adrenaline, cortisol, aldosterone and testosterone. These are the hormones that are naturally secreted by the body when it is in a survival mode.

What really happens to the body when it is flushed with stress hormones?

The immune system is jeopardized.

The gastrointestinal track shuts down.

Memory becomes problematic.

Thinking becomes fuzzy.

All senses are dulled - touch, feel and smell.

Overall energy is depleted.

Blood pressure and respiration increase.

Water and nutrients are sent to the lungs and heart. The rest of the body is ignored. After all, the body is in a survival mode. Why bother nourishing the neurons? The connection between the effects of stress on the body and the symptoms of Parkinsons is stark.

When the body is preoccupied with making the stress hormones, cells throughout the system become seriously dehydrated. When cells become dehydrated, how can they get rid of the toxins and waste products? The answer is obvious. They don't get rid of the toxins.

Recovery for persons with the symptoms of Parkinsons involves helping the body remember the place of balance and helping the individual move out of a suspended state of stress. Most people are so stressed they do not even realize they are stressed!

When the body is on continuous alert year after year there is less and less demand on the body to produce dopamine. The natural ability of the body to manufacture dopamine withers away.

Note that the body is doing precisely what it was designed to do. It is not broken. It is working perfectly. There is no inherent demand to produce dopamine, so less and less dopamine is manufactured. The body is too preoccupied with producing the hormones that are needed when it is under stress.

Why again does the body stop producing dopamine? When we stop using any skill, proficiency declines little by little, day by day.

Consider a physical example. If you stop working out and exercising, it does not take long for the muscles in the body to turn to flab.

"Use it or lose it" is the name of the game. When you do not use it you lose it!

© 2013 Parkinsons Recovery

If you do not use the body's learned ability to manufacture dopamine, it will gradually lose the ability to produce dopamine in the quantities that are needed. The cells needed to produce the hormone die and are not replaced. The body says to itself:

"Why bother? There is no need for dopamine."

Although increasingly a young person's disease, the symptoms of Parkinsons do not emerge in many people until the later years. This is because there needs to be an 80% depletion in the body's capacity to make dopamine before the symptoms of dopamine depletion actually surface.

When it comes to hormones, they key issue turns on the question of balance. Is the delicate balance of the 40 or so hormones (one of which is dopamine) right? It is really not a question of too little or too much.

When too much dopamine is poured into the body using medicines or supplements other serious side effects can emerge: compulsive behaviors (addictions to gambling, shopping, food, sex, sweets) and uncontrollable jerky movements called dyskinesia by medical professionals.

It takes a long time for the body to give up its ability to produce any hormone it thinks it may need in the future. But it will give up, eventually. It obviously will take time to convince the body otherwise because its natural state is to maintain balance and harmony.

CALCIFICATION

Johan Boswinkel, the father of Biontology Sciences, argues that very few people actually have Parkinson's Disease. Why? He views evidence Parkinson's disease to be a calcification of the body due to a malfunction of the parathyroid gland which is responsible for the metabolism of calcium. Calcium is deposited in the tissues of the body rather than the bones. Muscles receive insufficient blood flow which induces trembling and tremoring. Arteries in the brain can also become clogged with calcium.

He has observed that women who take calcium supplements tend to have Parkinson's symptoms. If the body did not distribute the calcium before getting the supplement it surely will not know where to distribute it after. Calcium supplements will be distributed to the same wrong places, making the problem even worse. The body's ability to distribute calcium to the right places is restored once the parathyroid gland gets back on line.

In summary, the problem is not a dopamine deficiency. Johan Boswinkel argues it is a malfunction of the parathyroid gland. Other symptoms of Parkinsons are caused by imbalances in the liver, gall bladder and appendix. These problems persist because the body does not recognize there is a problem with these organs. Once the recognition system is reactivated, the body gets busy with healing the problems.

CAUSAL SEQUENCES ARE MULTI-FACETED

Sharry Edwards from Sound Health and I share a common perspective on the causes of symptoms associated with Parkinson's. It is a multi- faceted condition which involves very long string of causal sequences. On a general level, the symptoms of Parkinson's are caused by interference in the brain to nerve communication. This obstruction can be caused by a wide variety factors including toxins, inflammation, trauma, biochemical imbalances, particularly vitamins B1, B2, B5, B6, B12 and Choline, blocked receptors and malfunctions in genetic signaling. This list is a lot to chew on, but Parkinson's is anything but a simple condition.

Look at any chart of the biochemical chains in the body that are necessary to produce any of the hormones needed by the body to function. We are talking here about thousands of cause and effect links. When any of those links is degraded or broken, the effect on the body's ability to produce dopamine or serotonin or melatonin or any one of the many hormones necessary to sustain life is disabled.

Sharry has identified five cycles in particular that are the pathway to neurological health:

1. ***Urea cycle.***

2. ***Neurotransmitter cycle.***

3. ***Folate cycle.***

4. ***Methylation cycle.***

5. ***Transulfuration cycle.***

There are a multitude of causes and effect processes within each of these five cycles. A mutation, blockage or interference anywhere in any one of these five cycles will compromise a critical function of the body.

Acknowledge the complexity of the body. There is no mystery about why so many symptoms are associated with Parkinson's disease and why each person's experience is unique. Because there are dozens of reasons the pathway can be compromised, it becomes obvious that a single Holy Grail "cure" does not exist and will never be found. The road to recovery involves a series of adjustments to one or several of the processes in one or several of the cycles. A return to balance usually takes time and requires patience.

Voice profiling makes it possible to see where the link is broken in the complex chain of metabolic sequences. I believe Sharry Edward's research is at the cutting edge of where medicine is headed in the future. I also believe doctors will soon be using frequencies to diagnose and treat disease.

Many people hold dear to the mistaken believe that their bodies need more and more L-dopa and dopamine. As a guest on several of my weekly radio shows, Sharry discovered several listeners who volunteered to have their voice profile analyzed actually had too much dopamine in their body.   Most people believe that if they are experiencing symptoms, their dopamine levels must be too low. Sharry found that the problem for these individuals was that the dopamine was not being assimilated and absorbed. A critical link in their metabolic chain was deactivated or inoperable.

During her last presentation sponsored by Parkinsons Recovery, Sharry presented the results of a voice analysis for Michael J. Fox. Why does he currently experience the symptoms of Parkinson's? His issue turns on the unfortunate impact of the COMT gene.

COMT is the name given to the gene that codes for an enzyme called catechol-O-methyltransferase, one of several enzymes that degrade dopamine. Several pharmaceutical drugs have been developed that alter the activity of COMT. Inhibitors include tolcapone and entacapone which are commonly used in the treatment of Parkinson disease.

Some people are likely thinking – big deal. If Michael J. Fox' problem is genetic, then nothing can be done for him. He will just have to honor his fate. The sweet news for everyone (and especially Michael J. Fox) is that the belief of genetic immutability is mistaken. Any gene has a specifically identifiable frequency. You can activate a sleepy and inactive gene in the body by using a frequency that alters the function of the target gene.

© 2013 Parkinsons Recovery

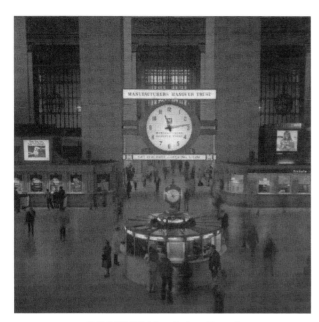

GCT NYNY by John Fasulo

CAUSES OF PARKINSONS SYMPTOMS

Some people who are diagnosed with Parkinsons believe that they "caused" the condition themselves. This is not true. People with Parkinsons did not do anything to cause their disease or create the condition. Symptoms are evidence that the body is a working miracle. The body is simply giving you information that something is out of balance and needs attention.

Recent research suggests that the symptoms of Parkinsons originate in the olfactory center of the brain. The sensation of smell is lost long before the neurological symptoms present themselves. Simple tests that evaluate a person's ability to smell specific scents have recently been devised as early screening diagnostics for Parkinsons. If the problem originated outside the area of the brain responsible for the production of dopamine, doesn't it make sense to suspect that the problem cannot be solved by the replacement of dopamine in the body?

Symptoms can often be temporarily reduced or eliminated with dopamine supplements (whether through prescription medicines or herbs). Medical doctors openly acknowledge however that dopamine therapy does not address the root cause of the condition.

Recent research also suggests that constipation is a predictor of Parkinsons. Infrequent bowel movements indicate a constipation problem. Studies have actually tracked the number of bowel movements people have over the entire course of their life. Incidence of Parkinsons (and other illnesses) has then been correlated with the frequency of bowel movements early in life.

© 2013 Parkinsons Recovery

Findings show that people with infrequent bowel movements early in life are more likely to experience the symptoms of Parkinsons later in life. If constipation plays a large role, doesn't it make sense to suspect that the problem cannot be solved by the replacement of dopamine?

Let's take a step back and consider how symptoms are interpreted by psychologist Steven Fenwick, Ph.D.

> *"As you look at the underlying meaning and purpose of the symptoms, what are they trying to tell you? It is like it has a gift for you."*

> *"Even though you may hate the symptoms - we all hate symptoms - but even though we hate them and we want them to go away and we do everything we can to make them go away, which is good, we also want to look at what the meaning is."*

> *"What is it trying to tell you about your life? What is it trying to tell you about your life's purpose and meaning? And as you unfold that and get more in touch with that and express it more in your life, often times the symptoms do get better. "*

> *"From a Process Work point of view, I would say ... instead of always trying to repress the symptom, experiment. Amplify the tremor or whatever your most disturbing symptoms are with just making them bigger and feeling what they are expressing. "*

> *"Maybe you could dance it some; of if you're sitting in a chair you could move various ways to express it. You could draw it. And just feel - If this had a message for me, what is it telling me?"*

The cause of symptoms is rooted in a multiplicity of sources: thought forms, trauma, stress, toxins, digestive system problems, pathogens and physical injuries to the brain.

1. *Unresolved trauma becomes trapped at the cellular level and mucks up all systems in the body.*

2. *Stress has a mainline connection to the symptoms.*

3. *There is extensive evidence in the research literature that toxins in one form or another (iron, pesticides, mercury poisoning, etc) are implicated in the symptoms of Parkinsons.*

4. *Digestive problems have a deleterious impact on the functioning of neurons.*

5. *Living critters of various shapes and origins (pathogens, mold, bacteria, viruses, Candida, etc.) can wreak havoc on our neurological system.*

6. *Direct injuries to the head can be a factor for some people.*

Any single factor or combination of factors taken together can overtax the body's immune system, the elimination organs and the body's ability to maintain a natural balance of hormones. Neurons are particularly sensitive little critters. It does not take much to traumatize them.

The key to recovery is thus to find ways to release the trauma, reduce the stress, release the toxins, improve the digestive function and regenerate cells. Depending on the individual, one or more factors may be the primary trigger for their symptoms. When given the proper nourishment and support the body is well equipped to rejuvenate itself. This is true even in cases of cellular destruction resulting from physical injury.

When ...

Trauma remains trapped

Reactions to stress persist

Fuel for the cells is insufficient

Toxins remain lodged in the tissues

Uninvited guests are left to build their own playground in our body

Elimination organs in the body are challenged

The body's cry for help will get increasingly louder. The body's struggle to maintain balance will become increasingly more difficult. With no relief in sight, the body becomes overtaxed, overwhelmed, and overworked. The body cannot succeed without help. Without help, the symptoms of Parkinsons will get progressively worse. Taking medicine to increase your dopamine level constitutes one small piece of a 50 piece puzzle.

The exciting news is that there is a long list of therapies and treatments which you can consider to address each problem. My interviews with medical doctors, naturopaths, homeopaths, osteopaths, EFT practitioners, herbalists, aroma therapists, energy healers and others provide rich insights into the many options for healing that are available.

The work we have been doing at Parkinsons Recovery focuses on a most fundamental question of all:

What seed thought lies at the root of the physical symptoms?

Once the seed thought that is driving a symptom is released, removed, detached, ejected and shielded, the core mechanism that creates the imbalance is no longer present.

© 2013 Parkinsons Recovery

Restorative statements replace the destructive seed thought with a positive intention to heal. Once the seed thought is released and replaced, the engine driving the symptoms is dismantled. Healing unfolds immediately.

SEED THOUGHTS

When I first started my research on Parkinsons I held the belief that it takes a minimum of two years to fully recover and that many people take much longer to return to a state of full health and wellness. I have since concluded this thought is dead wrong. I only got this insight after writing the Five Steps to Recovery book which is all about how our thoughts are always manifested to the nth degree.

My realization is this. If I believe it takes two years to recover, it will take two years to recover. I have a new thought and belief. Recovery can happen now if we so choose it to be so.

How in the world can this happen? By releasing the thought form itself that is creating the imbalance in the body. By thought form, what do I mean exactly? There is clearly no universally held thought form (at the unconscious level) for people with the symptoms of Parkinsons. Issues differ for each person. Here are some examples of thoughts that might sound familiar (or not).

- *I am afraid of trusting*

- *I am afraid of death*

- *I am afraid of responsibility*

- *I am afraid of success*

- *I am afraid of money*

- *I am afraid of intimacy*

- *I am afraid of love*

- *I am afraid of Loss of love*

- *I am afraid of rejection*

- *I am afraid of being abandoned*

- *I am afraid of failure*

- *I am afraid of being present to myself and others*

- *I am afraid of change*

- *I am afraid of living*

- *I am afraid of being disappointed*

- *I am afraid of being abused*

Any one or any combination of the thoughts above can be the engine that drives the symptoms. People can do all the detoxes in the world – with some modicum of success – but the toxins will be retained by the body until the relevant seed thought of fear is released. People can do all the healing work in the world to release the trauma – also with some modicum of success – but the trauma will be retained by the tissues of the body until the seed thought of fear is released.

It is a lot like trying to get rid of dandelions in your yard during spring. If you mow them down, they disappear for a day but return in full yellow bloom the next day. If you want to get rid of the dandelions, you have to cut out the seed that created them. Everyone knows you have to dig up dandelion roots to get rid of them.

The seed thoughts that nurture the symptoms of Parkinsons thus have to be released, removed, detached, ejected and shielded before the body will return to its natural state of balance, clarity, centeredness and overall health.

As long as the seed thought remains, you are cultivating a garden of low frequency organisms that promote ill health. All thoughts, all material objects, all colors, all sounds have a frequency that is specific to them. Medicine of the future will use frequencies to heal illnesses, not medicines and surgeries.

Low frequencies are conducive to illness and disease. Fears have extremely low frequencies that sustain the foundation that is needed to foster illness in the body.

Trauma always institutionalizes fear in the body. The embodiment of fear signals the body to retain the toxins for its own survival. After all, how can any living entity remain alive if they are suspended in a continual state of fear. The hormonal imbalances in the body become so large that all systems in the body eventually go off line. The organism cannot survive.

The universal rule of the universe is that "likes attract likes." Low frequency seed thoughts and low frequency toxins hang out with one another. It is a closed, private club with strict rules of admittance. No one is allowed to leave once they become trapped unless and until the seed thought is cleared. You have to extract the glue that bonds thought forms to the toxins.

© 2013 Parkinsons Recovery

A low frequency nursery is cultivated in the body through the fear that underpins the moment to moment babble of our thoughts. Imbalances in the body are the inevitable result when the thoughts of fear are cemented into the fabric of our being.

Seed thoughts can be connected to:

- *Self judgment*

- *Self worth*

- *Feeling not good enough*

- *Feeling unworthy*

- *Panic attacks*

In the work we are doing, it really does not matter what stimulus created the seed thought. Perhaps it was the look of a mother to a child at birth. Perhaps it was a physical trauma. Perhaps it was the premature death of a family member. Perhaps it is the accumulation of all of these events and more. The origins of the seed thought are of no consequence.

With quantum healings, you identify the seed thought that underpins the illness and release it. Once released, you develop a restorative statement to replace the destructive seed thought that was causing the illness in the first place. All of this happens when the work is done. You do not have to wait or moan or suffer or agonize or engage in intellectual back talk. You simply identify the seed thought, release it and create a new seed thought that is restorative.

There is nothing magical about quantum healing work. It is not mysterious or complex or contorted. It is straightforward and simple. We are dedicating our efforts this year to showing people with the symptoms of Parkinsons how they can do quantum healings for themselves with the hope they will teach others to do the same. We will accomplish this mission through interviews, the <u>radio programs</u>, the <u>newsletter</u>, the <u>blog</u> and our live <u>Jump Start to Wellness</u> programs.

When the destructive seed thoughts are released and replaced with restorative statements, the frequencies linked to the physical become very high indeed. Healing happens now in the context of these high frequencies. The best part of all is that low frequencies cannot exist in the presence of the high frequencies. This means the body will finally allow the release of the toxins and trauma trapped at the cellular level. Used in combination with the other therapies, the body can return to its natural state of health and wellness.

© 2013 Parkinsons Recovery

I will first address the palpable reasons why the symptoms are manifested in the context of stress, traumas, toxins, digestive issues and injuries. I will then explain how the seed thoughts that create the symptoms in the first place can be released.

STRESS

One of the most poignant illustrations of the damage done to cells by sustained stress is seen in the plight of salmon that fight their way upstream to spawn. We see these fish frantically meander through the waters of the Puget Sound and up the fresh water streams. The energy is frantic. You can see the pathway they carve through the waters of the Puget Sound in the fall because they churn up the waters like a high speed mixer.

Where do the salmon get all of this unrestrained energy? The same place we get this energy when we are stressed - the surge of cortisol secreted by the adrenal glands. Salmon are swimming to spawn. They destroy their bodies in the process. After they spawn, they die.

What actually happens to their bodies? Adrenal glands become swollen and stop functioning. The delicate balance of hormones is totally disrupted. Most acquire ulcers. Immune systems are destroyed. All become mentally disoriented. Tumors grow on their organs, especially their kidneys. Bacterial infections appear overnight. Parasites enter. The transformation from health to illness is quick.

When stressed, humans secret cortisol from their adrenal glands as well. The process of deterioration is the same. The difference is that humans take their sweet time before organs lose their ability to function, immune systems are totally compromised and hormonal balance is completely destroyed. The impact of stress devastates the ability of the sensitive neurological system to function properly.

Here is how John Briggs, ND[3], explains the effect unrelenting stress has on the chemistry of our body:

> "A lot of times I will see people who are dealing with issues of emotional stress, burdens, anger, frustration - all these will indeed have a biochemical effect on your body. When you are angry, there is a biochemical change that goes on in your system. You can usually feel how you feel after you get done. You feel poisoned.

---

[3] These comments were taken from my radio program interview with John Briggs, ND, on April 16, 2009 (http://www.blogtalkradio.com/parkinsons-recovery)

By the same token, consider the scenario of the little mother whose car falls on a baby and she gets out there and lifts the car off the baby. The little 98 pound mom does this. How does she do that? That is what happens at that point in time, the amazing adrenal response that puts the system into overdrive. You can only do that for a short period of time.

That is like driving one of the souped up roadsters that you have nitrous oxide in. You can use the nitrous oxide for a short period of time for quick burst of speed, but if you use it for any length of time - what are you going to do? You are going to burn out the vehicle. You will burn up the engine.

Some people ... whether they are carrying excessive burdens or stresses ... these chemistries stay at certain levels over extended periods of time and it can start affecting what is going on physically with their body."

What triggers stress? The answer is fear. Is a tremor one of your symptoms? When animals are afraid they shake their entire body. So do humans – but we call it a tremor that needs to be treated rather than a natural response to fear.

For many people, the tremor stops when they sleep. Why? A safety response is induced with sleep. The body has no reason to prepare for battle. When we release, remove, detach and eject fear, tremors have little reason to exist unless they are stimulated by toxins or triggered by injuries.

TRAUMA

What is meant by trauma? Virtually everyone with Parkinsons we have worked with is able to identify a traumatic event or a series of events in their lives. Some of the trauma that is reported to us is physical: difficult births, hospitalizations while an infant, falling out of a tree when young, head injuries, automobile accidents - you name it.

Traumas can also have strong emotional roots. I was discussing trauma with a Parkinsons support group when one woman raised her hand.

"I know an example of this. I have a friend whose son committed suicide. His Parkinson's symptoms flared up two months later."

For some people the trauma is primarily emotional, not physical. Examples include the early and untimely death of a parent of sibling, service during wartime, sexual abuse, verbal abuse, alcoholism, over controlling parents, etc. You name it. All persons who currently experience the symptoms of Parkinsons have encountered trauma in one form or another at some point in their lives.

© 2013 Parkinsons Recovery

When trauma is unresolved it remains trapped in the body, literally. This is not some strange esoteric phenomena. The effects of trauma can be seen in the twists and knots of the physical body itself.

Recent longitudinal research demonstrates that children who have been exposed to violence at an early age show a significant erosion of their telomeres, a key indicator of aging. Trauma is absorbed by the cells. The long term damage to health is shocking, even among children. Imagine the effects for adults who were traumatized as children and have lived for several decades.

Of course it looks differently depending on the person and the trauma they have experienced. Bodies always show the trauma regardless of the origin: a left shoulder lower than the right shoulder or a right eye lower than the left eye or a twist in the trunk of the body or ...

Jaclyn Gisburne, Ph.D. has observed a strong connection between the specific location of symptoms and the nature of the trauma. People who have issues with their arms or legs or face will have experienced a trauma that is in some way related to their arms or legs or face.

> "If we look at the pattern of the tremoring and the other symptoms you can see how that pattern fits with the trauma story that comes up. There is a clear correlation between people who are unable to walk and their trauma story about not being able to go forward or having gone forward and having the trauma".

Jaclyn Gisburne has discovered one early trauma in particular for persons with Parkinson's symptoms. She finds that many people as children experience a loss of support of one or both parents. The child is placed in the position of having to take care of their parent(s) at a very early age, as young as five years old or less. Effects of early childhood trauma materialize many years later in the form of the neurological problems of Parkinson's.

Fascia, the delicate tissues in the body that connect all of the body's systems, become physically entangled with trauma. The site of the trauma becomes "wound up" like a wash rag after being rinsed and hung up to dry. Tissues become dehydrated. The trauma is trapped at the cellular level because the person has not had an opportunity to release it.

So what is the big deal if the body is twisted and wound up? The stress and trauma that is suspended in the tissues leads to ill health and degenerative diseases of one type or another. That is the big deal.

In state of perpetual tension and stress, the body has no opportunity to relax and produce the luscious hormones such as dopamine that make us feel good. Instead, the body turns the switch onto continuous alert, pumping out more adrenaline than is required.

Without being conscious of it, people begin to anticipate day in and day out that a new trauma of one form or another is about to haunt them or their family. The feeling of anticipation becomes so familiar that the person is not even aware of the stress that is being created in their body. Is it any secret to anyone that perpetual stress eventually causes serious damage to their nervous system?

What does the body do when the signal of fear is perpetually present? The body prepares itself for battle. It moves all of the critical resources to the only organs that matter - the organs that we need for survival. Nutrients, oxygen and water are dispatched to the lungs and heart.

The heart rate increases. Respiration increases. Adrenalin is furiously pumped into the body. Our arms and legs are primed for action. Our mental function is put on hold. We become confused and disoriented. Don't these outcomes sound a lot like Parkinson's symptoms?

What does this mean for the rest of the tissues in the body? Without oxygen, without water and without proper nutrition, the neglected cells gradually become unable to renew themselves. It becomes more and more challenging for the body to get rid of unwanted waste products and toxins.

The person eventually becomes constipated. Cells that make up the building blocks of the nervous system become less able to rejuvenate themselves. The system gradually shuts down. Nerve endings become desensitized.

Regardless of its source, trauma freezes up tissues throughout the body. Muscle tissues in many people with Parkinsons feel much like concrete after it has hardened.

CONSEQUENCE OF TRAUMA
Many adults (myself included) have held the belief that if we are able to function in the world as adults by educating ourselves, getting good jobs, and making a contribution in our respective fields, we have successfully overcome any and all traumas we experienced as a child.

I personally convinced myself for 50 years that I could "will" traumas from my own childhood to vanish into thin air. Speaking from personal experience, I must confess this plan was a big flop.

What I now know to be true is that traumas from childhood (and traumas we experience as adults) have a permanence about them. Trauma resides inside our cells as we age. They get stuck in our tissues and settle in for the long haul. Trauma accelerates the aging process. Like it or not, our issues are indeed in our tissues.

Everyone is familiar with the feeling of chronic stress that is perpetuated by fear, but not everyone is aware of the toll it takes on our physical body. Under conditions of chronic stress, cells interrupt their normal function. Instead of nurturing healthy aging, the production of life sustaining proteins is altered to produce the hormones that are required for survival. Under stress, adrenaline pumps out of the cells with the enthusiasm of flood waters that caress the crest of Niagara Falls. The body ages much more quickly when in survival mode.

When a threshold level of trauma and stress is reached the body becomes less and less able to tolerate it. It takes time for the hormones in the body to become seriously imbalanced. It should thus come as little surprise that it also takes time for hormones to return to their natural state of balance and harmony.

TOXINS

To be clear at the outset - it is well documented in the research literature that the symptoms of Parkinsons can be caused by toxins. Which ones? There are so many varieties. There are so many types. There are so many sources. Each of us is exposed to thousands of toxic substances over the course of our lifetime.

There is no way to avoid them. Exposure to toxins comes from the foods we eat which contain pesticides, the chemicals we use to clean our homes and even from the products we use to clean and beautify our bodies.

The body's natural defense to an overwhelm of toxins is to dispatch them to the extremities of the body – the legs, arms and head. They body will do everything possible to maintain the integrity of the vital organs which are all located in the trunk of the body. The body will take any steps necessary to keep the vital organs from becoming toxic.

One of the ways to approach the problem of toxins in the tissues of the body is to detox. Just as important, however, is to reduce (or even eliminate) your current exposure to toxins. Many people are not aware that they are exposing themselves to deadly toxins every day. What toxins you ask?

Toxins are everywhere. We live in a toxic world. The hard reality is that we have to be careful about what substances we touch, what substances we put in our bodies and what substances we put on our body.

The source of toxins may well be one that you never imagined, wine. Are you a wine drinker? Recent research found high levels of copper, nickel, zinc, chromium, manganese and vanadium in both red and white wine. Prolonged ingestion of wine will eventually overwhelm the body with a continuous assault of toxins that cannot be removed naturally by the elimination organs: kidneys and liver. Wines from Hungary and Slovakia were found to have the highest level of heavy metal contamination. French wines were third on the list. Wines from Argentina, Brazil and Italy appeared to pose no risk of heavy metal contamination.

We have to be especially careful about soaps, detergents, cleaning agents, shampoos, make up, skin care products and sun screen. You would be surprised to discover how many toxic substances are probably hanging around your household.

I think there is a strong possibility that Parkinsons symptoms for some people are caused by exposure to a product a person has used their entire life – makeup, soap, detergent, shampoo, garden pesticides, toothpaste – you name it. If you have used the product for decades, you do not suspect it is the culprit.

This is precisely how moles (or spies) become so dangerous. They enter into the secret service of a country (CIA, FBI, Scotland Yard) at an early age. They move up the ranks. They become one of the big wigs. All along, they are passing secrets to the enemy. Everyone trusts them because they have been hanging around so long and because they have status.

Do you give a certain "status" to products that you put onto your body that have toxins? Do you want to use a personal care product because you are convinced it is the only one for you, even though it contains substances with long complicated chemical names that sound toxic?

I suggest that everyone conduct an audit of everything they put on their body or in their body. If the product contains an ingredient with a long, complicated, scary name – throw it out (or do some research to discover what that substance is). The chances are good that if you are unfamiliar with the name, it is toxic or your body is allergic to it.

I recently had an experience that is a reminder of the harm a product can inflict on our body. I have been having a problem for the past four months with chapped lips. My lips have become so dry that they have been bleeding. I have never had a problem with chapped lips – ever. I have lived in cold climates – Michigan and New York – but never needed to use Chap Stick to moisten my lips.

What is up here?

I began to wonder. What have I done differently in the past several months? My initial suspicion was a supplement I have been taking to reverse my hair color back to black. Perhaps I was taking too much? I reduced the daily dosage and the problem continued to worsen. I bought Chap Stick. It did not help.

My next step was to realize I am a researcher and perhaps I could actually use those skills to help myself. I did a search and found that one possible cause of chapped lips is sodium lauryl sulfate in toothpaste. My daughter had given me toothpaste she purchased in Italy that I have been using for the past – you guessed it – four months. I looked at the ingredients and sodium lauryl sulfate was on the list. I stopped using the toothpaste and presto – the problem was solved. My lips have returned to their normal self – moist, soft and free of cracks and fissures.

Instead of thinking you have to put something on or in your body to feel better, you may need to stop putting something on or in your body. The skin is the largest organ of the body. Anything we put on our skin becomes food to the body. If the soaps, shampoos, lotions or skin cleansers that you put on your body have toxins, you are feeding toxins to your body every day. It is possible your body can not keep up with the work of removing toxins The bottom line is that you may be creating a New York City garbage strike in your own body because of the lotions you are putting on your face every day.

Toxins can also proliferate throughout the home. Storage areas underneath sinks are usually toxic waste dumps. Open the sink door and you get toxic exposure from inhaling the toxic gases.

A comprehensive audit of your entire house is a must for anyone with the symptoms of Parkinsons. It is worth a weekend commitment to rid your household of noxious toxins that may be making you seriously ill.   There are several excellent books that can help you create a toxic free, healthy home. Check them out. It is a good time for a spring cleaning.

Karen Logan. Clean House. Clean Planet.

Jeffrey Hollender, Naturally Clean: The Seventh Generation Guide to Safe & Healthy, Non Toxic Cleaning

TESTS SHOW I DO NOT HAVE TOXINS
I talk with many people every week who currently experience the symptoms of Parkinson's. When I ask if they think toxins might be an issue, I frequently hear the following response:

> *"I thought toxins might be an issue for me but I went to the doctor and was tested for toxins. Tests did not show any evidence of any heavy metal toxins. I know now that toxins are not my issue so I am considering other possible influences."*

I ask what diagnostic test was used and learn that the lab analyzed a urine sample. If you are interested in whether you have been exposed to heavy metal toxins over the past 48 hours, a urine sample is valid. But after a few days – heavy metals do not show up in the urine. They become nested in the brain cells and throughout every organ of the body.

Joe Hickey, MD, explains during my radio show that there is an approved diagnostic test that most medical doctors use to determine whether heavy metals are an issue for a person. This diagnostic test (which is the accepted protocol) shows invalid results because it analyzes urine. He used this test for 10 years and found no evidence of toxins in any of his Parkinson's patients.

© 2013 Parkinsons Recovery

After 10 long years, Dr. Hickey began to question the results of his own testing. Really, he asked himself? The research clearly shows toxins are a formidable factor for Parkinsons. He began to question his own diagnostic protocols. Once he switched to using analyses of hair samples, toxins began to show up in record numbers.

Lawrence Wilson, MD, reported during my radio show that even analyses of hair samples do not necessarily detect toxic levels of manganese in Parkinson's patients. He has discovered that once a person's elimination systems get back on line – kidneys and livers begin functioning well – massive evidence of manganese is detected in hair samples. Manganese is not stored in hair. It is buried in the brain cells and only begins to creep out of the body when natural elimination organs begin to function properly.

So, you have been told you do not have toxins? From what I now know, I must say to you – I do not buy it. Everyone in a body in the 21st century has toxins whether they currently experience symptoms of Parkinsons or not. The correlation with Parkinson's symptoms is far too strong to be ignored by any single diagnostic test which presumes toxins are not an issue.

Summary

Consider the possibility that something you have been exposed to over the years is the primary cause of your Parkinsons symptoms.

- Perhaps it is something you put on your body like soaps or shampoos or toothpaste.

- Perhaps it is something you are exposed to like the toxic laundry detergent you use to wash your clothes.

- Perhaps the culprit is the food you eat because it contains MSG or other additives.

SOLVENTS

John Briggs, DC, explains the consequence of exposure to solvents for Parkinsons:

"There are so many solvents in our environment. We find that a lot of these solvents are in our water, especially if we are on a municipal water system. A lot of the chemicals they are treating our water with are solvents. If we look at a lot of the colorings and preservatives - what do we find there? We find things that have a solvent activity.

Solvents break down fats. When we look at the coatings around the nerve we have this thing called a myelin sheath around the nerve. That myelin sheath is a fatty tissue that insulates the nerve and assists in the transfer of electricity. Being a fatty material - anything that is a solvent has a potential of breaking that down.

Since solvents break down fats, there is potential of creating imbalance with Parkinsons ... where we see a nerve building up a charge and then discharging, building up a charge and then discharging. It is like a bad capacitor. It can't hold a charge.

If you stripped out the insulation on the wires on your radio and you turned it on, what is going to happen? You are going to short circuit. With something like Parkinsons, what are we seeing? Short circuiting.

A 2012 study has found a compelling link between TCE (trichloroethylene) and PERC (perchloroethylene), common industrial solvents, and Parkinsons Disease. TCE is used for degreasing metal parts in the manufacturing process. In the past it has been used to decaffeinate coffee and as a general anesthetic. Exposure to these solvents is highly likely for electricians, carpenters, dry cleaners, artists and photographers.

Laurie Mischley, ND, recommends that anyone with Parkinsons symptoms never dry clean your clothes. Most commercial dry cleaners use these highly toxic solvents. When you wear clothes that have been cleaned using dry cleaning solvents you are ingesting toxins directly into your body through your skin. You might as well drink Agent Orange and say to hell with it.

DRINKING WATER

We are exposed to toxic solvents in the tap water that we drink. Twenty-two year veteran of Parkinsons Cynthia Gilbertson comments on the critical importance of water filters:

"A decent water filter is critical. A carbon granular filter is not enough. With Parkinsons there are so many thousands of chemicals in the water that are not even measured that can affect us. It is really important to get a good filter."

MSG, ASPARTAME AND COLAS

Symptoms of Parkinsons are caused by the diet colas you drank when you were 12 years old. OK, I admit it. This is an exaggeration. Or maybe not.

Michael J. Fox's symptoms were caused by all the colas he drank as a child. OK. I admit it. This is farfetched particularly in light of his vocal profile. Or, maybe not.

Consider the possibility there is a grain of truth to these two farfetched assertions that the symptoms of Parkinsons may have been planted in your body during childhood.

Do you suspect that your symptoms are not related to toxic exposure because you have never been exposed to deadly toxins? Read on. No one escapes from exposure to deadly toxins or from the nasty strategy they use to invade and ultimately destroy the organs and systems in our bodies. Toxins have a mind of their own.

© 2013 Parkinsons Recovery

Toxins have a way of creeping into your body gradually and ever so slowly so you do not even notice what is really happening. The first stage of damage occurs during childhood with exposure that - at least on its face - looks benign.

Consider by way of example a common toxin that is sneaked into all processed foods, sodas and diet drinks - Monosodium Glutamate. MSG is found in virtually all processed foods. No one escapes from exposure. No one.

Most children put soft drinks into their bodies. I certainly did. MSG is found in all diet soft drinks.

Reactions to MSG exposure in children appear as skin rashes and general problems with the mucous membranes. Symptoms vary from child to child but will include coughing, sneezing, nose drainage, digestive bloating, gas and stomach upset. Symptoms are temporary.

The child becomes a teenager, then a young adult. Not satisfied with skin deep penetration, the MSG toxins dig in deeper. They invade the muscles, joints and connective tissues, creating arthritic type pain, overall weakness and malaise. After all, there is more tissue mass to dominate.

Young people who are tired all the time believe their fatigue is due to the demands of jobs or family. It may be more likely that their fatigue is caused by the MSG in diet colas they drank as a child and that they continue to drink today.

Enter phase three at middle age. Happy with their success, the toxins squirrel their way into the major organ systems. Some toxins favor particular organs - like the heart or lungs. It is not uncommon for middle aged persons to encounter hormonal problems or heart attacks.

Toxins are now snugly and comfortably lodged in your tissues. End of story? Afraid not my friend. If there have been no interventions to release the toxins from the tissues of your body (such as homeopathy or other natural detox therapies) the MSG toxin becomes more and more settled, more and more comfortable as they snuggle deep inside the tissues of your body.

To be snugly lodged in your tissues and organs is not satisfying enough for the MSG toxins. By no stretch of the imagination have the MSG toxins retired. They want the homerun of a lifetime, the Snickerdoodle of Snickerdoodles.

Enter the final phase - the grand finale. Some people call this the senior years. I prefer to think of this period of life as a time to renew your youth and vitality. MSG toxins now attack the neurological system with their sophisticated weapons and stealth fighter bombers.

Neural impulses are weakened. The entire neurological system is compromised. The central nervous system and spinal cord is affected. The spinal fluid becomes contaminated. Muscles spasm. Arms twitch. Conditions such as Parkinsons and Alzheimer's are diagnosed.

To summarize, the path to destruction of the neurological system is poisonous and destructive. The effects work slowly over a life time. The real damage to the nervous system may be caused by toxins that entered the body 40 years ago. When we drink that diet cola as a 12 year old child, the effects do not vanish in an hour, a day or a week. The toxic effects stick with us for a lifetime until we figure out ways to invite the toxins to find another home.

We know that symptoms are related to excessive free radicals. Aspartame and MSG, two of the chemical substances in colas, are well known to generate a huge volume of free radicals in the brain. What is one thing you can do now to get relief from your symptoms? Stop drinking colas today.

HEAVY METALS

There is no doubt from an examination of the research evidence that heavy metals wreak havoc on the neurological system. Perhaps you are thinking – this could not be your problem since you have never been exposed. Think again my friend.

A primary source of energy for many countries including the United States is coal. The fifty coal burning power plants in the United States that emit the most pollution poured twenty (20) tons of mercury into the air in 2007. The word you just read was tons, not pounds. Once released, mercury settles in lakes and rivers where it moves up the food chain to humans who eat contaminated fish.

Exposure to small quantities of mercury will cause symptoms to emerge eventually, though it may take several decades. Long term exposure causes tremors, inability to walk well, memory problems and pain. Hum – aren't these symptoms of Parkinson's disease?

AMALGAMS AND METAL FILLINGS

Some people experience a running flush of toxins from having metal amalgams that are used as fillings for teeth that have decayed. It is like having a broken thermometer in your mouth that leaks mercury into your body every day. Mercury destroys nerve tissue.

I advise that you do your own research on the impact of metals on your heath. The American Dental Association has declared that metal filings and crowns are safe. I have personally made the choice to have a biological dentist remove all of the metal fillings and crowns in my mouth.

Metal fillings and crowns can also interfere with the communication between the mind and muscles known as proprioception. I personally had been challenged with swallowing pills until I had all the metal in my mouth removed. Metal creates a battery effect in the body. The heightened electrical activity is not conducive to healing neural pathways. My motivation to remove a metal crown was charged after doing an interview for the radio show April 9, 2009 with Simon King. Simon has discovered that crowns and metal filings have a devastating impact on our health over the long term. He identified a metal crown in my mouth that was creating a serious interruption in the connection between my mind and my body.

If you decide to remove the metal in your mouth, I recommend you consider going to a biological dentist who has a specific protocol for removing the metals. The metal should not be removed too quickly. It is also important to do a cleanse before hand and during the actual removal.

Should you have all of the metal in your teeth removed? There is no simple answer. Some people with the symptoms of Parkinsons have had the metal in their teeth removed and all of their symptoms vanished! Others have gone to the expense and seen no difference. Still others have seen a surge of symptoms that might have been caused by a rush of metal into the tissues of the body when the metal was removed. I recommend that you learn muscle testing and ask your body for the answer as to whether you should have metals in your teeth removed.

If you are motivated to explore this option further, you can check out a listing of 147 holistic dentists (primarily in the US) who are have special training in the replacement of metal fillings or crowns with non-metallic material. This particular group of dentists call themselves holistic dentists. They are concerned about the potential health problems that metal crowns might be causing for people.

MANGANESE

Fumes from welding create a toxic source of manganese toxins. Studies have in fact reported significant evidence of Parkinson's disease among welders. These high concentrations of manganese become trapped in the brain cells and are virtually impossible to release from the brain tissues using standard detox protocols such as chelation.

The most effective detox approach is to strengthen the body's natural systems of elimination (the kidneys and liver) so that over time, the body can eliminate the toxins naturally. This is no quick fix, but you can count on the body to do the job if its elimination organs (including the digestive system) are fully functional.

PESTICIDES

Twenty studies have shown that the symptoms of Parkinsons disease are caused by exposure to pesticides. The longer the exposure, the more likely symptoms of Parkinsons will surface. Do we need twenty more studies to say there is "conclusive" evidence? I think not.

© 2013 Parkinsons Recovery

Research evidence also shows a correlation between living in a rural area and Parkinsons. There are a staggering number of agricultural pesticides and sprays that have been used in rural areas. Skin exposure is unavoidable. Pesticides also leak into the ground water, the sole source of drinking water. Do we need more studies of pesticide use in rural areas to conclude there is a connection to the symptoms of Parkinsons? I think not.

William Langston, MD, documented the case of a man who acquired the symptoms of Parkinsons overnight – literally. After a meticulous investigation, Langston and his colleagues determined that the man had taken a dose of heroin which was contaminated by Paraquat, a horrendously dangerous pesticide otherwise known as Agent Orange. This case is documented in this You Tube video: http://www.youtube.com/v/UTImkp1e9Uk?fs=1

Agent Orange, the herbicide used extensively in Viet Nam during the 1970s and in various counties to destroy marijuana plants, is officially acknowledged by the United States government to be extremely toxic and harmful to your health. The Veterans Administration now awards benefits to Viet Nam veterans who experience Parkinson's like symptoms and were exposed to Agent Orange during the Vietnam War.

Pyrethrins are insecticides that are used to kill insects. They are extremely efficient in penetrating the nerve system of bugs. This is why they are so effective as insecticides. Permit me to use a little simplistic line of reasoning here. Pyrethrins destroy the neurological system of insects but do no harm to the neurological system of humans? I think not.

The only difference as I see it is that we humans do not die instantly as is the case with insects. Of course Pyrethrins destroy the neurological system of any living organism. Research has shown a direct connection between exposure and the symptoms of Parkinson's.

Two other toxins have also been connected to the symptoms of Parkinsons: Rhodanine and Permethrin. The chemical agent Rhodanine is used in virtually all pesticides and herbicides. Incidentally, Rhodanine is a substance that is found in nature. It is for all practical purposes, "natural," "organic" but also highly toxic.

Permethrin is a toxic chemical used to soak US military uniforms. Future studies will undoubtedly show a much higher incidence of Parkinsons among the military.

Toxins enter the body through the skin, mouth and nose. No one escapes exposure today, even when they make a conscious effort to avoid exposure. Naturopath John Briggs gives just such an example:

"People may be spraying bug spray covering their mouth and nose because they do not want to inhale any of this. They do not want it getting into their body. But if it gets on the skin it will affect the nervous system."

Consider the variety of intended (and unintended) ways toxins muck up the delicate exchange of impulses that are fired throughout the body's intricate network of neurological pathways.

REFRIGERANTS AND DEGREASING CHEMICALS

Researchers have detected a compelling relationship between exposure to trichloroethylene (TCE) and Parkinson's symptoms. TCE is a chemical solvent that is used in metal degreasing solutions and refrigerants. The research contrasted the experience of 99 twins. One was diagnosed with Parkinsons. The other was not. Analysis of the data revealed a 600% higher risk of having symptoms of Parkinsons with prior to TCE. They also found an increased risk from exposure to tetrachloride (CC14) and perchloroethylene (PERC), both of which are also used as chemical solvents.

WARS

Soldiers are exposed to noxious toxins because of their involvement in wars or other dangerous work. Exposure is not always overt as in the case of exposure to the toxin Agent Orange in Vietnam.

The US military sent stocks of cola drinks to Iraq in 2008 which cooked in the scorching hot storage rooms. Toxins created from overheating the colas posed serious health complications for soldiers who drank them until the source of the problem was identified.

DENTURES

Consider one example of a source of toxins that most people do not think about: dentures. Here is what London Chiropractor Simon King has to say about dentures:

"Dentures have the potential to be toxic. Even denture paste has the potential to be toxic...Dentures are made from acrylics that have to be cured. Many people - especially if they are using denture cleaners – can destroy the coatings on a denture and expose monomer which is potentially very toxic.

People can solve this very quickly, either by sending it back to the lab to be re-cured or to get their dentist to wave their ultraviolet light over it and re-cure it. Ultraviolet light cures monomer. One really novel way of doing this is to go to a nail bar which use ultra violet light to cure the nails.

© 2013 Parkinsons Recovery

The denture paste is very important. There are types of denture paste that are gels normally. These gels contain ingredients like petrolatum which of course is made from petrol. These things will affect our bodies drastically."

DENTURE CREAMS

Perhaps the culprit is the denture cream you use. OK. OK. I know many people don't use denture cream, but stay with me here. This is just an illustration of an important idea which I believe affects every person in a body today. I have concluded from my own extensive research this includes everyone other than aliens we cannot see.

What is the big deal with denture cream? It can cause a toxic exposure to zinc which depletes the levels copper in the body. The body needs the correct balance of zinc and copper to function.

What is the consequence? According to a number of law suits that were recently filed against denture manufacturers, the side effects are:

* numbness or tingling at the extremities	* Decrease in stride of walking
* reduction in movement of extremities	* blood pressure issues
* pain in the extremities	* constipation
* episodes of stumbling while walking	* sexual dysfunction
* poor balance	

This list of side effects includes many of the same symptoms of Parkinsons. If you use denture cream regularly, I suggest that you conduct your own independent research and sort out the issues for yourself. Ask your doctor about denture creams.

If you do not use denture cream, this recent string of law suits raises a different question: Are you being exposed to toxic levels of zinc through daily exposure to other toxins? Perhaps over the years with regular use, a toxic build up has formed in your own body.

I personally have a rather simplistic approach to toxins. I never use a product that contains ingredients with long, complicated names that sound ominous. Look at the ingredients in everything you touch, everything you put onto your body and everything you put in your body this week. Take a minute to read the ingredients. You may be surprised to discover you have been adding a little poison to your body every day.

MATTRESSES, COUCHES AND CHAIRS

When I present the argument that toxins are one factor that causes the symptoms of Parkinson's, some people immediately reply,

> *"I have never been exposed, so toxins cannot be a factor in my case."*

Clearly, they may be dead right. Toxins may not a primary factor or even a contributing factor. But let me give you a reason why you may have been exposed to toxins and did not even know it.

For 30 years federal and state laws have required the application of fire retardants (polybrominated diphenyl ethers or PBDEs) in clothes, furniture and bedding to withstand 12 seconds of contact with an open flame. This toxin can be detected in the furniture and clothes in most homes in the United States.

What is the big deal you ask? This particular toxin causes a disruption in the production of thyroid hormones and, to make matters worse, interferes with functioning of the nervous system.

So you say,

> *"If the toxin is in the bedding of furniture, surely it is no big deal. If it is not disturbed, surely it can't cause me any harm!"*

I honor your optimism, but I am afraid it is unfounded. The chemical is released from the furniture in tiny dust particles that are released from normal wear and tear.

A reason this news is particularly problematic for Parkinsons is that functioning of the thyroid is primary to being able to balance the over 40 hormones in the body.

Now multiply these treacherous effects one thousand fold. My question is: why doesn't everyone who ingests processed foods, sits on couches and sleeps on mattresses have the symptoms of Parkinsons?

There is nowhere to hide from exposure to toxins these days, not even sitting down in the comfort of your own safety sealed home. You may be exposed to toxins when you sleep at night in your bedroom. Flame retardant chemicals are used to treat beds, mattresses and chairs. Simon King questions the value of flame retardants during my interview with him on my radio show on April 9, 2009:

> *"You might be able to get out of a burning building, but it is not much good if it is poisoning you over the years you have it.*
>
> *One of the keys to look for is how do you feel when you wake up in the morning.*

Do you feel better than when you sent to bed?

Or, do you feel worse?

If you go to bed feeling ok, and you wake up feeling lousy, there is a good chance that something in your bedroom is poisoning you."

CARPETS

Simon King sketches the results from a (Journal of Nutritional and Environmental Medicine, 1995, Volume 5, number 4, Pages 375-386) that examined the impact of toxins in carpets on mice:

Researchers put 300 individual samples of carpet in the air flow of four mice. They did that for two hours - half an hour twice a day for two days. In 10% of those carpet samples, all four mice died. In up to 60% of the carpet samples, they could see the toxic effects on the mice.

Perhaps you got ill shortly after you put a new carpet in your house. The cause and effect connection is strong. The carpet is installed. You then notice the symptoms. You do not notice the symptoms before the carpet was installed. OK. Perhaps the formaldehyde which is used in the manufacture of carpets could be causing the symptoms.

I believe a worthwhile question to ask is:

"What was new or different in my house (or my workplace) before you began noticing the symptoms"?

A family member of a woman with Parkinsons recently told me that a $20,000 very thick, very upscale carpet was installed throughout her house just before a presentation of her symptoms. Using my overly simplistic thinking, I offered the following observation:

"Since the symptoms showed right after the carpet was installed, perhaps her symptoms are being caused by exposure to the formaldehyde in the new carpet. Can the carpet be removed?"

The answer was no way.

"Can she live somewhere else for a few weeks to see if the symptoms resolve?"

No. She is close to being bedridden and cannot leave the house.

Was the formaldehyde the cause? We obviously will never know. But, if I were a betting man, I would put good money on the hunch that her symptoms were caused by exposure to the formaldehyde in the new carpet.

I know nothing about the chemical composition of formaldehyde, but I can tell you this. When I say the word out loud, it does not feel good to me. Who would choose to pour formaldehyde into your own hide to see what happens?

COOKING UTENSILS

What type of cooking pans do you use? Are they aluminum? Are they stainless steel? Are they iron? Are they Teflon? Are they copper? You can drive yourself crazy thinking about the potential for toxic exposure from doing something as simple as cooking a meal.

TOXIN TESTING

Nutritional Counselor and Pharmacist Randy Mentzer recommends hair analysis as a method to identify toxins:

> *"There might be a possible trace mineral toxicity with Parkinsons and that would be manganese. You can check all of those things with blood, urine or hair analysis. Hair analysis is a good way to check for toxic metals. We are exposed to toxic metals and toxic chemicals more and more each day in our culture.*
>
> *What if the concern is not what you think it is and it is something totally different that you have missed, but it shows up in a hair analysis. Maybe it is mercury. Maybe that is the problem. It is a good idea to check those things out."*

You can also get rich assessments of the presence of toxins in your body with bioenergetic testing and voice profiling. Both technologies identity the frequencies of toxins and evaluate whether these frequencies resonate in your physical body.

ALTERNATIVES TO TOXIC PRODUCTS

Exposure to toxins is the most formidable health treat of the twenty first century. Without realizing it, we are cleaning our bodies and our homes with products that contain deadly toxins. Some people experience neurological symptoms because they are exposing themselves to toxins every single day when they wash their hair, laundry their clothes, clean their bodies and scrub up their kitchens and bathrooms. Are you one such person? Read the ingredients of the products you currently use. If it contains a substance that has a long, complicated name throw it out and find an alternative. You may be excited to discover that your symptoms will dissolve when you stop poisoning yourself.

© 2013 Parkinsons Recovery

On my radio show December 12, 2012 Cassie Batt from a company called My H2O at Home (www.myh2oathome.com/cassie) discussed a number of green products that do not contain toxins. This French company has invented a wide range of cleaning products that are not only safe, but very effective.

TRAUMA - TOXIN INTERACTIONS

For most people toxins and trauma are found in combination. When both trauma and toxins are present in the body, the effects are multiplicative. The body becomes so overwhelmed that none of its systems are able to function properly.

Why do we often see both trauma and toxins in the same person? The body retains heavy metals (and other toxins) because they have a grounding effect for a person who is in a continuous state of fear. Isn't that clever of the body?

The wisdom of the body knows that toxins are bad for the maintenance of its systems, but the better choice for some people is to help a person who holds a great deal of fear feel safer and more secure. The low frequencies of the heavy metals bring people "down to ground" so to speak and help to relieve the troubling anxieties that are associated with fear that is sustaining the symptoms.

If you try to detox the body and remove the heavy metals, the body will resist unless you also release trauma that is trapped in the cells. The body will hang on to the toxins for dear life until the fear has also been addressed. This is why it may be more expedient to address the traumas first and attend to releasing the toxins as a follow up therapy.

For anyone under extreme stress or anyone who has experienced significant trauma, toxins will naturally cumulate in the physical body over a long period time. There is no way around it. This is a toxic, stressful world.

Jaclyn Gisburne, Ph.D. also sees a strong correlation between trauma and toxins which she eloquently explained December 30, 2009 during my radio show.

> *"When the body is traumatized many things become dysregulated - not just the brain. Intestines close down. You stop doing uptake on nutrients. Your body stops metabolizing properly. Your liver, your adrenals, your kidneys all get taxed to a greater extent. Oftentimes you will see yeast growth coming up in the intestines. Then you get toxins that wouldn't normally be absorbed through the digestive track.*

> *At that point, your whole body is very susceptible to toxins whether they come through the skin or whether they come through the lungs or whether they come through the*

© 2013 Parkinsons Recovery

digestive track. You become very vulnerable because as your body has to start detoxifying it is overwhelmed.

If you are suppressing a trauma - if you are suppressing a memory even for years - you are still suppressing the whole body which means that part of the body which is supposed to be detoxing is also going to be part of what is being suppressed...It is difficult to get rid of toxins if you just try to go at this as a fragmented equation. You really need to look at all of the things systemically that need to be restored in the body."

For some people - and particularly people who are eventually diagnosed with Parkinsons - the cumulative effect of toxins and trauma reaches a saturation point. The body becomes overwhelmed. The neurological system in the body screams back with warning signs that something is dead wrong.

What do I mean by trauma, toxins and time? By way of example, consider the story of a 58 year old man who exemplifies what happens when the combined effects of trauma, toxins and time overwhelm the body.

Fred (not his real name) was diagnosed with Parkinsons in 2004. Among his many other talents, Fred is a photographer and TV cameraman. He always develops his own photographic images in a dark room. It should thus come as little surprise that he has had years and years of exposure to noxious chemicals like glacial acetic acid and hypo fixer.

To create the perfect image Fred uses a photographer's trick. He rubs certain areas of a picture with developer chemicals using his bare hands. Why? You get a better image. That is why. Rubbing with the developer (and especially rubbing with your bare hands) gives sharper contrast to the image.

Was Fred exposed to toxins over a prolonged period of time? Is there any doubt?

Fred took his photographic developing chemicals to his doctor to ask if they might be a factor that contributes to his Parkinsons symptoms. After meticulously examining Fred's chemicals the neurologist concluded correctly that no direct research evidence exists that the photographic chemicals Fred brought to her for examination are connected to his symptoms.

I also have seen no research studies that make a direct link between photographic developing chemicals and Parkinsons. I have a different question than the question Fred asked. Why is it necessary to find a direct link between any specific chemical and Parkinsons? It is not necessarily any specific toxic chemical or substance that is in question here.

There are thousands of toxic chemicals that contribute to toxic overload in the body. A photographer's chemicals certainly satisfy the criteria of toxins, as do many other substances we are exposed to on a daily basis.

Toxins in the body compromise the immune system, bottle neck the digestive system and clog up neural networks. Can there really be any doubt that the body will rebel - eventually?

Of course we could consider the option of scientifically proving that Fred's photographic chemicals cause his symptoms. Let us see now. How many years would this take? Speaking as a researcher, my conservative estimate is 40 or 50 years. What is the cost of this research? It is staggering. We could feed all the starving children in Mexico. Researchers involved could retire from their university appointments early.

Would the conclusions help Fred or anyone who is diagnosed with Parkinsons? My rocket science guess is that it is highly unlikely.

Fred points out that many famous photographers have had Parkinsons, Margaret Bourke-White to name one. Is it really any coincidence she had Parkinsons?

Research does demonstrate direct links between toxic exposure and the symptoms of Parkinsons. In particular, pesticide exposure has been found to elicit the symptoms of Parkinsons. Again, the issue is overall exposure to toxins, not necessarily exposure to any specific toxin per se.

The second factor is time. The body is well equipped to eliminate waste through the kidneys and the digestive track as long as the body is not flooded with too many toxins. Fred was exposed to toxic chemicals over an extended period of time. There was thus a gradual build up of toxins in his body for years.

Toxins eventually become lodged inside the cells. The body does a good job of isolating the toxins so they do as little damage as possible. The body is very good at damage control. As the number of pockets of isolated tissue that encapsulate the toxins increase, overall function of the body becomes threatened.

Trapped toxins are like having unpleasant guests in your home who refuse to leave. As the weeks pass - and as the years pass – you become more and more enraged, less and less rational with your house guests. Nothing you do, nothing you say to your guests makes them leave. They like your house. They refuse to leave.

What are your choices here? Shoot them? This is not an option. They are family members. Besides, it is illegal and evil to kill someone.

© 2013 Parkinsons Recovery

Leave yourself? Wait a minute. This is your home. Why do you have to leave? Besides, one thing we are unable to do is leave our bodies (unless you happen to have that special skill of teleporting yourself to another reality).

Give your guests a break here. Look at it from their point of view. If you were a toxin, wouldn't it be neat to find a comfortable home inside a cell and just hang out there forever? It is safe there. It is warm and cozy. Why not be fat and happy?

Give the toxins a little consciousness here and what do you conclude? It is a lot cooler to hang out inside a cell than winding up in a sewer.

How about the third factor - trauma? Fred was working as a TV cameraman prior to his diagnosis with Parkinsons. During this time in his life he was having serious personal conflicts with several co-workers. The experience was prolonged and incredibly stressful. When stress persists day in and day out, it takes a nasty toll on the body's ability to remain healthy.

When the toxins and stress reach a critical level, the body reacts by exhibiting the symptoms of Parkinsons. The skeptic will say - you have not proved that any of this is true. This is all just a theory.

Know what? The critics are perfectly correct. All of this is just a guess. But it is a good guess.

Fred's story is not unique. My interviews with people who are diagnosed with Parkinsons reveal stories that contain the same themes. There is either significant exposure to toxins or to trauma. In most cases, there is exposure to both.

How do I know my theoretical explanation is correct? I have no direct evidence - yet. But I hold the belief that my theory is correct because it is what people tell me over and over. I am simply repeating the obvious by summarizing their stories.

ELECTROMAGNETIC EXPOSURE

Exposure to electromagnetic toxins can also do significant damage to the neurological system. Consider the many ways we are exposed to electromagnetic fields every day: TV's, computers, cell towers and electrical stations. Smart phones and cell phones are also a formidable source of exposure. Where is your cell phone or i-phone now? If it is near or even on your body you may be exposing yourself to a life threatening illness.

How do I know this? Simple. Read the small print instructions you received when you purchased the phone. You will see a warning to never place your phone near your body.

If you want more palatable proof, listen to the radio show that aired November 24, 2010 with my guest Compounding Pharmacist and Nutritional Counselor Randy Mentzer. He recounts his own chilling experience with hooking his cell phone on a chain that hung around his neck. In one short month Randy had to undergo an emergency medical procedure to drain 3 pints of fluid from his chest.

Avoid placing your cell phone or smart phone next to your ear. It is best to turn on your monitor so that you can hold the phone some distance from your body when you have conversations. Your neurons will thank you profusely.

I am not done here folks. Electromagnetic exposure is the health threat of the century. Do you live near a cell phone tower? I recommend you move to another home. At a minimum use a meter to evaluate the level of exposure in your bedroom. If you live near a cell phone tower, it will show dangerously high levels of exposure. The most susceptible time for being exposure is when we are asleep which is why it is so important to know the level of exposure in your bedroom.

Do you have a smart meter that monitors your electricity? Write a letter to your electric company asking them to remove it. If needed, ask your doctor to document the extent of your own electromagnetic sensitivity. The electric company will claim that the level of exposure is too slight as to be an inconsequential threat. Compelling research studies show this is precisely why electromagnetic exposure from a smart meter is so deadly to your health.

Dietrich K. Klinghardt, M.D., Ph.D. has a compelling 40 minute video on the problem with smart meters that explains the dangers involved. Watch this video. You will be convinced to take positive action if necessary.

Please take the problem of electromagnetic exposure seriously. Some people have neurological difficulties primarily because of electromagnetic exposure. Once the exposure is removed, their symptoms are reversed.

DIGESTIVE ISSUES

Logic suggests that neurological challenges are rooted in the neurons and the strained brain – body neural connections. In part this is obviously true. But another significant (and some would say key) factor are problems with the digestive system. If the food needed by the body is not being assimilated and processed, neurons do not have the fuel to maintain the energy required to fire the neurons.

How much fuel is needed? Much more fuel is needed to energize the neural connections throughout the body than most people realize. One very practical example is illustrated with the noise of neural firings that are heard by surgeons during Deep Brain Surgery.

© 2013 **Parkinsons Recovery**

It sounds like 4th of July. During DBS, surgeons move an arm when inserting a probe into the brain as they listen to the sound of neurons firing in the brain. It is this sound that instructs surgeons on whether they have the probe placed correctly or not. We are not talking here about subtle sounds. The noise sounds like chaotic static from a short circuited short wave radio.

Another analogy will hammer the point. When sitting around a campfire, the fun is to listen to the crackling of the wood burning as well as to nudge up closely so you can warm up on a cold evening. The crackling stops when the wood is burned up and turns into ashes. It takes a great deal of wood to fuel the crackling. The fuel thus has a very limited life span. Once the fire burns down, you have to stoke it with more fuel. The type of wood also affects the speed of the burn, the noise and the heat that is generated.

You can't eat live food once every 30 days and expect your neurons will be adequately nourished. Neurons must be fed every day with the right fuel in order to maintain their function, just as a fire must be stoked and nurtured during those cold winter evenings when warmth is sought. Neurons are a noisy organism that must be continuously nurtured.

Sources of Digestive Problems

> *"I've done everything right. I take supplements every day. I'm doing exactly what my doctor said I need to do. I'm eating well. I am exercising. Yet, I have very little energy. I'm depressed. So what's going on? What am I doing wrong?"*

Within these questions lies a clue to the imbalance that is aggravating the symptoms of Parkinsons. The answer to their questions falls in the belly (literally) of this person's digestive system. Yes, they are giving their body everything that it needs to perform efficiently and effectively.

The problem is this. While the right foods are being ingested, the digestive system itself is clogged. The transport system that sends food to the cells has malfunctioned. Cells are not being nourished. The question turns on,

> *"Why is my digestive system not working properly?"*

Let's preview now the factors that can shut down a digestive system and render your life force immobile.

GLUTEN

Neurological problems can be created by the food we eat. Comfort food in the form of breads, croissants and pastas is seductive and addictive. I love comfort food. Most people I know love comfort food. The difficulty with comfort foods is that they contain gluten which is found in

© 2013 Parkinsons Recovery

most grain products. When you go to any restaurant, it seems as though 80 or 85 percent of the foods that are served have wheat as an ingredient.

Grains such as wheat can destroy the villi in the small intestines for some people. Villi absorb the nutrients needed by the tissues in the body to function. This deprives the body of nutrition that is critical to health. The consequences to health and wellness are serious.

I will now discuss two compelling reasons why you would be best advised to stop eating wheat. Perhaps I am being un-American here, but making this change to your diet promises to have a positive influence on the health of your neurological system.

1. *When we ingest wheat our intestines get lined with a hardened paste. This paste like material is a formidable barrier that blocks the transfer of nutrients into the blood system and their subsequent delivery to the cells.*

   Remember what happened when you were a child and played with flour? You mixed water with the flour to make face masks or dolls or other play things. You molded the paste and allowed it to sit. Remember how it hardened over night?

   Well guess what? This is the very same process that takes place inside your body. Intestines become plasticized. A hardened cover seals off food from the blood stream. The body is unable to function properly because the cells are starving.

   Another consequence is possible. The walls of the intestines become weak and tear. The food you eat spews out into your abdomen. This is serious stuff folks.

2. *Sharry Edwards from Sound Health has written an article where she presents a convincing argument that genetically modified wheat (which is now found in most processed foods) distorts neural cell signaling and leads to symptoms associated with Parkinsons Disease. This turned out to be the reason for neurological symptoms she was personally experiencing. Her symptoms vanished after she stopped eating wheat. For more information, read Sharry's research report on the Parkinsons Recovery Blog.*

There are now at least ten stores across the United States that carry only products that are free of gluten. I interviewed the owner of one such store, Joe Spancic, who described his own personal battle with gluten. You can hear my interview with Joe on the Parkinsons Recovery Radio Show page by scrolling down to the program that aired October 15, 2009.

Part of the formula for recovering from Parkinsons is to eat healthy food. But healthy food is only a partial solution. The good food you are eating may not be sent to the cells where it is needed most.

Consider the option of detoxing your entire digestive system. Clean out the gunk in your intestines. Give it time. Cement in the intestines takes time to break up and clear out. Stop eating wheat. Clean out your gut. You will be amazed at how much better you feel.

LIVER AND GALL BLADDER ISSUES

Johan Boswinkel, inventor of the Chiren, a new biontology technology, said on my radio show September 26, 2012 that symptoms are just like the flashing lights on a police car. You can certainly see, feel and experience something is wrong. But what is it? Why are those flashing lights creating such a disturbance?

Most problems in the body are rooted in the organs found in our trunk, usually the liver and gall bladder. If mobility problems are connected to a lack of strength, the root cause is likely to be a liver problem. Even when the liver is diseased, it has a miraculous ability to suppress its own dysfunction and make it possible for the body to continue to function, though symptoms will eventually become evident. If mobility problems are due to a general lack of tension, the cause is likely rooted in a gall bladder problem.

If you currently experience neurological difficulties, the most important question to ask yourself is : *What is the cause?* Western medicine only treats symptoms, so that is not a question which addressed. I believe it is the most important question to ask. Once you have the answer you can treat the cause of the problem.

Johan Boswinkel has found the cause is rooted in the most unsuspecting places, even infected appendixes. If you are serious about getting well, then the ideal strategy is to think outside the box and ask: *What is the cause?* Once you have asked the question, you will find the answer.

DAIRY

Let's first be clear about what constitutes dairy. Many people think they do not consume dairy because they do not drink milk. If you consume any of the following foods, you are consuming dairy: butter, cheese, cream, half and half, ice cream, sour cream, cottage cheese, yogurt, frozen yogurt, whey protein and milk.

Laurie Mischley, ND, gave a beautiful summary of the research evidence on the association of dairy consumption and Parkinsons in her book, Natural Therapies for Parkinsons Disease. She explains that three different prospective studies have evaluated the association between dairy consumption and Parkinsons. Prospective studies are rich designs because they provide the opportunity to make causal inferences. All three studies found precisely the same thing: Consumption of dairy is associated with an increased risk of developing symptoms of

Parkinson's disease. More specifically, 3-6 servings of dairy per day results in a 60-80% increased risk.

What is one thing you can do for yourself that will save you money and help provide relief from the symptoms of Parkinsons? My answer is: stop eating dairy. Throw away the ice cream in your freezer that is screaming out to you to "eat me up" because the ice cream is literally eating up your neurons.

One of the reasons eating dairy inflames Parkinsons symptoms is that pesticides are often found in dairy products. When you eat ice cream, you may also be eating legal doses of pesticides that are known to cause symptoms of Parkinsons.

This is a hard sell for me. How can I convince you to stop eating dairy when it is one of my most favorite foods? One of my favorite foods to eat is whipped cream. I love whipped cream. It makes me happy. It reminds me of the best of times from my childhood. If any dessert has whipped cream, I want to eat the dessert to enjoy the whipped cream.

Eating whipped cream also makes my intestines bloat. My entire digestive system screams out in pain. My spleen is not a happy camper. I pay a heavy price for days because I indulged myself in a few minutes of pleasure. I am not out of the woods yet from eating pumpkin pie and whipped cream several days ago. End of story. If I eat dairy, I pay the price.

Why? The body needs acids to breakdown and digest food, but too much can do great harm to the tissues and organs. Dairy is highly acidic. Each time you eat dairy products, lactose sugar is fermented which results in the production of lactic acid.

When the digestive system is blasted with acids from dairy products like ice cream, milk and cheese, the body responds by coating the intestinal track with mucus. This is an eloquent response actually. Mucus provides a natural defense against the damage that is done by the accumulation of too much acid.

Too much acid burns away at the cellular structure of the body. Too much acid burns holes in your tissues and organs. Too much acid reduces life spans and creates disease. If it were not for mucus, your organs would be riddled with holes and fissures.

Visualize what the intestinal track looks like when it is coated with layer after layer of mucus. How can healthy food be digested properly? It cannot. There is a thick barrier of slimy gunk that prevents the nutrients from being assimilated by the blood stream.

Do you take a barrel full of supplements every day but still do not feel better? Your supplements are sliding down a slippery slope of mucus throughout the digestive system. It is like flying down a tubular water slide at the park. Your body is flying though an enclosed tube just as food travels through your intestinal track. But at the water park you enter the tube, fly down for the ride and are ejected. You leave nothing behind. You come out the other end intact.

This is what happens to supplements when the digestive system is compromised. They enter the tube, fly down in tack and are ejected. You might as well stop spending money on the supplements and pay for visits to the water park. At least you will get some exercise and have fun.

With an accumulation of thick mucus in the lower bowel, transit time of fecal matter increases. The fecal matter is encapsulated with gobs of mucus. Digestive problems are inevitable including constipation, gas, bloating, ulcers, nausea and irritation of the intestinal walls. Is whipped cream worth these agonies? I think not.

The accumulation of mucus goo on intestinal walls is the ideal home for unfriendly microforms and parasites. The microforms and parasites are also travelers. Who wants to stay home year around? They travel throughout the body by boring holes in the intestinal walls and dancing through the blood stream, stopping here and there to take side trips in the heart, kidneys liver or, of course, neurons. How can a neuron fire when there are hundreds of uninvited intruders obstructing the electrical pathway? The electrical distortion is monstrous.

Unchecked microforms burrow themselves deep inside the structural fabric of neural networks. How well would you function if your home were overtaken by uninvited strangers who demand to be fed, housed and nurtured? Cynthia Gilbertson is a congressional coordinator in New York for the Parkinsons Action Network. What is one of Cynthia Gilbertson's key recommendations for anyone with the symptoms of Parkinsons?

"Have yourself tested for parasites. I didn't know. I had all sorts of parasites."

Unwanted microforms are not family members. They are intruders. They are breaking into your home and robbing you of life force. I assure you if this were a court of law, this is sufficient cause for fatigue and depression. Guilty as charged.

Still want that whip cream? My addiction is beginning to waver, but I am not done. Our body is a mass of intricate neural networks. Key connections to every major organ in the body are found in the bowels. If the bowels are obstructed with yucky, gooey mucus all of those connections are compromised. There is a Trojan in the neural network of the body which is forcing an eventual shutdown. Is it any wonder that some people have significant mobility challenges?

© **2013 Parkinsons Recovery**

I have one more thought to pass on which helps me avoid eating whipped cream (though I still have relapses). The origins of all dairy products are living animals. Animals (including humans) are factories for puss, mucus, blood and infection. All dairy products contain puss, mucus, blood and (often) infection. When you eat that whipped cream you are also putting the mucus, blood and puss from other animals into your body. This is a gross thought to be sure, but it helps me avoid the temptation to eat ice cream and whipped cream.

I have convinced you (and myself) to avoid eating dairy products? In part, I am writing this to remind myself about the consequences of what I put into my body. How about you? Are you convinced?

What about the mucus that is already present in our digestive systems? I suggest that you do digestive cleanses and take probiotics as a matter of routine. Probiotics put the healthy organisms into the digestive track that are required for digestion. I have had several people with the symptoms of Parkinsons tell me that taking probiotics regularly has provided significant relief from their symptoms. Different probiotics are needed for different segments of the digestive system. Some probiotics work well on the stomach, others on the small intestines and still others on the large intestines. Consult with your doctor or nutritional counselor to obtain probiotics which will do a thorough job.

You would not think that digestive issues are a cause of the Parkinsons symptoms, but I believe that for many people they play a leading role in causing the symptoms.

SUGAR

Sugar is a dangerous toxin that poses shocking obstacles to reversing the symptoms of Parkinsons. Some people do all the right things to heal the symptoms of Parkinsons but see little result from their efforts. This is because their bodies are swamped with heavy doses of one toxin that is entirely legal and found in virtually all processed foods. This toxin is sugar.

Sugar is a deadly toxin that we put into our bodies because it is pleasurable. We don't just touch it or smell it. We eat it. The cell damage that is directly caused by sugar has a Hurricane Katrina effect on your neurological system.

I have interviewed people with Parkinsons who told me their doctor recommended that if they wanted to start feeling better, they had to stop eating sugar. Some people can't refuse the cravings. Those who do stop eating sugar tell me that they do feel a lot better. The doctor was right all along.

Sugar cravings may well be a signal that your immune system has crashed. You will never be able to fight off viruses and bacterial infections unless you can get your immune system back on track.

Your body will not begin to address neural issues if bacterial infections or viral threats are screaming for attention. When the body is overwhelmed with hosting unfriendly critters, it responds accordingly. It prioritizes what problems need to be addressed first. Infections are at the top of the list. Neural abnormalities hide out in the cellar of the body's priority ranking.

Sugar is the food of choice for bacteria and viruses. Imagine if you will that the bacteria and viruses are a household of children who scream at you 24-7 to be fed sweets - candies, sodas, cookies and cakes. When you refuse to feed the children sweets, they become more obnoxious and certainly more unruly. They become a veritable pain in the ass because they never stop screaming they want to be fed - not vegetables or protein - but sugar.

If you eat sugar and desserts as a matter of habit you guarantee your body will be a host an overgrowth of infections and viruses. It is a vicious cycle. More sugar leads to more bacterial and viral infections. More infections trigger more sugar cravings. Those bacteria demand to be fed. And yes, they do have a consciousness that is compelling.

Permit me to explain more vividly what you are doing to yourself when you insist on eating foods front loaded with sugar. Imagine if you will that you have been kidnapped by a very nasty group of criminals who have demanded a $100 million ransom from your family. Your family has turned down this request because they do not have $100 million, much less $1 million to offer. Unknown to you, it is the practice of these kidnappers to free their victims if they are unsuccessful with milking money out of the families.

To ease relations with your abductors, you have been baking them pies -blueberry, blackberry, chocolate, strawberry and custard. The pies of course are front loaded with sugar. Your captors loved eating the pies so much every evening that they decide to keep you around - forever.

Your captors are analogous to the nasty little critters that are hanging out in your body - the harmful bacteria and viruses. You are never going to get rid of them until you stop making (and eating) the pies loaded with sugar.

Perhaps you are thinking that: "*Sugar is not that big of an issue for me.*" Perhaps, but humor me for a minute. Look at your finger nails. Do you have white spots on them? The white spots are a marker when you ate a large quantity of sugar (and represent one of the ways the body eliminated it). Your nails take about 6 months to grow. If the white spots are in the middle of a nail it means that you ingested a large quantity of sugar three months ago. Check it out. Finger nails do not lie, but we are all fond of lying to ourselves from time to time. For some it becomes a habit that is difficult to break.

OK. So sugar is bad for you. How can you (or I) reduce our own sugar cravings that may have haunted us our entire life? We can address nutritional deficiencies, assess food allergies and strengthen our immune systems.

There are alternatives to sugar. Why not investigate the alternatives that can be used in place of using raw cane sugar. Then, start using an alternative to pure sugar that is right for you.

Know in advance that you may not be able to tolerate one or more of the alternatives. That is, the alternative may be worse for you than raw sugar itself. Why not celebrate in advance how much your body will thank you if you can find a natural and safe substitute for sugar that your body can tolerate?

Three natural alternative substitutes for sugar are agave, stevia and zylitol. Here is a sketch of information about each of the three alternatives.

Agave

Agave syrup is a sweetener commercially produced in Mexico. Agave syrup is sweeter than honey, though less viscous. It consists primarily of fructose and glucose.

Agave has a fructose content that is higher than is found in high-fructose corn syrup. Agave is notable in that its glycemic index and glycemic load are seemingly lower than most other natural sweetener alternatives.

Recent concerns have been raised by researchers about methods used to manufacture Agave that are creating a toxic residue. Be sure and do your homework before deciding which sugar substitute is best for you and your body.

Stevia

Native to subtropical and tropical South America and Central America stevia is also known as sweetleaf. The taste has a longer duration than that of pure sugar. Stevia however can be associated with a bitter after taste at high concentrations.

Xylitol

This alternative sounds like an expensive prescription medication, but it is not. It is a five-carbon sugar alcohol that is used as a sugar substitute. Xylitol is a naturally occurring sweetener that can be found in the fibers of fruits and vegetables such as berries, corn husks, oats, and even mushrooms. It is extracted from corn fibers, birch trees, raspberries, plums, and even corn. Xylitol is by all accounts as sweet as regular sugar. Xylitol has been around a long time. It is used as a sweetener for diabetics in some countries and it is used in various products like gums and toothpaste to reduce tooth decay.

Check out the possibilities. Do an extended search on the internet for more information. Experiment. You can buy xylitol, stevia and agave from most health food stores, food co-ops and even some grocery stores.

I think a safe and natural food sweetener is a delightful choice for people like me who love to eat a delicious dessert every now and then. If you are like me, consider a switch from sugar to a natural substitute.

There is no direct research evidence to indicate that using alternatives to sugar will help relieve the symptoms of Parkinsons. Based on pure logic, it makes sense to me that using a natural substitute for sugar has the potential to unclog neural pathways.

SUGAR CRAVINGS ARE CAUSED BY NUTRITIONAL DEFICIENCIES

Sugar cravings mean that you are not giving your body the nutrition that is necessary for it to function optimally. We are certified body abusers. The abused victim in this case just happens to be our own body.

You can approach this challenge in two ways. You can set about to determine what nutritional deficiencies contribute to the imbalance. Is it too little of vitamin D3, or B6, or B12 or magnesium or ...?

You can ask your doctor to order an exhaustive series of tests that evaluate nutritional deficiencies in the body. Specific prescriptions of vitamin and mineral supplements will remedy the deficiencies in time and reduce the cravings.

This approach works well for some people. The downside it is expensive, time consuming and time limited. The tests have to be repeated again and again to maintain the balance that is needed.

Or, you can focus your intent and energy on giving your body all the nutrition it needs to heal. This means eating fresh foods that are free of pesticides and additives. With the later strategy, what does it matter whether you are deficient in one vitamin or mineral or another? If you eat nutritious, fresh food every day, you will eventually give your body all the nutrition it needs to heal whatever imbalances are present.

In summary, pay attention to the basics and your body will heal itself. Eat live food. Stop eating foods you are allergic to. Strengthen your immune system.

© 2013 Parkinsons Recovery

Set your intention to no longer allow sugar to control you and your life and the problems of fatigue, depression and sleeplessness will become memories of the distant past. You may well be surprised as well at how your overall mobility and agility improves.

INJURIES

For some people, the primary culprit is trauma. For other people the primary culprit is toxins. For still other people, the primary culprit is a malfunctioning digestive system. For a small number of people, the primary culprit is physical injury to the brain.

Injuries obviously can have a profound impact on the cellular integrity of the brain. The nature of the physical injuries varies widely. Research shows that traumatic injury to the brain – whether from falls or boxing matches or automobile accidents or other accidents – is associated with an increased incidence of Parkinsons. It is no surprise that heavy weight boxing champion Muhammad Ali has Parkinsons.

Some people have experienced injuries to their jaw bones and suffer from TMJ Disorder – or Temporomandibular Joint Disorder. One nonprofit organization – the Parkinsons Resource Organization, has been focusing their investigative efforts on evaluating the improvement in symptoms once jaw misalignments are corrected with a dental appliance.

Acupuncturist Janice Walton-Hadlock has discovered a connection between foot injuries and the symptoms of Parkinson's disease. She finds that foot injuries interrupt the normal flow of energy through meridians of the body. Her nonprofit organization is dedicated to teaching people gentle therapies that encourage healing of such an injury, including the Chinese treatment of Tui Na.

The words Tui Na translate into "push-grasp" or "poke-pinch" in Chinese. The therapy uses a series of pressing, tapping, and kneading with palms, fingertips, knuckles or implements that help the body to remove blockages along the meridians of the body and stimulate the flow of qi and blood to promote healing. The therapy has some similarity to the principles of acupuncture, moxibustion, and acupressure. Her website includes information material about the cause and treatment of Parkinsons which have been helpful to many people, especially with regard to issues regarding medications. The website (http://www.pdrecovery.org) is a rich and useful resource.

Four other challenges can cause neurological havoc in the body: low cellular energy, dehydration, inflammation and critters. This is why people often experience significant relief from their symptoms from:

- Taking COq10 (which addresses low cellular energy)

© 2013 Parkinsons Recovery

- Using the Aquas (which are homeopathic medicine designed to hydrate the body)

- Taking antioxidants (which reduce inflammation in the body)

- Clearing bacterial infections.

I will next preview each challenge with special attention to the challenge of Parkinson's.

LOW CELLULAR ENERGY

Movement that involves slow starts and abrupt stops is a troublesome symptom for people who have been diagnosed with Parkinsons Disease. Many explanations are offered for mobility difficulties. At the core of them all lies low cellular energy.

The goal of every cell is to stay alive. Cells get energy from what you eat. They use raw materials like magnesium, selenium, ribose and CoQ10 to create energy.

How do they do this? You are probably wondering whether you really need to know this answer. Perhaps not, but I am going to proceed with a little more detailed explanation for one reason. The ability of the body to sustain life is truly a miracle. It is far more complicated than pouring fuel into an engine and turning on the ignition switch. More directly, it is not simply a question of filling up the tank in your body that holds and manufactures dopamine.

At least one miniature cell known as mitochondria is found within each cell. Mitochondria are the power plants of the body in the sense that they manufacture ATP (adenosine triphosphate).

ATP has three phosphates. When a cell needs energy it breaks one of those bonds to create a blast of energy. This is what keeps the cell alive. This is what makes movement possible. If the cell does not have that blast of energy - if the mitochondria do not have the raw materials needed to manufacture ATP - the cell dies. Cells are dying all the time, but the body suffers when there are too many cell deaths too quickly. It does not get the window of opportunity to manufacture new cells to replace the ones that died.

It should come as no surprise that when a sufficient number of cell deaths occur, movement will become difficult as will many other functions of the body. If the mitochondria do not have the raw materials they need to fuel the power plant, any and all functions will eventually become problematic: walking, talking, thinking, swallowing, eating and even having fun.

Researchers are now investigating ways to revitalize the mitochondria for persons who currently experience Parkinson's symptoms. Why? Two pesticides in particular – rotenone and MPTP – have been implicated as two nasty culprits that devastate dopamine cells. They also ravish mitochondria.

It is intuitively smart in my book of logic to focus resources on revitalizing and reenergizing the mitochondria power plant of the body if you are currently experiencing the symptoms of Parkinson's. Cellular energy can be revitalized through an infusion of oxygen and/or the substances used by the mitochondria to manufacture ATP. A supplement known as Corvalen combines ribose and magnesium to provide the fuel that is required to ignite more energy at the cellular level.

DEHYDRATION

If your body does not have sufficient water, cells are unable to get rid of the wastes that naturally accumulate. Cells cannot create energy without creating waste. How is a neuron supposed to release waste through its delicate cell membrane that is dry and brittle? It can't.

Dehydrated cells are just like New York City during a garbage strike in summer time. Garbage workers do not pick up the garbage because they are on strike. Garbage on the sidewalks grows each day until the entire city becomes a toxic dump. The stench is nauseating. The potential for disease is assured.

Cells of neurons by their nature are juicy. When neurons become dry and brittle from lack of adequate hydration, waste cannot be efficiently released from the cell interiors. Waste backs up, hardens and obstructs the ability of the cell to conduct its job of generating energy.

No cell can survive in such an environment in the long run. If the garbage in New York were never picked up, everyone would eventually have to evacuate the city.

When a body becomes dehydrated, cell deaths rise and symptoms flare. Some people find they get incredible relief from their symptoms by hydrating their bodies. People sometimes take supplements or herbs or medicines to counteract the symptoms, but this can create more of a waste log jam if there is not sufficient water to remove the waste that accumulates naturally.

You are probably thinking, OK. The solution is simple. Drink more water. Unfortunately, it is not as simple as drinking more water as Jaroslav Boublik, Ph.D. explains:

> *"If it were as simple as drinking more water, a lot more people would be a lot more hydrated than they are. It is pretty clear to me looking at the people around me in the world that it is not that simple. Forcing yourself to drink more water may have a short term impact on your state of hydration but it will do little to address your baseline hydration state.*
>
> *The analogy I make is many people who work in office spaces will be familiar with the sad and sorry potted plant in the corner of the board room which really gets neglected*

pretty badly. The fact is that if you water that potted plant chances are that most of the water will simply flow through it and end up in a puddle on the floor.

I think many of us are like that potted plant. We have been neglected so long in terms of providing adequate amounts of hydrating fluids into the system that when we do pour a large amount of water into our bodies most of it simply flows through.

Certainly when people have an epiphany and decide they are going to get really hydrated by drinking their 8 or 10 or 12 glasses of water a day they find that the only real impact on them is that they spend a lot more time going to the bathroom. This suggests to me (and has been long supported with research) that there are two pathways of hydration in the body.

There is short path and long path hydration. Short path is into the mouth, into the digestive tract, into the circulation, straight to the kidneys then down to the bladder and out. Very little of this fluid impacts the hydration of individual cells.

Then there is long path hydration. Here that circulating fluid does manage to get into extra cellular fluid, then into the cells where it carries nutrients in and then back out of the cells where it carries toxins out back into the circulation and then through the kidneys and bladder. Long path hydration is what we are looking for.

Long path hydration unfortunately does get switched off with neglect. Simply pouring more water into the system doesn't switch it back on again. You need to take a proactive step. We believe Aquas are a good example of that but there are probably other things you can do to provoke long path hydration.

The analogy I like to make here is to think about the ebb and flow of the tide. The water that is available in the body is the most significant amount of matter that is able to move in and out of cells. It is in fact the mechanism by which all nutrients are brought into cells and also all toxins are taken out of cells.

If the mass of water that is moving in and out of cells is low then the ability for nutrients to be taken into the cells is reduced and the ability of toxins to be removed by the cells is reduced. So, simply increasing the available mass of fluids that can move in and out cells will both improve the uptake of nutrients and also the clearance of toxins. It is very important for the body to be well hydrated to facilitate the clearance of toxins.

© 2013 Parkinsons Recovery

INFLAMMATION

Many scientists now look at inflammation as a contributing factor to many chronic conditions. In the case of Parkinsons, it makes logical sense to speculate that neural networks function poorly when the tissues connected with the neurons are swollen.

Think about how you feel when you eat too much. I personally feel bloated, sluggish, blocked and immobile. All I can do until some of the food is digested is to sit up straight and pray I do not have to move for a while. Meditation is a choice, but I usually fall asleep.

This is precisely how neurons feel when they become swollen. Give your neurons a break. They have feelings themselves you know. There is not enough room for the neural networks to function when the tissues are swollen. Electrical pathways become obstructed.

The distribution of hormones to your muscles and tissues also becomes difficult when inflammation is present. The tissues throughout your body are busy handling an emergency. They have little space to receive the sweetness of any uninvited hormonal visitations.

It is like seeing two friends having a huge fight. They are both furious at one another. As their friend who is witness to the fight, you try to squeeze in a word or two, but your friends ignore you. They are too preoccupied with their own fight. In a similar fashion, hormones have difficulty squeezing themselves into tissues that are inflamed.

When all of the healthy cells function at their peak levels, you will feel better and find relief from the symptoms of Parkinsons. Conversely, you will certainly feel worse when the tissues in your body are inflamed. Depression creeps in. Fatigue becomes a way of life.

Nutritional Counselor and Pharmacist Randy Mentzer offers the following observation on how inflammation plays a key role in contributing to the symptoms of Parkinsons.

> *"If we back up and ask what causes Parkinsons - we don't know. But nutritional scientists know this. The basis for all chronic, degenerative disease starts with an event. We don't know what that event is with Parkinsons, but we know that something happens. Whatever happens causes inflammation. This process of Parkinson's disease ... all starts with an event that causes inflammation.*
>
> *You want to eat foods that are anti-inflammatory. You want to avoid the foods that cause inflammation. You want to take supplements that are anti-inflammatory. Omega-3s are anti-inflammatory. We use Omega 3's for a number of anti-inflammatory processes including arthritis. Omega 3s are very essential."*

Infections are also the source of inflammation. Symptoms may not solely be due to hormonal imbalances. Here is John Briggs, ND, [4]perspective on inflammation and Parkinsons:

> "If we are looking at Parkinsons and we are looking at the fact that we have nerve transmission that is being interrupted, being altered, anytime a nerve is not functioning correctly we can say - is there pressure against that nerve? There could be swelling and pressure against the nerve if there is an infection."

ASSESS ALLERGIES

Why then are the tissues in your body always inflamed? You may be allergic to a certain food (or foods) that you love to eat. A hidden source of inflammation for most people is allergic reactions to something they put into their bodies.

How do you know if you are allergic to any foods? And, if you are allergic, how do you figure out which foods they might be?

It is very easy to know. Stop eating the foods you suspect may be causing the inflammation for two weeks. See if you feel better. This sounds easy, but it is anything but easy. Let me explain why.

Let's consider one food by way of example: ice cream. I love eating ice cream myself. Here is my conversation with myself (and I am not making this up).

> "Maybe the inflammation is being caused by eating ice cream. Oh, I think not. After all, when I eat ice cream I do not get sick. I do not have rashes. I do not have stomach aches. I do not sweat or puke or turn purple. It must not be ice cream."

Being the logical person that I am, I continue eating ice cream. I stop eating turnips instead to see if turnips might be the problem. They are not. All is well. I still get to eat the ice cream.

There is a double twist to my logic. My body has become acclimated to processing and digesting ice cream. If you also love to eat ice cream, you have probably liked eating ice cream since you were a child. As an incredibly clever living entity, the body quickly learns how to turn on systems that reduce the allergic reactions to ice cream. In other words, the true symptoms are masked when we eat ice cream regularly. I thus conclude:

> "I do not feel that bad when I eat ice cream."

In one sense this is true. In another sense you would be feeling so much better if you stopped eating ice cream and started eating healthy substitutes.

---

[4] Taken from my radio interview with John Briggs, ND, on April 16, 2009.

© 2013 Parkinsons Recovery

Because you have always eaten ice cream your entire life, the truth is that you have actually always felt lousy. You just did not know it. It is the only way you have ever felt - lousy.

Ever heard yourself say,

> "I seem to be so depressed all the time."

> "I drag every day of the week."

There it is. Because you become acclimated to feeling tired and depressed, you forget what it is like to feel good. The only way to know if a food is causing fatigue, inducing depression and entangling neural networks is to stop eating that particular food for at least two weeks. In my example, the test is to stop eating ice cream for two weeks.

Then, eat a lot of ice cream one day. Indulge yourself. Reward yourself for doing the test. Eat a quart or two of your favorite ice cream. Make it three. Then see how you feel. If you notice a flare up of fatigue and depression after eating the ice cream you can almost certainly conclude that ice cream is causing inflammation in your body.

I report this truth with such detachment as if it has never happened to me. But it has and it did. My naturopath muscle tested me for various food items and suspected that I had allergies to dairy. I love eating cheese. I love chocolate milkshakes.

> "I am OK when I eat these foods. I love them. That cannot be the problem."

Did I stop eating milkshakes for two weeks? Of course I did not. I convinced myself that I was actually very healthy and that I deserved a little pleasure in my life.

After fighting this battle for years, I finally did the gold standard test for allergies. I did not drink milk shakes for two weeks straight. The anticipation of being able to have a milk shake became more and more intense with each passing day until day 15 arrived when I ate two milk shakes, one chocolate and one vanilla. They were thoroughly yummy as always.

I paid a dear price for those few minutes of bliss. I became seriously depressed for several days. The fatigue was overwhelming. I really just wanted to sleep and forget about working or playing. I was miserable.

The truth is that I did not realize how tired and depressed the ice cream was making me until I gave my body a chance to detox itself from dairy. After 14 days of not eating ice cream the inflammation that was literally always present in my tissues had subsided.

© 2013 Parkinsons Recovery

My experiment was a success. When I added dairy back into my body, it became obvious that my body cannot tolerate dairy. I now know this is why I had constant ear aches as a child. Of course I did not like the outcome, but excellent substitutes for dairy do exist.

If you have Parkinsons you need energy to feel better. It is hard to do the things that will make you feel better if you are depressed or if you are tired all the time. It is thus highly probable that a big reason why you feel bad is because of food that you are eating.

My problem is dairy. Your problem may be wheat or corn or soy or whatever. Give the experiment a try and see what you can discover for yourself. Most people are allergic to something. They just do not know it.

There is no better test for food allergies than to apply the gold standard as I have described above. Make the assessment systematic. Before you begin the test prepare a chart which lists all of the symptoms you currently experience down the rows of your chart. Mark off three columns. Denote the first column as the level of severity before making any changes. Denote the second column as the level of severity at the end of the two week elimination period. Denote the third column as the level of severity after adding the food back into your diet.

Rate the level of severity for each symptom as one (1) for minor to five (5) for severe. Before starting the gold standard test, record the level of severity for each symptom. Eliminate the food that you suspect may be an allergen for two weeks. This is the hard part of the test for most people. Record the level of severity for each symptom at the end of the two week abstinence in column two.

Add the food back in. Splurge! Record the level of severity for each symptom after eating the food again in column three.

Believe me, you do not have to know any statistics to see immediately whether you are allergic or not to the food you have just tested. The food allergy test is free and superior to any other test for allergies on the market. The gold standard test does demand a strong dose of determination, commitment and discipline. The end result can have a huge impact on how you feel. Say goodbye to depression and fatigue. Say hello to life.

Naturopath doctor Ivy Faber explains the increasing problem of allergies for people today:

> *"We have become very allergic to different foods because of how the soil and foods are compromised. Also, there are phenols which are naturally occurring chemicals that are within the structure of the food itself. Different foods can have the same naturally occurring chemical ... but if you get a lot of that chemical in your body - it can become a*

toxin. Then you start being reactive. All the sudden you start reacting to foods in ways that you may not have before.

A lot of time people are allergic to their vitamins, like the B vitamins, vitamin C, vitamin A. These are all allergens. They may need vitamin C but they may not be absorbing it or utilizing it the way it needs to be because of the blood brain barrier or the information is just not getting to where it needs to."

When sugar is added to foods you are allergic to, there is a multiplicative effect that is horrible. Sugar ravages our neurological system and inflammation caused by an allergic reaction shuts down the neural pathways. It is a double whammy that causes havoc with your ability to walk, talk and think. The potential for neurological destruction is indescribable.

A snow storm analogy helps illustrate the impact that inflammation has on the function of the neurological system. Travel on Interstate highways is problematic during heavy snow storms. Snow plows shovel snow from the main thoroughfare onto the shoulders. Width of the passable lanes narrows. Accidents narrow the access room further, so that you have to travel at a snail's pace.

Narrowing of the highway lanes and obstructions caused by the snow and accidents are precisely what inflammation does to your neurological system. Neural pathways are restricted and blocked by inflammation. Transmission of electrical impulses is distorted and obstructed.

Inflammation in and of itself will make you feel lethargic and depressed. The short lived euphoria from eating sugar is followed up by profound bouts of depression. Stop eating sugar and there is a good chance the depression will lift.

If you really want to feel better, stop eating sugar – all sugar. This therapy is absolutely free. In fact, it will save you money on food that is making you ill.

Alternatively, you can take anti-depressants and many different prescription medications that will mask the effects of sugar. It is much less trouble and certainly less expensive if you simply stop eating sugar.

CRITTERS

Bacterial and viral infections create horrible problems for the body's neurological system. Most people have critters and parasites of one type or another that are hanging out in the tissues of their organs. Critters that create formidable challenges for the neurological system are Candida, a yeast infection, and mycoplasma, a deadly bacteria without cell walls that is undetectable by most medical tests. Critters that cause Lyme disease create symptoms that are virtually identical to those of Parkinson's disease.

© 2013 Parkinsons Recovery

LYME DISEASE

I suspect a surprisingly large number of people have been mistakenly diagnosed with Parkinsons instead of Lyme disease which is reported to be the fastest spreading infectious disease. The bacterial infection comes from a nasty spirochete spread by ticks that have been feeding off of infected deer. The infection causes inflammation which impairs neural functioning.

Lyme is incredibly difficult to detect. If you have tested negative for Lyme disease, it does not mean you do not have it! The tests are horribly inaccurate and the bacteria are incredibly sneaky critters. A rich source which previews the diagnosis and treatment of Lyme can be found on Dietrich K. Klinghardt's website: www.klinghardtacademy.com

As with most diseases, there is an underlying event which obstructs the body's ability to eliminate the Lyme infection. In the particular case of Lyme, the underlying factor is often abuse that was experienced at some point in a person's life, often at an early age.

Here is John Briggs, ND perspective on Lyme disease:

"Lyme disease is the great imitator...You can find it affecting almost anything. If Lyme disease is involved, then obviously we need to go after that in particular. If a person had Parkinsons and they are not seeing benefit from whatever protocol they are doing, it would be wise to be tested for Lyme. We are finding there is probably a whole lot more Lyme disease out there than people realize because it is going undetected. A product called Samento is a TAO-Free Cat's Claw that is excellent for knocking out Lyme disease."

I have heard reports from people the using a herb from Asia has proved helped. The name of this herb is Artemisinine. Dr. Zhang (www.dr-zhang.com) recommends using a garlic extract with a high concentration of Allicin. Bee Venom is also used to address the pain from infections like Lyme.

TETANUS

Voice profiling for Parkinsons Recovery radio listeners by Sharry Edwards has revealed a fascinating discovery. Evidence of a Tetanus infection was found in over half of the voice profiles that were analyzed. These listeners did not have Parkinson's. They were infected with the Tetanus bacteria.

- *Tetanus is characterized by a contraction of the skeletal muscles which makes movement difficult. Mobility challenges are symptomatic of Parkinson's.*

© 2013 Parkinsons Recovery

- *Tetanus usually begins with spasms in jaw muscles. A surprising number of people with Parkinsons have found their symptoms have resolved after being treated for TMJ disorder (which is a jaw misalignment).*

- *Tetanus is an infection of the nervous system. Everyone agrees Parkinson's is a nervous system condition.*

- *Symptoms of Tetanus include drooling, excessive sweating, hand or foot spasms, swallowing difficulty and anxiety. All of these symptoms describe Parkinsons Disease.*

In summary, there is a reasonable possibility you do not have Parkinson's disease. You have a Tetanus infection. Heal the infection and presto - your symptoms will vanish.

CRITTERS STICK TOGETHER

Most people follow a simplistic protocol for addressing infections. Their idea is to identify the specific bacteria that is present in their body. Once identified, the ideal therapy that can treat it successfully can be pursued with the help of their doctor. For example, if tests show they have a Lyme infection, they will discuss with their doctor the optimal treatments for Lyme.

If only it were this simple! Critters are crafty. They are devious. They have a persistent ability to survive. When antibiotics are taken, some of the critters are eliminated so that the body can function again. This is a good thing. Unfortunately, most of the critters sneak away into the nicks and crevices of the body and hide out – literally. They are dormant until they decide time is right to strike out again and multiply.

There are hundreds of mutations of critters. Most people have a collection of many different forms and mutations hanging out in the tissues and organs of their body. For some people, these infections have been present for decades. There is rarely just one bacterial infection present.

To make matters even more complicated, critters will sometimes glob together in clusters. This is a sneaky strategy that helps insure their survival. Just image looking at a high powered microscope that shows a town meeting of critters who are all connected to one another as if they were family.

The ideal strategy for eliminating critters is to strengthen the immune system so that the body can heal itself. The body knows precisely what do to. We just need to give it a little support.

CANDIDA

Candida is essentially a yeast infection and an overarching label for many varieties of yeast infections that grow in our bodies. Where does yeast come from? Bread products almost always contain yeast. Most processed foods include yeast as an ingredient. Just look at the labels sometime.

Candida initially starts as a yeast overgrowth in the intestines and mucous membranes. It is fed by taking antibiotics, corticosteroids and oral contraceptives and eating a diet that is rich in sugar and carbohydrates.

Too much Candida in the digestive track gobbles up the healthy flora we need for digestion. Without healthy flora in our gut (which are also living organisms) we cannot digest our food. It goes in. It comes out - unaltered.

Without healthy flora the body also cannot absorb supplements. Everything slides through our digestive system like a 5 year old at a water park. You may be spending $30 a day on supplements everyone says should help, but if you have a yeast overgrowth, most of your investment is winding up in the toilet, literally.

The frontal assault of Candida has just begun. When the healthy flora are extinct, Candida critters leak into the blood stream through the intestinal walls. There are no guards standing at the gate to stop them. The little critters have a grand time traveling throughout every nook and cranny of your body. Just listen in to one of their conversations.

> *Ah, there is not enough sugar to gobble in the heart. Let's move on to the lungs.*

> *Ah, there is not enough food to eat in the lungs, how about the brain? The brain is filled with sugar on a good day. Good. Let's go there.*

The army division lines up and marches onward. The army of organisms grows and multiplies. It soon begins to overwhelm. Are you feeling overwhelmed? You can thank Candida overgrowth for that unpleasant feeling.

CANDIDA AND PARKINSONS

Am I off the track here? Isn't this supposed to be a book about Parkinsons? You must be wondering what Candida overgrowth has to do with the symptoms of Parkinsons? I believe it plays a supporting role in the destruction of the cells that produce dopamine in the body. Here is a technical explanation.

People with an overgrowth of Candida exhibit elevated levels of acetaldehyde in their gastro intestinal track. Acetaldehyde is one of fifty different toxins that is produced by the Candida organism. And you thought I was talking about a harmless pinch of yeast?

When concentrations of acetaldehyde become too high, the liver is no longer able to remove it successfully. Acetaldehyde has no other choice than to hang around the tissues of the body with a special preference for the brain.

What happens next comes as bad news for the nervous system. Acetaldehyde combines with dopamine to synthesize a substance called Salsolinol. Hang on to your seats:

Salsolinol destroys dopaminergic cells in the substantia nigra. Internally manufactured by the body, Salsolinol itself is a neurotoxin. Increased levels of salsolinol have been found in the cerebral spinal fluid and the urine of people who have been diagnosed with Parkinsons.

The sequence of causal events is the following:

1. *Candida produces acetaldehyde.*

2. *Acetaldehyde causes the synthesis of Salsolinol.*

3. *Salsolinol kills off the cells that produce dopamine.*

The above causal sequence is what scientists call a theoretical argument. It is a causal sequence of very complicated events that have not been proven empirically. We may have a definitive answer in 50 years if you are willing to wait that long. I personally think the theoretical possibility is compelling enough for anyone with the symptoms of Parkinsons to take Candida overgrowth seriously.

CANDIDA AND THOUGHT FORMS

I have another causal sequence I believe is at play here. There is no proof for this argument I am about to make, but my intuitive powers tell me I am dead on target.

Candida are living organisms that colonize. They do not work independently like professors at universities who talk to themselves and a few other liked minded Ph.D.'s who have no connection to reality. Candida critters text each other on their cell phones. They connect with every other like minded fungus in sight and out of sight. They are more organized than the Teamsters Union. If there is a shortage of sugar or carbohydrates to eat, they know where to go in the body to get it because everyone reads the news on their cell phones.

Candida have a very low vibrational frequency. If you have Candida overgrowth in your body, you are ensconced with a continuous vibration that is very low. There is no escape.

The consequence? Negative thought forms are also associated with very low frequencies. The overgrowth of Candida sustains, supports and nurtures our own negative thoughts that we express to ourselves and others day in and day out.

© 2013 Parkinsons Recovery

It is critical to sustain positive thoughts for healing to happen. It is also virtually impossible to sustain positive thoughts moment to moment, day in and day out when an onslaught of low frequency Candida critters are dragging us down into the dust bowl of gloom and doom.

Have you ever asked yourself:

Why do I fall into the gutter of negative thinking all the time?

Why do some negative thoughts glue themselves to me?

Why can't I unglue negative thoughts from the control center of my brain?

When I asked myself this question, I hypothesized it might be because of a Candida overgrowth in my body. I suspected that the Candida fungi had invaded my brain, my ears, my eyes, my toes. I suspected that regardless of how intensely I wanted to have high frequency thoughts, my thinking was continuously undermined by low frequency, unwanted and uninvited hosts in my brain.

So I decided to undertake a six week Candida cleanse which was very elaborate and intense. What happened?

1. Mental confusion is caused by Candida and is a symptom associated with Parkinsons. One of my challenges has been brain fog, poor memory and some confusion. I handle a lot of detail day in and day out. It is excessive. Some days I could not remember what I was working on the day before. After my Candida cleanse the brain fog lifted. My thinking is now as clear and coherent as it ever has been.

2. Depression is a consequence of Candida. Many people with Parkinsons experience depression as do I from time to time. It moves in and hangs around for a few hours or days. Since my Candida cleanse I have not had a minute of depression.

3. Dark blotches and spots on the body are caused by Candida. Most of the dark spots on my arms and hands - which I always thought were freckles since I was a teenager - have vanished. I am not freckly any more. The surprise is that the spots were never freckles. They were always evidence of the Candida that has settled into the tissues of my body at a very early age.

4. One of the symptoms of Parkinsons is excessive sweating. Sweating is the body's way of attempting to release something it does not need or want. I believe

© 2013 Parkinsons Recovery

sweating is the body's way to release the Candida (and other unfriendly critters) that are partying on the skin of our bodies.

5. Many people have problems with excessive salivation. There it is again - the body's natural response to removing the fungi critters.

6. Candida overgrowth is known to be associated with anxiety attacks, the ominous feeling that something bad is about to happen. Many people with Parkinsons tell me about their own horrifying experiences with anxiety attacks.

7. Constipation is a symptom of Parkinson which can be caused by a Candida overgrowth in the intestines. Candida rubs out the good flora. It takes over the field of play in the intestines and provokes inflammation in the intestinal track.

8. One of the symptoms of Parkinsons is fatigue. After my own Candida cleanse, my energy soared.

In summary, if I were to ask 100 medical research scientists whether they thought Candida overgrowth contributed to Parkinsons I suspect only a few would raise their hands. I for one do believe it plays a significant role in causing symptoms - or, at a minimum, aggravating many of the symptoms.

Why not investigate doing a Candida cleanse if you suspect an overgrowth might be an issue for you? Do you have evidence of any fungus growth on your body? Is your tongue white? If so, you probably have a yeast infection (known as Thrush) in your mouth.

You can heal a Thrush infection by emptying the contents of a probiotic capsule (which contains digestive enhancing ingredients as Acidophilus and Bifidus) on your tongue, swish it around your mouth for a minute and then swallow it. Do this three times a day until the infection clears. Change the acidic conditions that support the infection and the living yeast fungi will not be able to survive.

You may succeed in eliminating Candida from your mouth, but chances are good it has crawled into the nooks and crevices of your tissues. Candida is one of the most challenging infections to get rid of, primarily because for most people, the critters have leaked outside the digestive track and crawled into the organs.

The potential damage that Candida can do goes hand in hand with the degree of its retrenchment into the body. Once Candida critters settle into the crevices of our tissues, they do not willingly leave. It is like asking a two year old to leave their birthday party early.

© 2013 Parkinsons Recovery

Most Candida cleanses on the market have limited (if any) effectiveness. It is a continual, uphill battle and the reason why many people have such low energy.

One approach will prevail in the short run but few people can pull this one off: A strict diet which includes a long list of prohibited foods: This list includes:

- *No fruit juices and dried or candied fruits.*

- *No sugar.*

- *No melons – including watermelon, honeydew and cantaloupe.*

- *No cheese and dairy products (exceptions are kefir, eggs and butter).*

- *No antibiotics.*

- *No yeast.*

- *No condiments, sauces and dressings containing vinegar and sugar.*

- *No processed foods.*

- *No alcohol or malt products.*

- *No condiments, sauces and dressings containing vinegar and sugar.*

- *No processed and smoked meats.*

- *No coffee and tea (exception is green tea).*

- *No food leftovers (that may contain mold).*

Whew! Are there any foods on this list that you love to eat? The agonizing challenge of a Candida cleanse (whether it is a dietary cleanse or a herbal cleanse) is that you never get rid of all the Candida because they serve a useful and important function in the digestive track. Candida cleanses are a question of balance – which incidentally is the same issue that Parkinson's symptoms present. Some people have way too much dopamine; others too little just as some people have too many Candida critters crawling around in the playground of their body. What is needed is to maintain the correct balance.

The more you are able refute those sugar cravings, the more likely it is that you will maintain the correct balance. If you have an overgrowth of Candida, consult with a knowledgeable health care professional who can help you identify a cleanse protocol that will be successful. Candida critters are a lot smarter than we are. You can count on it.

MYCOPLASMA

One of the primary causes of many illnesses is the presence of Mycoplasma bacterial infections throughout the organs and tissues of the body. What is so damaging about this particular bacteria? They have no cell walls. Any one of 100 different species of Mycoplasma attach to the power generator of the cells – the mitochondria.

Mycoplasma are the terrorists of the body. They are so well hidden no one can find them, much less destroy them. Because they have no cell walls, medical tests rarely detect their presence.

They have been given varying names by researchers: stealth viruses, sub-viral bacterium particles, prions and Mycoplasma/Brucellosis. Sounds scary eh? The damage they are capable of doing is no illusion.

Why are Mycoplasma so dangerous? They slowly and meticulously eat away at the tissues, muscles and cells in various organs and cells of the body. When the immune system is depleted, trauma is present (as in the case with Parkinson's), cellular oxygen is limited and the body is too acidic. Mycoplasma destroy the mitochondria, the primary source of energy for the body. Once mitochondria die, the vital production of ATP is disabled. Our life force is sucked dry.

Mycoplasma are smart little devils. They attach themselves to the cells found in the weaker organs and systems. If a person is challenged neurologically, neurons are the preferred target.

They survive by taking proteins, sugars and cholesterol from neighboring cells to survive. It is no wonder that they prefer to hang out around neurons and brains. Both have an abundance of cholesterol.

Sometime dormant for decades. Mycoplasma are activated by physical or emotional trauma and toxins. Why do many people with Parkinsons have low energy? They probably have an abundance of Mycoplasma.

They thrive off sucking the life force of its host. Once it invades the neurons, the chance of reinstituting a healthy neural communication signaling system is impossible. The only solution is to eliminate them.

How do you destroy them? Some doctors recommend a 6 month to year regimen of antibiotics. This will not eliminate them altogether and it also destroys the immune system. Other doctors prescribe certain herbal remedies such as Samento to support the immune system. Effectiveness of either approach varies widely across persons.

I have challenged some of the most advanced researchers in the country to assess the frequency of the various species of Mycoplasma. Once the frequency of each species is known, they can be destroyed using acoustic therapies.

© 2013 Parkinsons Recovery

To summarize, the trigger for your symptoms may not be a deficiency of dopamine. Rather, it may be the aggressiveness of the Mycopasma bacteria that are terrorizing your cells, your neurons and your substantia nigra. They will obstruct your recovery.

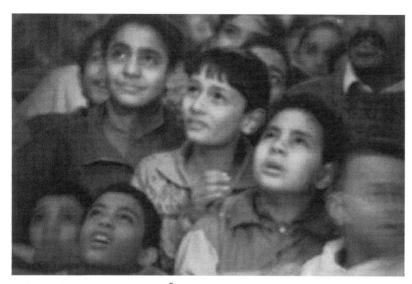

Photo by Donne Willett[5]

Is there a common thread with regard to what people do to feel better? Most people talk about diet - but not everyone. Most people talk about exercise - but not everyone. Many people talk about ways they go about detoxing their bodies - but not everyone. Most people talk about ways they relieve stress in their life -but again, not everyone.

My interviews with many people who have found ways to get relief from the symptoms of Parkinsons have unearthed a wide variety of approaches and therapies that help. Some of them I have not even heard about! What works beautifully for one person does not necessarily work at all for someone else. This makes perfect sense to me because the factors that cause the condition vary considerably across persons.

For some people the primary cause is stress. For other people the primary cause is toxins. For still other people the primary cause is lack of exercise and the absence of a healthy diet. A combination of factors often plays a role.

So what is the answer to this question? Is there a common thread among people who have figured out ways to feel better? My answer is unequivocally yes! There are two common threads.

First, people who are feeling better hold the unwavering belief that they are recovering. Instead of saying to themselves:

---

[5] "Enchanted' was shot in Alexandria, Egypt. These young people were watching a sort of magic show as part of Ramadan festivities late in the evening. The photo was juried into the San Diego International Photo Show, 1999, as part of the San Diego Fair. It received a second place ribbon in the Open Photography category in the Los Angeles County Fair, 2000." Donne Willett

© 2013 Parkinsons Recovery

"Poor me. I am on a slow path of deterioration."

They say to themselves

"Lucky me. I am on an exciting path to recovery."

Second, people who are feeling better are committed and determined to try anything that their intuition tells them may help. They are always on the lookout for therapies and approaches that have helped other people with Parkinsons or have helped other people with chronic conditions. They are always experimenting. They will give anything a chance if their intuition tells them it is worth a try.

My impression is that most people have a good sense about the likely cause of their symptoms, whether it is stress or trauma or toxins or an unhealthy lifestyle. For many it is too much stress and trauma in their lives. For others it is exposure to toxins. For still others it is diet.

There are many excellent therapies that help to relieve stress and release toxins. Information about healthy living is readily available.

People who are feeling better are constantly on the lookout for therapies to try and activities to do that offer a promise of relief. They search the Internet. They talk to other people with Parkinsons. They investigate. They make phone calls. They ask me questions and I research the answers.

They don't just read about therapies or talk about them. They actually try some of them out. Only then do they know whether any particular therapy works for them.

They keep the ones that work. They discard the ones that do not work for them. By the way, there is no single approach, medicine, therapy or remedy that does the trick. A combination of approaches is necessary.

Do they experiment with everything they hear about? Of course not! But if their intuition tells them a particular therapy might offer relief from their symptoms, they go for it. After one or several sessions they know whether the therapy will help.

I do not believe that there is one daily routine that can help everyone. And, I do not believe that there is one set of drug therapies, body work, or natural approaches to healing that works for everyone.

I do believe the answers are highly individualistic. The daily routine, the therapies, the diet, the type of exercise that can help you find relief from your symptoms is yours to discover. Carl, one of the Pioneers of Recovery, agrees:

© 2013 Parkinsons Recovery

"Well, my experience with this disease, whatever underlies it is so unique to the individual that you have to do a sort of serious self assessment about your lifestyle, about your approach, your thoughts about this disease."

"I would certainly recommend trying to stay away from the traditional drugs as long as you can and still function at a level that allows you to be happy with life. In hindsight I think, I wish in the early, early stages, I had known a little bit more about energy work. Maybe that would have delayed some of the symptoms on-setting. But then again, who knows?"

"I don't know what to say because when I talk to people, different people have different reactions to different therapies. Things that have worked for me, I've noticed that other people have tried it but have not had as good effect and vice-versa. There seems to be a very, how do I say - individualistic (if that's a word) component to this disease or this condition."

"You have to sort of figure it out. There's no magic formula as far as I can tell, I mean, there's no magic cure. It may take a multiple healing approach. One thing I should mention, that I do feel strongly about in terms of trying to heal or recover from this disease, is that I think it really takes an intensity of treatment that our traditional medical system is not set up to handle. Certainly not cost wise."

"I recall a story that <u>Toby Christiansen</u>, the drummer, told me. He was trained in Africa by a very powerful shamanic healer in East Africa. And he said,"

> *'Carl, if you had Parkinsons and you lived within the tribe that I was trained in they would work on you every single day until you recovered.'*

"And that was part of their society. That's the way they treat people. They didn't care what it cost or what the burden was to the tribe but that's the way they would treat people. We're not set up that way."

The mission of Parkinsons Recovery is to identify the modalities, therapies, drugs and approaches that help people with Parkinsons feel better. There are a multitude of possibilities to consider. The good news is that with a little trial and error, it is possible to find your own "individualistic" combination of approaches that will help you feel better.

No one likes to have the symptoms of Parkinsons. They are horrible. A usual response is to launch a battle against the symptoms or to find ways to suppress them through medications, drugs, herbs, supplements or other therapies. I am suggesting here that you consider a counterintuitive approach that is embodied in process work:

- *Acknowledge the symptoms as gifts in disguise.*

- *Set the intention to explore what they are really about.*

- *Listen to what your body is telling you.*

- *Your body is not broken. It is working perfectly.*

The best way to figure out the daily routine, the therapies, the natural approaches and the lifestyle that works for you is to learn about the many alternatives that offer the promise of relief. Then - when you have a sense one might help - try it out. Take a risk.

I can guarantee you that not everything you try is going to help. But, some of what you try will help. You will be the beneficiary of exciting rewards for your commitment and dedication to travel down the road to recovery.

If you do not experiment with a new way of living, you will in all likelihood not get better. If you do experiment you will have something to look forward to and, better yet, you will eventually begin to feel better. It is a choice.

Enjoy the ride. You are on the road to recovery. It is a lot more interesting than watching TV all day long.

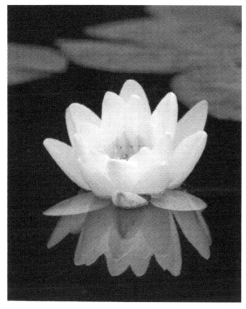

Lotus Blossom by Judith Giddings[6]

THE HIDDEN SECRET TO RECOVERY

Exciting discoveries are on the horizon for how anyone can recover from chronic imbalances and illnesses like Parkinsons. Scientists have already acknowledged that imbalances in the body can be detected by measuring frequencies that are present. Even more exciting is a future where the body can be nudged back into balance with machines that adjust existing frequencies.

The most exciting news for me is that since healing is all about raising our frequencies, we can all help ourselves get well now. We do not have to wait for the new diagnostic instruments and treatment therapies to be invented and approved for use.

Low frequencies are associated with imbalances, illness and disease. High frequencies are associated with balance, health and wellness. If you are being pestered by symptoms, it means that your body is oscillating at a frequency that is too low to sustain health and wellness. Raise that frequency and you will begin to feel better. Put simplistically, that is why we begin to feel better when we eat live food and exercise.

ABOUT FREQUENCIES

What do I mean when I say "frequencies"? I am talking here about physical phenomena that are measurable with scientific instruments. This is not esoteric nonsense.

Radio signals are a good example. All FM radio stations transmit in a band of frequencies between 88,000,000 and 108,000,000 cycles per second. AM radio transmits in a band of

---

[6] "Lotus Blossom has also been on the cover of a meditation CD (The Meditation Experience by Judith Pennington) and was featured in the 2007 Creativity and Parkinson's calendar (June)." Judith Giddings

© 2013 Parkinsons Recovery

frequencies between 535,000 to 1,700,000 cycles per second. In other words AM radio stations transmit at significantly lower frequencies than the FM stations.

Every tissue, cell, organ, hormone, bacteria and virus transmits a frequency that is specific to that particular organism. Existing instruments can diagnose illness and imbalances in the body as a function of the various frequencies that are emitted. Bioenergetic testing has been around for 40 years now. Diagnostic instruments that use frequencies to detect imbalances will become much more sophisticated over the coming years. In the near future, doctors will manipulate frequencies to treat the imbalances that have been identified through the diagnostic testing.

Many of you may be familiar with the enormous interest in "hands on healing" that has taken various forms such as Reiki, healing touch, Zen massage, acupuncture, acupressure, homeopathic medicine, the course in miracles and so forth. All of these therapies are successful because they help to elevate our frequencies.

ALL TOXINS HAVE A FREQUENCY

- *Why do I emphasize the importance of cleansing our bodies from pathogens - those obnoxious critters that hang out in our organs and tissues?*

- *Why do I write about the issues associated with unfriendly bacteria in our digestive system?*

- *Why do I write about the challenge posed by Candida, viruses and molds that are trapped deep inside our tissues?*

- *What does all of this have to do with Parkinsons? Am I just trying to fill up the airwaves with garble?*

All such organisms oscillate at extremely low frequencies - so low that they do not emit a frequency that even matches the frequency of an AM radio station. If you have an abundance of unfriendly critters hanging out in the nooks and crevices of your body, your body cannot help but oscillate at a low frequency. It is no wonder that imbalances persist when low frequencies are present. Symptoms will continue to haunt us.

Heavy metals and pesticides also have very low frequencies. That is why it can be helpful to detox your body. Once heavy metals and pesticides have been purged, the body can instantly jump up to a higher frequency. If you don't remove the low frequency metals, you are hosting a heavy metal rock band in your body that is blaring its "head banging", low frequency vibrations throughout every cell of your body ad nauseum.

© 2013 Parkinsons Recovery

ALL THOUGHTS HAVE A FREQUENCY

All thoughts have frequencies which get translated into chemicals that shake, rattle and roll through every cell of your body. Thoughts alter the chemical composition and behavior of your cells for better and for worse. Production of hormones can be stimulated or obstructed depending on the nature and frequency of each thought you generate. There is nothing simple about the mechanism at play here.

If you think symptoms are destined to get worse next week, you are calling in a very low frequency to be present. If you think:

"I am on the Road to Recovery."

You are calling in a high frequency to be present. This is why attention to your own moment to moment thoughts is critical to recovery. Transform your thoughts and you instantly transform your health. This is the foundation of the *Five Steps to Recovery*.

What do you say when you are unable to remember something? Do you say:

"I am just having a senior moment."

The thought that underlies that statement has a very low frequency because the statement suggests your mind is not functioning well. Something must be wrong with your body. Heather MacTavish recommends a replacement thought form.

> *"It takes time to sift through all the facts, information, knowledge, and wisdom stored inside your head. Go ahead. Take your time! It is worth the wait."*[7]

All of the therapies and treatments that help people with Parkinsons recover share one feature in common. They restore new, high frequencies that override the low frequencies that have been sustaining the imbalances.

The big picture of recovery is simply this. Increase your frequency and you will get well. High frequencies always win out. It is not even a "war". Low frequencies cannot exist in the presence of high frequencies. They scram like scared sissies.

So, all things said, what is the hidden secret to recovery? Raise your own energetic frequency. All imbalances can come back to center in the presence of high frequencies.

---

[7] Heather MacTavish with Zubin Balsara (2009). Songs, Science and Spirit: Musical keys to open special doors of ability. Provident Publishing. Tiburon, California, p. 73.

© 2013 **Parkinsons Recovery**

RECOVERY CAN HAPPEN NOW

Healing can happen now when we are successful with revving up our frequencies and giving our bodies the boost they need to heal.

I find this to be true with the work I have been doing on myself. Deborah reports the same result. We see the same result with our clients.

Healing can happen now when we clear out the low frequency drain on our energy and replace it with high frequency thoughts, positive intentions, yummy food, exciting activities, fun friends, endless laughter and with work that nurtures our souls.

I have put into place three support systems that can help you shift your frequency to higher and higher levels.

> 1. Jump Start to Wellness is a two day event that I have designed to jump start everyone's frequencies. When the frequencies are high enough, I believe that any imbalances in the body can be healed.
> http://www.parkinsonsrecovery.com/jumpstart.html

> 2. Parkinsons Recovery sponsors a member website that is updated every day with high frequency thoughts, transmitting an infusion of positive energy every day. For this support system you will have to like using computers, since you have to access the information on an Internet website: http://www.parkinsonsrecovery.org

TREATMENTS OF THE FUTURE

What will medicine of the future look like? Diagnostic instruments of the future will assess frequencies and use biophoton tracking to diagnose and treat imbalances. Medical treatments of the future will manipulate frequencies in the body through sound and light. Once the frequencies have been adjusted and the light of the body has been aligned, the body will come back into balance. In one sense the various therapies that are helping people reverse their symptoms today are a crude version of what we will see unfold over the coming years.

In another profound sense, I believe it is possible to make all of this happen without the technology of the future. I am not talking here about sophisticated technology of stem cells implants or hormonal medicines or surgeries, all of which by the way have frequencies of their own. I am suggesting we know now what is needed to make the frequency adjustment that is necessary to heal ourselves.

You can wait on the sidelines for the machines to be invented and approved. Or, you can make the frequency shift yourself. I prefer the latter option myself because I am basically an impatient person who wants to see it happen now. Not tomorrow. Now.

Science is much too slow for me. Waiting for research evidence is like waiting for Godot. I am ready to see recovery happen now for everyone.

I obviously do not have a shred of evidence for what I am about to say, but I personally do not believe anyone has to agonize several years for their symptoms to resolve. These are historic times for everyone who is alive today. It is my personal belief that symptoms can resolve now with a jump start in frequencies.

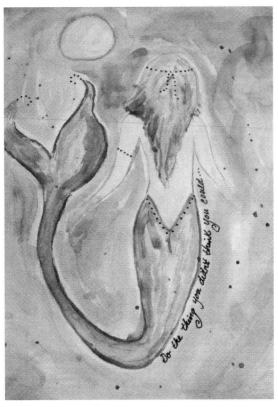

THERAPIES THAT ADDRESS
SPECIFIC CAUSES

Mermaid's Journey by Cindy Deluz

The good news is that there is something that can be done to release toxins and trauma from the body.

- *The key to feel better is to find ways to release the toxins and trauma that have been trapped and encapsulated in the cells.*

- *The key is to release the stresses in your life.*

- *The key is to address digestive backups and malfunctions.*

It takes a little time. It takes a little patience. In our book of good deals taking time and having patience is a cheap price to pay if you want to see long lasting relief from symptoms.

THERAPIES THAT RELEASE THE TRAUMA

I will now preview different therapies that are useful for releasing trauma: craniosacral therapy, Bowen therapy, Myofascial Release (MFR), Intramuscular Stimulation (IMS), Emotional Freedom Technique (EMT), Feldenkrais™ and laser therapy. Which therapy do I recommend for persons who currently experience the symptoms of Parkinson's? I do not have a clue how to answer that question for you – but your body can give you the answer if you ask it.

Some people tell me Bowen therapy is a life saver. That was certainly the case for John Bowman. Others say they notice no difference. Other people tell me craniosacral therapy is a life savior. Others say the opposite. Factors that underlie symptoms are so varied that the particular therapies that can help depend on our own individual circumstances.

I will say this however. If you know trauma is an issue for you – and frankly speaking it is an issue for most people – then begin to take seriously the challenge of finding a therapy that can help your body release the trauma that obstructs your ability to function.

CRANIOSACRAL THERAPY

Results of the Parkinsons Energy Project in Portland, Oregon showed that craniosacral work does help to relieve symptoms. Study volunteers were able to do things that they had previously been unable to do. Here are some examples:

↓ Cook Thanksgiving dinner	↓ Attend business meetings
↓ Take weekly nature hikes	↓ Swing arms freely
↓ Go out on a date	↓ Blink eyes
↓ Travel	↓ Hang out with friends
↓ Be assertive	↓ Drive without anxiety
↓ Take off a coat without assistance	↓ Handle stress better
↓ Stand up to brush teeth	

We also observed other positive changes from one treatment session to the next including:

↓ More flexibility getting on and off the treatment table

↓ Better posture

↓ Greater ease walking

↓ Enhanced mental clarity and expressiveness

↓ Greater flexibility

↓ More smiling, better skin color and overall vibrancy

↓ More vitality and youthfulness

Craniosacral therapy clearly had a positive impact on the overall health and well being of the study volunteers.

I have posted videos of persons who gave us permission to make them public. You can see them perform basic tasks before receiving the craniosacral treatments and afterward. The improvement is obvious. You can view them at www.blog.parkinsonsrecovery.com

Since I have personal experience with this particular approach, I would like to explain more about what craniosacral therapy is, why it helps to reduce stress and how it is used to release trauma that is held in the body.

One woman with Parkinsons who found relief using craniosacral therapy summarized the nature of the treatments beautifully:

> *"It is hard to believe anything is really happening, but it works."*

The work is very gentle. The person typically lies down on a comfortable table such as a massage table. Craniosacral treatments are not like a massage. The nature of the touch is very, very light and gentle. The person remains fully clothed.

Craniosacral therapy facilitates the body's natural ability to unwind and release any tension that is trapped throughout the body. It helps the neural system to rest and rejuvenate.

The intent of craniosacral therapy is to work with the body so that tension and trauma that is trapped at the cellular level can be released. Therapists are trained to "follow the body" as they allow tension and stress to be released from the muscles and tissues. The process is best described as one of unwinding tissues that are tightly entangled with too much tension.

Trauma to the body is analogous to a wet wash rag that has been twisted so many times that all the water has been squeezed dry. After the rag is exposed to the hot sun it dries out and becomes hardened and inflexible. This is what happens to tissues that have been traumatized. Craniosacral therapy softens and helps hydrate the tissues so that they can be properly nourished.

After talking with many, many people with Parkinsons I have concluded that stress is a key factor that aggravates symptoms. When stress can be relieved, symptoms get better. Person after person in my interviews tell me the same thing: There is a direct and immediate connection between their stress level and their symptoms.

When their symptoms flare up, people report they are always under more stress. When they are able to find ways to get relief from the stress, symptoms become less worrisome.

© 2013 Parkinsons Recovery

Stress creates inflammation throughout the body which is the basis for many chronic diseases. Reduction in inflammation is a key reason for the improvement in symptoms. Here is the sequence:

1. *Craniosacral work releases stress.*

2. *Inflammation is reduced.*

3. *Symptoms are relieved.*

Craniosacral therapy may or may not be your cup of tea. Results of the Parkinsons Energy Project (PEP) study clearly suggest that you will benefit from finding a way to reduce stress in your life and release the trauma that is trapped in your tissues.

Any way of reducing stress that works for you will help you to feel much better. Craniosacral Therapy is one way to help get relief from stress, but it is only one way. There are other natural modalities that are also useful to consider.

BOWEN THERAPY

The Bowen Technique uses a series of adjustments that are gently applied to muscles and to connective tissues. The therapy commutes vibrations to parts of the body that are out of balance. The adjustments release energy that is blocked due to trauma. These releases facilitate a healing of the entire neurological system. Bowen therapy helps balance the Autonomic Nervous System.

The basic therapeutic approach targets muscles and tendons that have been restricted as a result of trauma and stress. The Bowen therapist challenges the tissues and muscles to move in opposite directions. Brief pauses after each adjustment make it possible for an adjustment to stabilize as the blocked energy is released. The released energy travels through the body fully before the next adjustment is done.

John Coleman in Stop Parkin' and Start Livin' recommends Bowen therapy for people who currently experience the symptoms of Parkinson's. It helped him and he has found it has also helped his clients who currently experience the symptoms of Parkinson's disease.

MYOFASCIAL RELEASE (MFR)

Myofascial Release focuses on fascia, the thin, delicate layer of tissue that is found throughout the body under the skin and elsewhere. It involves application of gentle pressure on the fascia connective tissues throughout the body that are twisted, knotted and crumpled.

What do fascia distortions look like in a physical sense? Pull out a single thread from a wool sweater and what happens? The entire sweater crunches up, twists and contorts. If you pull

© 2013 Parkinsons Recovery

enough thread out, the sweater loses its shape altogether. The sweater's job to keep you warm is disarmed. The body's neurological system is compromised if fascia are distorted.

Mobility challenges are aggravated by fascia restrictions. Arms or legs can be severely restricted in the range and ease of motion. Tissues become so constricted that muscles feel like concrete. If your muscles are tight and you are having difficulty walking, it is very likely due in part to restrictions in your fascia.

What causes these restrictions? They are created as a result of traumas to the body that take various forms: emotional (such as abuse) physical (such as accidents) and inflammation. Bacterial and viral infections can be problematic for fascia.

The MFR therapist applies gentle pressure to the skin without oils or creams which elongates and moisturizes. A trained therapist senses the condition of the fascia and applies the appropriate degree of pressure in the appropriate locations. .

Occupational Therapist David Howell is a Myofascial therapist who offered an eloquent description of the therapy and the treatment during my radio show that aired April 15, 2010

INTRAMUSCULAR STIMULATION (IMS)
Neuropathic pain occurs when nerve endings become overly sensitive. Inconsistent signals become the norm. Some of the misdirected signals are interpreted by the brain as pain. Shorted muscles often found with Parkinson's, cause innocent, harmless signals to be exaggerated and misinterpreted as painful. Standard medical tests show nothing is wrong, but the patient knows otherwise.

Angela Wensley has obtained welcome relief from her symptoms using Intramuscular Stimulation therapy (IMS). Here is her description of this therapy:

> IMS is a form of myofascial release that involves needling, sort of "scientific acupuncture"... I have been receiving IMS for 3 months with profound results. I have totally regained my range of motion of my right shoulder and the intense pain in my right hip has been considerably lessened. My posture is much improved.

> This is the single most effective therapy I have encountered for my PD. I understand that it originated in Vancouver but that there are practitioners all over the world. See http://www.intramuscularstimulation.com/2.htm especially the last paragraph.

EMOTIONAL FREEDOM TECHNIQUE (EFT)

Parkinsons Recovery is all about identifying approaches and therapies that give relief from the symptoms of Parkinsons. One among many such techniques I have identified from my research is the Emotional Freedom Technique (or EFT). EFT is a marvelous, easy to use technique that has provided relief to some people with Parkinsons I have interviewed.

Can it help you? Maybe. Maybe not, but why not find out more about it?

EFT can be self-administered. Anyone can use it. It is free. You do not need to hire a therapist, though some people prefer to go this route. In my opinion it is well worth giving EFT a try. There is really nothing to lose.

Emotional Freedom Techniques (EFT) involves tapping on acupuncture points along the face and collar bone (and other acupressure points on the body) while a person focuses on a specific issue they wish to address. EFT is useful when a person has an unwanted thought, feeling or belief they wish to shed.

Most people find it convenient to shove unpleasant feelings into the closet. Feelings about having poor balance, inaudible speech, lousy handwriting, enhanced anxiety or intensified fears are unpleasant. If you cram them in the closet and shut the door you no longer have to confront them. EFT takes unwanted feelings and negative thoughts out of the closet and brings them into consciousness as the person taps on acupuncture points and practices accepting themselves. The template of EFT is:

> *Even though I resent [insert name of feeling here] and it feels absolutely horrible, I completely and totally accept and love myself.*

You can learn to do EFT on yourself when symptoms flare. Or, you can use EFT to prevent symptoms from amplifying. Anyone can use EFT throughout the course of the day to address little frustrations and irritations. It is easy to do and takes only a minute or two. Or, you can devote a block of time during the day to release a feelings such as resentments, grief, hurt, anger or separation from family and friends.

EFT creates a fundamental change in the chemistry and physiology of the cell receptor sites. Bernadette Hunter, an Emotional Freedom Technique (EFT) Performance Specialist, says that EFT helps drag our skeletons out of the closet from yesteryear so we can come to peace with our unresolved traumas.

Bernadette says EFT is a no nonsense method. You do not have to know all the science behind it. You also don't necessarily need a practitioner to help you learn it though it is helpful in the beginning to get at the root issues that are creating the symptoms.

Bernadette explains,

> "When we have a thought, chemicals are released by the hypothalamus which are experienced as emotions. They lock into the cell receptor sites. We have 1-2 trillion cells in our body, all of which have a lot of cell receptor sites. If we don't process an emotion, it stays in the cell receptor sites. It blocks that site from getting the nutrients and protein that it needs to be healthy. Over time, cell receptor sites shrink up and die."

What happens to the cells that remain? They divide. If you haven't cleared out the fears (or anxieties or resentments or anger or rage or guilt or ... that are trapped in a cell, that one cell becomes two cells. You now have two cells that have a comfort zone for resentment. The natural process of division unfolds as the feelings begin to consume our thoughts.

Have you noticed that angry people often become more and more angry as time marches on? Bernadette explains why.

> "On a physiologic level, if they haven't released that anger from their cells. The chemicals - the emotions of anger- don't have a chance to release. The cell divides. Now you have twice as many cells feeling very comfortable with anger."

> "EFT unlocks the emotion chemical out of the cell receptor sites. I watch it before my eyes. Oh, the anger is gone. Oh the sadness, the deep grief is gone. There is this lightness in the body. It is literally happening on a cellular level."

Neural networks are the most sensitive cellular structure in the body. EFT helps to cleanse the emotional blockages that muck up neural networks.

A key benefit of EFT involves ending our own internal struggles and resolving the fights that we instigate with ourselves. Bernadette explains:

"It is really easy to fight against having a serious illness.

- *I hate this.*

- *Why Me?*

- *I can't believe this is happening.*

- *This is awful.*

© **2013 Parkinsons Recovery**

- *My life is going to go downhill from here on out.*

- *The prognosis is horrible.*

I have worked with a lot of people with physical pain. There is something beautiful about saying:

"Even though I have pain, I deeply and completely love and accept myself.

There is something about saying that – I can't explain how this shift in the brain happens – but I can feel it and see it shift in front of my eyes. There is something about the acceptance of what we find is unacceptable."

With physical illness, your body is already working overtime. Bernadette explains that EFT is innocuous but powerful. If you persist, if you find a daily EFT regimen, you can make major shifts in your recovery.

Monica, an individual with the symptoms of Parkinsons, received a live Emotional Freedom Technique session with Bernadette during my Parkinsons Recovery Radio Program which aired May 21, 2009.

Monica worked on the issue of anxiety with Bernadette. The following week she reported that her anxiety issues had been for the most part resolved.

"I had a vet appointment this a.m. and I wanted to advise you of the outcome. On a scale of 1 - 10, the experience was a 0 - 1. I noticed also while driving there was more relaxation. I felt very happy inside, very relieved that I could feel this way after 2 years of fighting and worrying about nothing. I think it may be carrying over to improving my walking in confined areas, like inside the house. I was so tense inside the house. Something has released but I can't put my finger on it, something to do with fear...

Tomorrow I have an even longer drive to meet a girlfriend for brunch...I have no anxiety about it. There's no fighting going on in my head. I actually am looking forward to the whole event".

What follows is the email Monica sent to me after her brunch:

"I had another longer driving trip 2 days later with continued good results...Also noticed the longer I drove the more relaxed I became as far as more relaxed in the forearms vs. tightened contracted muscles".

Listen to the radio program if you are interested in getting a first hand, close up preview of how EFT is done. It obviously helped Monica. It may help you too.

© 2013 Parkinsons Recovery

EMOTION CODE™

Emotions can linger decades after a trauma. The longer it lingers, the more difficult it has been to release – until recently. One technique that has received an enthusiastic response is the Emotion Code™, an effortless approach for releasing emotional stress and trauma. As many as 60 different emotions can obstruct recovery. This approach identifies which emotions specifically are standing in your way from recovering.

Developed by chiropractor Bradley Nelson, the approach uses a systematic method of identifying the underlying emotions that pertain to a particular issue you may be having. The origin is identified using muscle testing and a powerful technique is used to release it. John O'Dwyer, a certified Emotion Code™ practitioner, demonstrated precisely how this technique is done during my radio October 17, 2012.

Some people commented after the show that they appreciate the roll play we did. It was not a role play. John was working on an actual issue that I have confronted my entire life. If you are called to pursue this approach for clearing out dead energy which is obstructing your recovery, listen to the radio show first. Then, if you are so inclined, contact John.

FELDENKRAIS™

A challenge connected to the symptoms of Parkinson's is rigidity of movement. Mobility of the eyes decreases. The head, neck and trunk move as if they were one rigid unit almost like a frozen bull dozer about to dump a load of dirt. Moving the body as a single, rigid unit becomes habitual.

Feldenkrais™ helps the body remember how to use sequences of movement that gently guide the body to move in a more organized, coordinated manner. A larger range of motion and greater flexibility become the norm rather than the exception.

Why not experience the possibilities for yourself? During the first part of my radio show that aired on December 8, 2010, Irene Paskernack, guided listeners through a series of gentle movements that increase the range of head movement from left to right. Don't take my word for it. Give the exercise a whirl yourself.

A free set of written instructions that are similar in their intent to Irene's exercise can be followed by visiting the easy movement website. These exercises increase the range of head movement with several gentle movements that invite the body to activate a sequence of movements to turn your head. Feldenkrais™ lessons in general help you body to reorganize the sequence of movements that can be lost when hormones are out of balance.

A guiding principle of Feldenkrais™ is to always move your body in the direction of ease rather than resistance. Some practitioners refer to this highly valuable practice as unwinding. When feeling muscle tightness and rigidity, some people decide they must use force and will to overcome the resistance. This strategy is destined to backfire. When movement is forced in the direction of resistance, the body becomes even more rigid and inflexible.

Feldenkrais™ taps into the neuroplasticity of your brain. The motor cortex communicates with your muscles. The sensory cortex receives feedback from the sensory nerves. Research shows that a mapping of these connections reveals a typical pattern of big hands, big face, big feet but a small torso.

Feldenkrais™ exercises increase the size of these maps to the torso and other underutilized muscles of the body. Irene Pasternack explains it is like increasing the bandwidth of a computer. Locate a practitioner in your area by visiting the Feldenkrais™ website.

LASER THERAPY TO HEAL SCAR TISSUE

One formidable source of trauma to the body is surgery. I have interviewed many people with the symptoms of Parkinsons who have had multiple surgeries. Scars from surgeries interrupt meridian pathways in the body. It is important to heal the scar tissue so that all channels of energy that nourish your organs and tissues are unobstructed.

What do I mean by channels? There are well documented energy pathways in our bodies that are given different names in acupuncture: The stomach meridian, the liver meridian, the spleen meridian, etc. You can find charts of these pathways in the library.

Surgery on your foot or hand or any part of your body for that matter interrupts the flow of vital energy across any one or more of these pathways. Acupuncturists place needles along the meridian lines that need a jump start. It is like recharging the battery of a car. An acupuncturist may place needles in your foot or neck to address issues with your digestion or mood.

For example, let's say you have had surgery on your hip recently. There is a big scar on your upper thigh that is located at the center of your body. This scar tissue from hip surgery creates a systematic interruption in the energy pathways that nourish one or more of your vital organs.

Check out the meridian charts to see if any surgeries you may have had lie on a key meridian. Do not be surprised to discover you may be having difficulty with an organ that is connected with the meridian that happens to cross the scar tissue.

Let me be clear that no one in the research literature has identified scar tissue as a factor that is related to the symptoms of Parkinsons. I personally believe that it can aggravate the symptoms, so why not address the problem?

The remedy is cheap and easy to do. No expensive tests are needed. No prescriptions need be written by a medical doctor.

© 2013 Parkinsons Recovery

Simply find wheat germ oil in a co-op or health food store. Apply the wheat germ oil to the scar tissue twice daily. The treatment takes 15 seconds.

I personally purchase wheat germ oil in capsule form. I then apply the wheat germ oil directly onto the scars on my body that resulted from surgeries. That is all there is to it.

THERAPIES THAT RELEASE THE TOXINS

It is wise to pull out any and all toxins that are hanging out in the tissue of your body whether you live on a farm or in the city. The good news is that the body is designed to rid itself of toxins through the good work of the kidneys, the liver, the lymph system and the digestive system. The bad news is that when toxins reach a critical level, the body becomes overwhelmed. It is no longer able to function as it was designed to function. Toxins literally become backlogged in the body.

The lymph system becomes clogged. The kidneys and liver become diseased. The digestive system shuts down.

The entire body becomes constipated. Your body cannot remove toxins if you are constipated. It is thus no mystery why nerve impulses become entangled and signals to move muscles are miscued. A critical point is reached when the body becomes saturated with too many toxins.

When the critical tipping point is reached the body is no longer able to release the toxins that have accumulated. Nerve cells become clogged with metals and chemicals that are harmful to your health. After a certain point, symptoms of Parkinsons emerge.

The effect of toxins on the ability of the body to maintain balance is similar to the effect of unresolved trauma. Muscles in the body tighten up and dry up. Cells die. Nerves no longer function as they were designed.

There are a wide variety of approaches for removing toxins from the body. I personally detox every six months to a year and usually adopt a different program each time. I figure if the last detox program did not get it, the new one will.

It is also critical to acknowledge the importance of facilitating the release of electromagnetic pollution and radiation from the body. Sodium alginate is a good chelator for pulling radioactive toxins from the body such as iodine-131 and strontium-90. I take nine drops of iodine (www.thyroidnascentiodine.com) every day to insulate against exposure to radiation which is problematic for persons living on the west coast of the United States due to earthquakes in Japan that damaged nuclear reactors.

© 2013 Parkinsons Recovery

I also believe it is important to solicit the help of a trained professional. Some medical doctors specialize in helping people remove toxins from their bodies. You can always count on naturopath doctors as a valuable resource. Below are several examples of the detoxification protocols that are recommended by very knowledgeable and experienced health care professionals.

John Briggs, ND recommends a detox program to his patients that he says has produced remarkable results:

> "I use a detoxification program that _Standard Process_ has put together that nourishes and restores the entire system. It cleanses the liver, the kidneys, the spleen, the blood, the bowel. As you are doing so, you are giving the body an outlet for removing stuff.

> It is a powerful cleanse. It takes 21 days. During that time it is a partial fast or modified fast. What you get to eat during this time besides the nutritional shake that is rich in antioxidants and other components - and it is also quite filling - you get to eat fresh fruits, vegetables and salad. That is the extent of what you get during that 21 days. The change can absolutely be life changing."

INFRARED SAUNAS

Infrared saunas help remove toxins. They come in many different styles. You can stand up in an infrared sauna or lie down in it. Some are like a shower stall.

When you use a regular sauna you start to perspire. The heat from infrared saunas penetrates from deep inside the body. The heat from deep inside the tissues pushes the toxins out of the body. Ivy Faber, ND recommends that if you use an infrared sauna on a regular basis you want to be sure and replenish the minerals you are losing from the detox. Lawrence Wilson, MD even has a blueprint on his website that makes it possible for you to make your own near infrared sauna for as little as $20-$30. He suggests using near infrared saunas rather than far infrared saunas because they have twice the penetration and emit no electromagnetic radiation.

Some people can tolerate the heat. Others cannot. As with any therapies, be sensitive to the needs of your body.

DMSA

You can do a DMSA detox which is a homeopathic approach that utilizes various herbals. Naturopath doctor Ivy Faber, ND explains the success with DMSA depends on the functionality of the person's organs. If they have good kidney function, they may do really well with the DMSA. If their kidney function is compromised, they may need help with some extra kidney drainage. She also recommends that when using DMSA you would also want to be taking a mineral supplement.

© 2013 Parkinsons Recovery

It is possible that any detox program can make your symptoms worse until the body realizes:

> *"This junk isn't going to continue flooding in and muck things up more. It is finally on its way out."*

ZEOLITE

Lyn Hanshew argues that accumulation of heavy metals in the body is one of the key reasons why so many people are developing chronic diseases like Parkinson's these days. Dr. Hanshew recommended a natural therapy called Zeolite that has been shown to be effective in removing heavy metals from the body.

Liquid Zeolite is derived from a volcanic mineral that has been found to remove heavy metals and toxins from the body's tissues. It has a crystalline structure much like a honeycomb. This unique molecular structure traps heavy metal toxins, making it possible for the toxins to make a painless "parting" from your body rather than being chased into the crevices of your brain which actually happens with some detoxification programs that wind up doing more harm than good.

Detox programs are not created equal. Heavy metals that hang out in the delicate tissues of your brain can obviously do significant damage to your neurological system very quickly. You do not want to choose a detox program thinking it will release heavy metals from the tissues of your body, only to discover that it corralled the metals into your brain tissue. Selecting the right detox program is clearly an important decision.

Robert Bonham reports several success stories from people with Parkinson's who have used Zeolite to detox heavy metals from their body. Robert was so impressed with the potential of a natural product called Natural Cellular Defense derived from Zeolite that he is now a distributor of the product. For more information about Zeolite you can contact Robert directly through his Natural Cellular Defense website at: http://www.mywaiora.com/859333. In my humble opinion, Zeolite is a detoxification method worth considering.

Healing Crises from Detoxes.

Ivy Faber, ND explains that a detox program can trigger a healing crisis. When your body begins to release toxins it retraces how the information came in.

Let's say at one time you had really bad knee pain. You are now detoxing. You begin to experience excruciating knee pain.

> *What in the world is going on?*

The knee pain may simply be evidence of the retracing process. This type of pain shouldn't last more than a day or two. If it goes further than that, then something needs to be readjusted.

© 2013 Parkinsons Recovery

ELIMINATE EXPOSURE TO NEW TOXINS

When I ask people the question:

"What do you suppose caused the symptoms you currently experience?"

I am continually surprised by the number of definitive responses.

- *I was exposed to Agent Orange in Vietnam.*
- *I was a professional photographer. The chemicals obviously did me in.*
- *I have been a gardener all my life. It was exposure to those herbicides that I used to use.*
- *I used to dry clean my clothes until I discovered that the chemicals the dry cleaners used contained dangerous toxins.*
- *I have been a painter all my life. It was the toxins in the paint I used.*

Many of these recollections occurred decades ago. Why are the symptoms popping now, so long after the initial exposure?

The body knows precisely what do when a dangerous substance invades it. The body's intelligence is far beyond anyone's comprehension to understand. If your body succeeded in getting rid of the toxins when you were initially exposed, why do you have the symptoms now?

1. Most people report that in retrospect, they realize that their symptoms did emerge at the time of the exposure. The symptoms were not debilitating and did not handicap the person in any way. They got on with their life expecting the symptoms to go away as many do.

2. I seriously doubt the toxins were eliminated. The molecular structure of toxins of all types makes them well suited to sneak into the nicks and crannies of the body's tissues and hide. What better place to hang out if you are a toxin? Everyone in a body these days has toxins that are buried deep inside their tissues.

3. The problem over time is the accumulation of toxins. No one can avoid exposure today. No one escapes the invasion of deadly substances through the food we eat, the water we drink, and the toxic air we breathe.

Yes, the body is well equipped to eliminate any and all substances that are harmful. There is a limit to how much of this work the body can do at any given time. The kidneys and bowels can handle only so much capacity every day. The problem turns out to be toxic build-up. Layer after layer of toxins accumulate over time.

Envision if you will that each toxin is a gummy substance with a different color. Consider just one example for one person who I shall call Tony. An initial layer of Agent Orange is tucked away in the tissues that cannot successfully be released by the body at the time. Imagine that layer as orange in color. As time passes on for Tony, layer after layer of one toxin after another is laid down on top of one other into the delicate carpet of his tissues. A gooey layer of brown toxin is piled on top of the orange toxin. Next a gooey layer of gooey blue toxin is lumped on top of the brown toxin.

Each toxin has a long complicated name that is scary enough in itself. Each comes from a different source. And, each has a markedly different molecular structure.

Like Tony, most people – especially those with Parkinson's symptoms - have a wide assortment of toxins that are layered deep inside their tissues. They hide out with absolutely no intention to escape. Impenetrable barricades are constructed so they will not be detected.

The challenge thus does not turn on the simple observation that, for example, you have a toxin like mercury or manganese. These two toxins are likely to be one among many others that corrupt the ability of your body to function.

Imagine that you have the eyes of your body. You now inspect this multi-layered carpet of toxins that are smothering your tissues. You know (as the body always knows) that toxins need to be eliminated. What do you see (as your body) when you look?

You see the top layer. The other layers are buried under the top layer. You do not acknowledge or notice the orange layer on the bottom. Your attention is directed only to the layer that you can see; the top layer - the most recent toxin that was ingested. All other layers of toxins remain and continue to interfere with the delicate function of your neurological system.

Some of you I know are terribly frustrated because you have done one detox protocol after another and the symptoms continue to persist. Why?

My answer is simple. You are being exposed to new toxins every day. If you do not eliminate the new exposures, there is no way in the world that your body will have the capacity to dig down into the lower layers of your toxic carpet and eliminate the toxins which entered your body at earlier points in time. What is the most important action you can take right now?

Do a thorough inventory of your household to identify any and all toxins that you are currently exposing yourself to. You have to stop the exposure to new toxins before you can heal.

- Your cleaning products may be toxic.

- Your soaps may be toxic.

- Your shampoos may be toxic.

- Your makeup may be toxic.

- Your laundry detergent may be toxic.

- All of the above may be true.

Today is the perfect time to throw out all of the toxic substances in your household that are harming the delicate tissues of your precious body. Today is the perfect time to replace them with alternatives that are green and toxic free.

Think about it. Once you realize that a product you have been using every day is toxic, how do you dispose of it? Do you give it to a friend? No! You do not want them to be exposed. So, why allow this product to harm you?

A Therapy that Helps Chase the Critters Out of Your Body

Low Dose Naltrexone (LDN)

LDN has been a miracle drug for some persons with neurological symptoms. It is a safe, inexpensive prescription drug that can be beneficial for persons with an immune dysfunction. It has been used for several decades to help patients recover from addictions though is not well known among most medical doctors as a treatment for Parkinson's.

Several decades ago New York City physician Bernard Bahari discovered that low doses of Naltrexone (which is why it is named Low Dose Naltrexone) offered welcome enhancements to the immune system. His patients - including some with Parkinsons - began to show remarkable improvements. LDN is recognized as a highly effective therapy for conditions including cancer, autoimmune disorders, autism, Parkinson's disease and even MS.

An excellent resource on LDN is: www.ldnscience.org. On the website you can preview a video that demonstrates how LDN works in the body by boosting endorphin levels. Peptides, produced in the brain and in the adrenal glands, are best known for relieving pain and enhancing well-being. Peptides modulate the immune system. LDN temporarily blocks endorphins from producing. This signals the body to increase the production of endorphins. What you get over time is a more functional immune system. It is not a quick fix.

Why should this help with Parkinsons symptoms? If one of the causes involves critters (and the list of critter candidates that are problematic is very long), then any enhancement of the immune system will eliminate critters and, in turn, reduce neurological symptoms.

Lexie, one of the 2012 Pioneers of Recovery, experienced remarkable results using LDN over a four year period. She continues to reduce her medications and is now virtually symptom free. Lexie was a guest on my radio show October 5, 2011.

Should you consider talking with your doctor about trying LDN? If you suspect critters are at play in your body, it would likely be a good idea.

A Natural Therapy for Electromagnetic Exposure

It will certainly help to reduce exposure to electromagnetic exposure. Never put your cell phone or smart phone up to your ear; listen with the speaker phone turned on. Talk on a land line whenever possible. Request all smart meters be removed by your electric company. Work as far away from a computer screen as possible.

Buy lavender plants and place them everywhere in your home. Set a plant next to your computer. Place several plants where you usually talk on your cell phone or smart phone. Put several plants in your bedroom. Why? Lavender eats the radiation. You will be sorry when one of your lavender plants die, but they have given up the good fight for life after eating too much radiation which would have been absorbed into your body instead. Thank them for the sacrifice and buy another plant.

Why People May Not Recover

Two entirely unconscious processes explain why some people flounder in their recovery programs. The first is a "child consciousness" association of pain with pleasure. The second is an entirely unconscious wish to take on the pain of a family member out of love.

Negative Pleasure

Every person endures hurts and pains as a child. An intricate process unfolds when we experience pain as a child pain regardless of its origin. We actually associate pleasure with the pain.

Why? It is a child's birth right to have pleasure in their life. If there is only pain, then the child concludes (quite illogically) that the pain must be pleasurable. All of the emotions associated with the original pain are thus hard wired in the brain to pleasure. This is called negative pleasure.

If you are like me when you search deep inside yourself, you will likely conclude:

> *"This has certainly not happened to me."*

After all, who in their right mind would find Parkinsons pleasurable? The stark reality, however, is that the association of pain with pleasure is an entirely unconscious process. Every person to a certain degree has a connection of pleasure with the pain that they have endured in their lifetime. This is their attachment to negative pleasure.

How can the connection of any pain with pleasure that resides deep within you become conscious and thus healed? First, simply acknowledge the possibility that this may be true for you. Second, the following exercise will help. Declare that you have decided not to heal from Parkinsons. Say out loud to yourself and your friends for one full day:

> *"No. I will not heal from this disease. I like feeling this way."*

The only route to your "yes" - I am ready to heal from the negative pleasure that is unconscious - is to acknowledge and honor your "no" - I refuse to heal. This brings the "no" voice that may reside deep inside you out in the open.

If you decide to do this exercise and if you wind up feeling a tinge of pleasure, you have come a long way toward making the association of pain with pleasure formed in childhood a conscious one. Once it becomes conscious, it can be healed.

Remember .... negative pleasure is not a conscious process. It evolved from your child consciousness which is anything but logical. At the time of your childhood, you survived because you found pleasure in the pain. As an adult however, holding onto negative pleasure no longer serves a useful purpose because it has the power to fuel the unpleasant symptoms of Parkinsons.

TAKING ON PAIN OUT OF LOVE

The bond of love that connects all members of a family system is profound. It is sustained in the energy field of each family member.

There is also a cellular connection from mother to child. This process, known as maternal microchimerism, has been well documented in research by Lee Nelson, MD, who finds the cells of mothers in cells of children that have survived for decades. The statement "*I am just like my mother*" is grounded in biological similarities as well as the shared history of family systems

The truth is that a child will do anything for a parent, a sibling, a grandparent or sometimes an uncle or aunt out of love...absolutely anything. If any member of the family system becomes critically ill, the child will say:

> *"Better that I have this disease than you."*

If any member of the family system dies prematurely, the child says:

© 2013 Parkinsons Recovery

"Better that I die than you."

The stark reality is that if any member of your family had a disease (whether Parkinsons or not) or died prematurely at a young age, you may be carrying an unconscious wish to take on their disease or die for them. Note that this is entirely illogical.

The family member has already died. Still, out of love you may be carrying the belief that it is better to take on a disease ... again ... out of love. The energy of this process is captured by the statement:

"Better that I become debilitated than you Dear Dad (or Dear Mom or Dear Brother or Dear Sister or ...)"

It is thus important to acknowledge any member of your family system who experienced an untimely death or debilitating illness. Then make the following statement to them in your thoughts:

"I honor and accept your fate."

This statement releases the energy that ties you (who is now an adult with Parkinsons) to a fate that is not your fate but the fate of someone else in your family system.

The process of taking on the fate of other family members is entirely unconscious. Simply acknowledge the possibility that you may have taken on the fate of another member of your family out of love. Once acknowledged, the entanglement can be released.

© 2013 Parkinsons Recovery

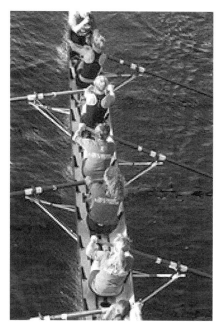

Rowing by Peter Thompson

NATURAL THERAPIES

People we work with are often perplexed by what constitutes a "natural therapy" for Parkinsons. The fundamental question is this:

> *"How do I know the difference between a 'natural treatment' and an 'artificial treatment"?*

That is to say, how do I know whether or not what I am currently doing to treat my Parkinsons is what my body needs and wants? As it turns out the answer is deceptively simple: Your body knows what it needs.

The body needs nourishment to perform the intricate function of balancing hormones. For example, if your body has a vitamin A deficiency and you are taking a vitamin A supplement, your body will say to you,

> *"Thank you very much. You weren't giving me the nourishment I needed to do my work before, but now you are. "*

Consider a simple analogy. You need to drive a nail into your living room wall. Consider a few choices. Use your finger? Or your big toe? Or your elbow? Or your neighbors head? Some of these alternatives might work half heartedly, but the chances of hammering the nail completely are pretty slim.

How about using a hammer? Most people would agree that a hammer is the tool of choice, given this simple task.

© 2013 Parkinsons Recovery

To balance hormones, the body needs more than a simple tool like a hammer. It needs nourishment to do its own work. If you are not giving your body the nourishment it needs, you might as well be hammering a nail into your living room wall with your big toe or little finger.

Some substances that are taken to relieve the symptoms of Parkinsons are "artificial" in character. They may be medicines that, while accomplishing useful functions, can have deleterious side effects. In this case the body will instantly recognize the substance as "artificial" in character.

The body inevitably rebels by sending you messages of pain and discomfort. More simply put, the body is unreceptive to any substance that is "artificial." The answer to a complex question is that your body is always able to differentiate a "natural remedy" from an "artificial remedy."

The first order of business is to listen to your body when you take any new substance. If your body rebels - if your body gives you any indication that it doesn't like what you are giving it - pay attention. Something needs to change.

Talk with your doctor. Consider the possibility that whatever you are taking may not be in the best interest of helping your body to recover from Parkinsons.

Natural Aging

What exactly happens to our bodies when we age? Let me highlight a few of the consequences of living a long life.

First, the part of the brain that tells us when to drink water does not work very well when we age. Many older people are seriously dehydrated.

Second, oxidative damage caused by free radicals increases with age. Free radicals are linked to stress, environmental toxins and the type of food we eat. Our bodies eventually become toxic waste sites unless we take positive action.

Third, immune system activity becomes excessive. To stay healthy you have to keep the immune system in check. This can feel like putting wet blanket after wet blanket on top of a raging fire.

Fourth, the ability of the digestive system to absorb nutrients is compromised. Many people take supplements. Why don't they feel better? The supplements are not being absorbed by the digestive system. If they are not being absorbed, they cannot be transported to the tissues where they are desperately needed.

© 2013 Parkinsons Recovery

Deficiencies in many critical vitamins and minerals are commonplace among older people. For example, most people over the age of 65 are deficient in vitamin B6 which is the key to maintaining a balance of hormones in the body.

Is there any way to escape the consequences of aging? I am afraid not. Given the dire consequences of aging, it should come as little surprise that our bodies may not function on all four cylinders.

If our digestive system is compromised ...

If our immune system is overtaxed ...

If oxidative damage is out of control ...

If we are chronically dehydrated ...

If we are critically deficient in key vitamins and minerals ...

Is there any doubt about why the symptoms of Parkinsons present themselves?

The good news is that while the consequences of aging are problematic, something can be done about each problem. When all systems in the body are brought back on line, the symptoms of Parkinsons will scurry to the sidelines. They are still in the game and will inevitably appear on the field again if we do not flood our body with the nutrients it needs to heal. The challenge gets more difficult with age.

Why do you eat? Let me answer this question for myself. If I am sad, I eat. If I am nervous, I eat. If I am hungry, I eat. If I am depressed, I eat. How about a different reason for eating good food? I eat good, fresh organic food because my body needs it to be happy.

A compelling body of <u>research</u> shows that neurological symptoms are reduced significantly by cutting food intake by as much as 30%. The shear act of eating produces free radicals that are terribly unkind to the vitality of your neurological system. Fasting is not only effective – it saves you money. You feel better and put money in the bank at the same time.

VITAMINS AND MINERALS

There is a body of research that asks the question: Does taking supplements contribute to health and wellness? Some studies report that supplements are not effective. I want to be very clear about my reaction to this body of work. It is a silly question that has an obvious answer. Of course supplements can help your body heal. Supplements are nothing other than food. The body needs food to survive and heal. Without food we die. Would any rational person argue that we should stop eating food?

© 2013 Parkinsons Recovery

Of course supplements can help when the body has a deficiency in the supplement that is taken. If there is no deficiency, the supplement will wash through the body and have no effect because the body does not need it. End of story.

Needless to say, there is considerable variability across the quality of supplements that are available on the marketplace. Many supplements are manufactured in China with no quality controls. For example, you may decide to take a calcium supplement. Many calcium supplements are made from crushed limestone that has been processed with citric acid. Your body cannot absorb this form of calcium. Its molecular structure is much too large. You really can never be certain what you are getting when you purchase a supplement.

Keep in mind that most supplements require processing of some form or another. Processing dilutes their efficacy. The highest quality supplements are harvested in the wild and are subjected to no processing whatsoever. This standard is rarely if ever met.

More disturbing is the presence of toxins and lead in some supplements. Supplements are no different than food. Some foods have toxins too!

How can you really know which are the high quality supplements that are free of toxins and which ones are not? There is an objective assessment of supplements which you can access by visiting the Consumer Lab website at: www.consumerlab.com.

Consider the possibility of ordering tests to assess mineral and vitamin deficiencies. After getting the results, make it a point to work with your doctor to bolster up your deficiencies so that your body can return to full health and wellness. Or, the simpler and more straightforward and less costly approach is to eat live foods every day that contain the fuel your body needs to maintain balance and nurture your cells.

There is a compelling reason why you may be feeling lethargic. That reason, simply put, is that your body is not getting the nutrition that it needs to function. According to USDA studies, nutritiously rich foods were readily available 100 years ago. The hard reality today is that people do not get the nutrition their body requires. Food today is nutritionally deficient even when that food is labeled to be organic. Depletion of the soils has made even organic foods energetically deficient. This is why supplements are necessary for most people.

Which ones? It obviously depends on your body and your metabolism. Larry Wilson offers a nutritional balancing program which involves a hair analysis. Recommendations are developed on the basis of the hair analysis of the supplements and specific foods your body needs to come back into balance. Given the general deterioration of our food supply, Dr. Wilson suggests a general list of supplements he has discovered most people require: Calcium and magnesium,

Omega 3 fatty acids, Vitamin D3, Kelp (which provides iodine), digestive aids (or Probiotics) and a quality multi-vitamin.

How can this be true particularly if you are the kind of person who eats healthy food? We do not get some of the vitamins and minerals our bodies need to function from the food we eat. In the particular case of Parkinsons, there is recent research evidence to suggest that the symptoms may be connected to a deficiency of folic acid, vitamin B6 and vitamin B12.

Folic Acid

Researchers have found that some people with Parkinson's symptoms have a disruption in their methylation process. This is a biochemical process in the body which takes folic acid and uses it to help cells repair themselves and divide into new cells. If cells are unable to rejuvenate, they die. The body eventually exhibits neurological symptoms. For some people, folic acid may be one of the keys to recovery.

Researchers injected a substance in mice called MPTP which causes the symptoms of Parkinsons. (May we all say a prayer of gratitude to the mice who sacrificed their lives in the interest of advancing science). The group of mice was then split in two groups.

One group of mice received folic acid in their diet. The other group did not receive folic acid. The mice given the diet with folic acid exhibited mild symptoms. The group that received no folic acid exhibited severe symptoms. Conclusion: folic acid is good for mice.

What about humans with Parkinsons? Mice are mice and humans are humans. Why should folic acid make a difference to your symptoms?

A deficiency of folic acid creates a chain reaction in the brain that is triggered by an overabundance of homocysteine. Too much homocysteine in the brain damages brain cells in the substantia nigra.

Research shows higher levels of homocysteine are associated with an increased risk of acquiring the symptoms of Parkinsons. Ask your doctor to assess the homocysteine levels in your body. If they are high, you need to take positive action to reduce the level.

How? Eat lettuce and spinach. (Many other foods also contain folic acid.) Folic acid converts homocysteine to a substance called cystathionine which is excreted through urine. Vitamins B6 and B12 are also important to the natural metabolism of homocysteine.

The bottom line is that folic acid, vitamin B6 and vitamin B12 are all important to everyone's health. Consult with your doctor about how much to take of these supplements. The mice experiment suggests they may be particularly important for persons with Parkinsons.

Folic acid is found in leafy green vegetables, citrus fruits and egg yolks. I personally like to juice leafy green veggies and then drink the juice to give my body the folic acid it needs. Taking supplements in pill form is a pain for me and swallowing pills every day is a chore I choose to avoid.

OMEGA FATTY ACIDS

Omega fatty acids nourish those sensitive myelin sheaths which provide insulation for neurons which can become brittle and thin. Both omega 3 and omega 6 fatty acids are needed, but most people have an abundance of omega 6 fatty acids. It is ideal to maintain a ratio of one to one between the two types. Several foods are excellent sources of omega 3 fatty acids: flax, hemp and walnuts and fish including sardines.

B VITAMINS

Vitamin B metabolism is "off line" for many people who currently experience Parkinson's like symptoms. This metabolic insufficiency compromises the body's natural ability to eliminate toxins. Several B vitamins are implicated: B3, B5 and B12.

VITAMIN B6

What follows is compounding pharmacist and nutritional counselor Randy Mentzer's perspective on vitamin B6.

> "Vitamin B6 *reduces the side effects of L-dopa but also reduces the effect of L-dopa. It is not a good idea to supplement with vitamin B6 when you are taking these medications. That creates a problem because B6 is really very important. If you are going to take Parkinsons medications like Sinemet or Stalevo or Maripex then you should try to get B6 in your foods and not take it as a supplement."*

Good nutrition is the most important thing you can do for yourself to feel better. What we put into our bodies makes all the difference in the world.

Production systems for food have changed dramatically over the last several decades. Food processing strips out some of the minerals and vitamins our body needs the most. What our body needs to function well is usually not available in the food that is sold in grocery stores. Consider now several examples: D3, Iodine, magnesium, potassium and sodium.

VITAMIN B12

A compelling body of research demonstrates that most people with Parkinson's symptoms have a serious deficiency of B vitamins, especially vitamin B12. This particular nutrient is only available from animal sources, so people who eat meat tend to have fewer problems that those who are vegetarian.

A protein rich diet however may need to be modified. Protein intake interferes with the effectiveness of Levodopa which is a Parkinson's medication. Protein blocks its absorption. Many people are advised by their doctors to reduce their intake of protein to insure that their medications continue to function as intended. A consequence for some people is a dip in energy levels as the B12 resources in the body are depleted. Some people can feel like, sound like and even look like a car running low on oil.

The body is an intricate, living organism that functions well because of the interactions of a multitude of causal pathways. Everyone's body jerks out of balance from time to time whether they have Parkinson's symptoms or not.

Vitamin D3

Vitamin D3 deficiency has been found in 55% of patients with Parkinsons[8]. Do I have your attention?

Why might vitamin D3 deficiencies be a factor with Parkinsons? Vitamin D3 is a potent antioxidant. It increases the expression of glutathione in the body which is a scavenger of free-radicals. Vitamin D3 also regulates nerve growth factor (NGF) which plays a critical role in the healthy function of the nervous system. NGF affects the plasticity and transmission of neurons. The bottom line is this: if you have a vitamin D3 deficiency, your nerves can not function normally.

Everyone gets vitamin D3 when they are exposed to sunshine. The effects of sunshine last about 2-3 months. In the wintertime - particularly for those of us that live in the Northwest - almost everyone has a serious vitamin D3 deficiency. Naturopath Laurie Mischley reports that less than 2% of her patients fall within the normal range. She advises that everyone with Parkinsons get tested for the level of vitamin D3 in their body. The blood test (25-OH Vit D) costs only $50. It is also important to be tested because vitamin D3 can be toxic if you get too much exposure.

Even people who live in sunny climates may have vitamin D3 deficiencies. As we age, the ability of the skin to synthesize D3 becomes more and more difficult and less effective. Vitamin D3 deficiencies cause depression. Vitamin D3 is available at pharmacies.

People who live in the Pacific Northwest who take D3 supplements in the winter are unlikely to get depressed. Those who do not take D3 supplements are very likely to get depressed. Some

---

[8] "Prevalence of vitamin d insufficiency in patients with Parkinson disease and Alzheimer disease," Evatt ML, Delong MR, et al, Arch Neurol, 2008; 65(10): 1348-52.

© 2013 Parkinsons Recovery

people solve the problem with anti-depressants. A more cost effective and safer alternative is to try vitamin D3 first.

IODINE

A second common, but overlooked deficiency in the body is iodine. Interestingly enough, processed foods don't have enough iodine for our bodies to function well. Eating table salt does not give you the iodine that you need. Iodine used to be included as a key ingredient of bakery products until it was replaced with bromide. Bromide offers no therapeutic value to the body. Worse yet Bromide displaces iodine and poisons the thyroid.

One hundred years ago iodine was the medicine of choice that was used to treat many ailments. Did your mother always paint iodine on your wounds as a child? It is the best antiseptic, antiviral and antifungal imaginable which is still used in emergency rooms today. It also insulates the body against the treat of toxins.

Iodine is a vital mineral which supports the thyroid. The thyroid is a critical organ of the body that regulates metabolism. Without a decent metabolism rate, your energy will dip into the cellar every day and lull you to sleep often. If you have low energy or know that infections are a factor, talk with your doctor about taking an iodine supplement. You can drink iodine or apply it to your skin. I drink nine drops of Iodine in a glass of water every day which I purchase from www.thyroidnascentiodine.com.

Magnesium

Magnesium in particular is a fundamental building block of the body. Deficiencies cause a myriad of symptoms. I suggest everyone consider a simple approach. Try eating foods that are high in magnesium.

Remember Popeye the sailor man? Popeye ate spinach and he was certainly strong. Spinach is enriched with magnesium. Black beans and pumpkin seeds are good bets too. Of course, magnesium and potassium supplements can also be tried as well. For our own use we purchase pure magnesium oils and sprays from www.ancient-minerals.com.

If your symptoms improve, chances are good they may be aggravated or even caused by something as simple as magnesium and/or potassium depletions. Deficiencies are a primary reason why people are often fatigued. A wide range of health problems are actually caused by magnesium deficiencies. Many times simple solutions work beautifully.

Followers of my work sometimes drift away because they get well. Here is an example of a reader who figured out that her problem was linked to a deficiency of both magnesium and potassium:

"I have enjoyed reading your posts, but my neurologist determined I did not have Parkinsons. Symptoms (muscle twitches) were apparently due to potassium depletion and low magnesium caused by blood pressure drugs and also Carpal Tunnel Syndrome (numbness in hands). Symptoms are mostly gone now."

POTASSIUM AND SODIUM

John Briggs, ND recommends the following remedy for enhancing the transfer of electrical impulses across the neurons:

"Obviously when we start looking at the electrical transfer … we have to look at what allows that electrical transfer? Potassium and sodium are a couple of things that are necessary. We have to have potassium. Where are you going to get your potassium?

Your fresh vegetables: Carrots are rich in potassium. If you need potassium, carrot juice is excellent. If you need some good sodium, celery is dynamite. If you need both sodium and potassium, I will suggest carrot juice with celery juice. It is dynamic. It brings it into the body quickly and it is a living food."

VITAMIN K2

Researchers have observed that the activity of mitochondria in persons with Parkinson's symptoms is compromised. Energy for the body is fueled by electrons which have been disrupted. This slows the process required to generate energy. Neurons and cells die off, creating a deficit in the critical mass of cells needed for the body to function properly.

Research using fruit flies with compromised mitochondria found that the administration of vitamin K2 restored the function of mitochondria. The subjects (fruit flies) were able to fly once again.

Will vitamin K2 work the same magic for humans as it did for fruit flies? Who knows. But if you have little energy, it would make sense to talk with your doctor about taking a Vitamin K2 supplement to see if you can float across the dance floor again without tiring. If it worked for fruit flies it just may work the same magic for you too! Such a decision must be taken mindfully, since K2 might be contraindicated with other medications you may be taking.

NADH

The fuel used by the body to generate energy at the cellular level is NADH. The following is an explanation provided by Steven Fowkes on the potential role of NADH in helping people with Parkinsons get relief from their symptoms.

"Mitochondria are little power plants, little blast furnaces inside our cells. They burn fuel and generate energy for us. ATP is the primary energy that comes out of them.

There is a secondary fuel that most people don't think of as a fuel, called NADH, which can be described as reducing power – the opposite of oxidation power. NADH powers the antioxidant defense mechanisms, which turns out to be a critical factor for both Parkinsons disease and Alzheimer's disease, mainly involving regeneration of a substance called glutathione.

Glutathione has sulfur in it. Sulfur is the pivot for all biology. Our entire chemistry is defended by a sulfur defense system. The sulfur intercepts all of these free radicals and oxidizing agents and protects us from oxidative damage.

In Parkinson's disease, the sulfur system is protecting against a long term kind of cumulative damage. The Substantia Nigra is named "Nigra" (which means black) because when you do an autopsy on the brain and look at those particular cells, they are colored black. There is a pigment in those particular cells. It turns out that pigment is caused by the polymerization of compounds that relate to dopamine which is a neurotransmitter in those particular neurons. This pigment is called melanin. It is black. It is produced from that specific neurotransmitter.

That is why those particular neurons die. The antioxidant defense system fails to defend that neurotransmitter. It becomes compromised. It polymerizes into the black pigment. Those particular cells become stressed. Then they shut down and die.

It all comes down to antioxidants. Those are defended by the NADH that comes out of the mitochondria and they are defended by the ATP that comes out of the mitochondria. So, the mitochondria are the "power grid," or electrical outlets, for our brain.

One out of a hundred "normal" persons will notice something from taking NADH, maybe not even that many. NADH with somebody with normal metabolism is already sufficient. Adding any more is like filling up your gas tank after you have gone 10 miles. It doesn't make any difference in how your car works.

With Parkinsons disease the positive response to NADH is probably 40%. This is something that I would put at the top of the list of therapies just because there are several aspects of mitochondrial metabolic function that are known to be associated with NADH. We know from the scientific literature that Parkinsons people respond more strongly to NADH.

NADH is not available by prescription. You have to get it from your health food store.

© 2013 Parkinsons Recovery

It comes in sublingual pills and it comes in enteric-coated pills. It is a relatively pricey thing, considering the fact it is just an activated form of vitamin B3. One gram of NADH sells for the price of a kilogram of niacin or niacinamide. It is very expensive and tends to be one of the higher-expense items on your supplement list.

That is the nice thing about testing something like this out. If you take NADH and you have no improvement in

- *your memory*

- *your cognitive function*

- *your tremor*

- *your freezing behavior*

- *and your body temperature doesn't change*

Then it is like – OK. That is it. You tried one bottle. It doesn't work. Give it up. Don't waste your money. Don't waste your time.

To test it:

1. *Take one pill the first day,*

2. *Then two pills the second,*

3. *Four the third,*

4. *Then eight the next,*

5. *Then 16,*

6. *Then take rest of the entire bottle.*

This stuff is so non toxic that the only way you can kill yourself would be to be a millionaire and spend all of your money taking NADH."

Steven Fowkes, 2008

5-HTP

John Schappi has found using 5-HTP, an over the counter serotonin-booster, has significantly enhanced the quality of his own life. His symptoms were alleviated including depression, insomnia and constipation. John has extensive information about 5-HTP on his blog: http://parkinsonsand5htp.blogspot.com. He was also a guest on my radio show May 4, 2011.

GLUTATHIONE

What follows is compounding pharmacist Randy Mentzer's perspective on Glutathione.

> *"As far as we know glutathione is your body's strongest antioxidant. In Parkinsons disease glutathione is deficient. Some studies have shown that the worse the Parkinsons, the lower the glutathione. Glutathione is very essential for the health of Parkinson's disease patients*
>
> *Glutathione does not cross the blood brain barrier. If you are taking glutathione the chances are not too much of it is going to be very helpful to you as far as Parkinsons goes.*
>
> *There are two forms of glutathione. There is the oxidized form and there is the reduced form. You have to make sure it is the reduced form. That is the active form of glutathione.*
>
> *Glutathione is something they call a tripeptide. It has three amino acids in it: cysteine, L-glutamic acid and glycine. The amino acids do cross the blood brain barrier. The most popular one and the most effective one that crosses the blood brain barrier is something called N-Acetilcystene. Your brain can take N-Acetylcysteine and add glutamime and glycine to make glutathione.*
>
> *If you are not getting the results that you think you should be getting when taking glutathione, consider taking N-Acetylcysteine. That is an amino acid that is available in health food stores or compounding pharmacies. Try to consult a compounding pharmacist and see what they say about it. Compounding pharmacists generally are more up on nutritional protocols than non compounding pharmacists."*

The Perlmutter Health Clinic in Naples, Florida treats Parkinsons with IV infusions of glutathione. The standard form of this glutathione therapy employs three IV treatments per week. This therapy is invasive and expensive, but the information I have gathered from interviews suggest that the treatments can help persons with Parkinsons get relief from their symptoms. People usually terminate the treatments because they are too expensive – not because they are ineffective.

Naturopath doctor Laurie Mischley is in the process of doing a study using a glutathione nasal spray. Because the glutathione is infused through the nose, it is not blocked by the blood brain barrier. Dr. Mischely said during my two radio show interviews with her in June, 2010 that she has seen remarkable improvements in her patients that use this application of glutathione. A high quality glutathione nasal spray (available only by a doctor's prescription) can be purchased through Key Pharmacy Compounding in Kent, Washington.

© 2013 Parkinsons Recovery

Marie Judd explains that after taking the glutathione enhancer Maxgxl, her husband Judd had an immediate positive reaction within the first two days. Maxgxl is a glutathione enhancer, accelerator and regenerator. It is not glutathione itself.

> *"We started the first of August. Within two days Judd had been having trouble with his eye lids wanting to stay closed even when he was trying to open his eyes. All the sudden his energy level was to a point where his eyes were wide open. That is a defined response.*

> *His talking for almost that whole week went up to about 80% of the time to a very normal tone. I have not heard his voice as strong or as regular as I did there for a while. This has been periodically off and on. He was able to talk complex sentences. He was able to pull together memories. The whole thing was coming together. That was exciting.*

> *We see it as an ongoing, positive effect. We have been seeing a higher energy level with ability to stand. He is 5' 11" and has been able to stand various times. "*

Marie also explained that while the effects have continued, the huge shift in the beginning was not sustained. One of her doctors had an interesting perspective on Judd's experience:

> *"Parkinsons responds to everything to start with."*

Now that is encouraging news!

CoQ10

People with the symptoms of Parkinsons have insufficient ATP (Adenosine triphosphate). Studies have found individuals with Parkinsons have a 44% reduction in symptoms when they take a CoQ10 supplement[9]. Many doctors routinely recommend that their patients take CoQ10.

CoQ10 plays a central role in helping the body generate energy in the form of ATP. Over 90% of the body's energy is generated this way. Organs with the highest energy requirements—such as the heart and the liver—have the highest CoQ10 concentrations. This is why cardiologists often recommend CoQ10 to their patients.

There is some uncertainly about the best dosage. A current study is evaluating the effectiveness of high dosages – whether 1200 milligrams or 2400 milligrams is best – or even more. I

---

[9] Shults CW, Oakes D, Kieburtz K, Beal F, Haas R, Plumb S, Juncos JL, Nutt J, Shoulson I, Carter J, Kompoliti K, Perlmutter JS, Reich S, Stern M, Watts RL, Kurlan R, Molho E, Harrison M, Lew M, and the Parkinson Study Group. "Effects of coenzyme Q_{10} in early Parkinson disease: evidence of slowing of the functional decline." *Archives of Neurology* , October 2002, Vol. 59, No. 10, pp. 1541-1550.

personally think everyone's body is different, so the best approach is to ask your own body what it needs!

I suggest that you take care to find a reliable source of CoQ10. If you do not get a high quality source, taking it will do you little good. Some people tell me:

"I tried CoQ10 and it did nothing for me."

There are two possibilities here as I see it. First, this person's body may not be deficient in CoQ10. They fall into the 60% category of people who receive no noticeable benefit from taking a CoQ10 supplement because their body already has enough. Second, this person may have tried a CoQ10 product that had very low quality.

Laurie Mischley, ND, recommends two reliable sources of CoQ10: Vitaline and Douglas Labs which offers a wafer version of CoQ10 which they call Q Melt. The cost of good quality CoQ10 can be as much as $200-$400 a month which is why many people search around for the lowest price they can find. Dr. Mischley explains you might as well not bother. Low quality CoQ10 will do your body little good and your pocketbook great harm.

In short, the quality of CoQ10 makes a huge difference. Be sure and shop around. Consult with appropriate health care providers before you make a purchase. Monitor the results closely in consultation with your doctor.

KETONES

A woman in her early fifties has early onset Parkinson's. During a 10 day fast she took no medications. Her symptoms improved significantly during the fast. However, once she began eating again, all of her symptoms returned.

Obviously, fasting is not a viable therapy for anyone. The brain constitutes only 2% of the body's weight, but consumes 20% of its metabolic requirements. If you do not eat, fuel in the form of sugar is not available to the brain. What does the body do in response to a fast?

It activates a backup system. The liver manufactures ketones by burning fat in the body. When blood-glucose concentrations get too low, the liver converts fatty acids into ketones. Ketones are a substitute for glucose as cellular fuel. Unlike fatty acids, ketones have the unique capability of penetrating the blood-brain barrier. In other words, they perform the same function for the brain as glucose.

Ketones are an alternative source of fuel for the brain. No insulin is required to facilitate the transport of glucose across the blood brain barrier.

© 2013 Parkinsons Recovery

Cells of the brain are very susceptible to fuel shortages. Without the fuel it needs to function, brain cells die in mass. Memory fades. Neurons deteriorate. Symptoms emerge.

My argument is straightforward here. Consider the possibility that for some persons who have neurological difficulties, the mechanism used by the body to transport sugar to the brain (so that it passes across the blood brain barrier) is defective. From a therapeutic perspective you can either repair the defective transport system the body uses to transport glucose to the brain or you can activate the backup system and rely on ketones.

Instead of attempting to fix a transfer system - transformation of glucose by insulin - which may have been sidetracked for whatever reason, why not rely on a system that is working properly? Why not simply encourage the body to make ketones? Once energy to the brain is restored, new brain cells form, memory returns, neurons regenerate and neural pathways are restored. This approach is being pursued with research by Richard L. Veech from the National Institute of Health using Parkinson's patients.

> *"More recently, a ketogenic diet has been shown to reduce tremor and rigidity in a small study of human patients by about 60% while improving mentation."*

Mary Newport, MD, advocates adding pure, non-hydrogenated coconut oil to your diet. She provided a lucid discussion of its benefits for persons who currently experience Parkinsons symptoms on my radio show May 9, 2012. She strongly advocates the use of coconut oil for persons with Alzheimer's symptoms and suggests it will also help provide relief to Parkinson's symptoms.

As an alternative you can also elect to eat a ketosis-inducing high fat diet by consuming butter, cream and carbohydrates. How about that for a recommendation? OK, I know. I know. Eating a high fat diet would obviously be silly and stupid. Well, maybe. Maybe not.

The two most popular oils used by people with chronic conditions like Alzheimer's to induce the body to make ketones: coconut oil and MCT Oil (Medium Chain Triglycerides Oil). Both have high fat content. Several people with the symptoms of Parkinsons have obtained relief using MCT oil (which is a part of coconut oil). MCT oil is available from any health food store and requires no prescription from a doctor. MCT oil is used by some people who do not want to gain weight from ingesting coconut oil.

What therapy do I use to trigger the manufacture of ketones in my own body? I was persuaded by Dr. Newport's argument. After hearing her discussion on the radio show I began eating my cereal with coconut milk which is yummy. I also began applying coconut oil directly to my scalp every morning which yields an invigorating wake up call. I place the oil in my hand and flop it on top of my head. My hot head melts the oil in a few seconds. Admittedly, my hair is greasy until I wash it so I must defer the treatment on days when I must go out in public unless I choose to look like a grease bag. Applying the oil directly to the skin is an easy way to take it into your body. The skin is a wonderful synthesizer. You do not have to eat it to get the benefit,

Obviously, we do not have the evidence or research to know precisely what will be the best approach for helping the body to make ketones. I suggest that you talk with your doctor about applying coconut oil (and perhaps a combination of coconut oil and MCT oil) on your skin after you shower or on your head in the morning. You can obviously also ingest the oils directly if you so chose. If you observe an improvement, your body is giving you a strong message: This may be one simply therapy that may prove highly successful.

CREATINE

Creatine is a nitrogen rich organic acid that also helps ameliorate symptoms of Parkinsons. It helps supply energy to the muscles and improves the overall health of mitochondria.

Creatine is naturally produced in the human body from amino acids in the kidney and liver. It is transported in the blood for use by muscles. Approximately 95% of the human body's total Creatine is located in skeletal muscles. The rest hang out in the brain or heart.

Creatine causes the body to become dehydrated. Serious side effects can result from taking Creatine. An advantage to taking Creatine is that it is very inexpensive – only $10 a month. Because of the potential side effects, it is important to consult with your doctor, pharmacist or health care provider before taking it.

LAUGHTER

When you laugh out loud, your body manufactures dopamine. It is the cheapest pill available because it is free.

Laughter Yoga Instructor Gita Fendelman (who finds Laughter Yoga helps her get remarkable relief from her own Parkinson's symptoms) tells a story about one of her students:

> "I have a student with Parkinson's. I always give homework to laugh for 10 minutes a day, every day. He and his wife did that every day for ten days. They came back to the next class. He said to me: You know Gita. I used to love to sing in church, but this Parkinsons robed me of my voice. I stopped singing because I could not hear myself. Do you know that after laughing once a day I could hear myself again in church."

Have you ever heard of Gelotology? It is the term given to the science of laughter. Laughter is so serious it has become a science in itself. In Anatomy of an Illness Norman Cousins used laughter to heal a presumably fatal disease (or at least so the doctors thought). Research shows that you can improve cardiovascular function with one minute of hearty laughter or 10 minutes on a rowing machine. I prefer the shorter alternative myself which is obviously more fun.

Gelotology research reports the following astonishing benefits from laughter. It:

• Improves cardiovascular health	• Purges stale air
• Shifts depression	• Invigorates the body with fresh oxygen
• Boosts the immune system	• Reduces blood pressure
• Improves communication skills	• Improves circulation
• Enhances creativity	• Drops the pulse rate
• Helps diabetes	• Raises endorphin levels which in turn reduces aches and pains
• Reduces stress hormones by 75%	• Lessons worries
• Releases muscle and emotional tension	• Gives aerobic exercise
• Massages organs	

You can obviously use a medication that is formulated to treat any one of the above conditions, but I can assure you that no one medication exists that can treat all of them. And, in contrast to prescription medications, there are no adverse side effects from laughing. You can only expect improved health on some level. Laughter is also free. Prescription medications can cost big bucks.

The truth is there are not many videos that make me laugh out loud. I often laugh quietly, inside. My body can manufacture a little dopamine with quiet laughter, but not a lot. However, a video of a Richard Simmons appearance on a game show made me laugh very hard out loud. I flushed myself with a welcome rush of dopamine. I thought you might like to try it out too.

A warning first: The video that plays when you click on the link below shows Richard Simmons doing a series of jokes that have implicit and explicit sexual content. He is a gay comic. If you are offended by gay humor, don't even think about clicking on the link below.

© 2013 Parkinsons Recovery

The neat part about this video is the infectious laughter from the audience. That in itself is enough to make you laugh out loud. The jokes actually don't even have to strike you as being funny. Your body just needs to laugh.

Join with the laughter of the audience even if what he does may not strike you as funny.

If you decide to click on the link below now and watch this 5 minute video, I hope it works as well as it worked for me to give you a dopamine "hit" today.

http://www.youtube.com/watch?v=ICJkuXSTymk

RIGHT NUTRITION

Terry Wahls, MD, argues that there are two underlying causes of chronic health conditions such as Parkinson's: (1) dysfunctional mitochondria and (2) too many inflammation molecules. Proper nutrition is the only long term solution to both problems. When we eat dead food, our energy plummets. When we eat live food, our energy soars.

Wahls proposes a raw food diet for persons with neurological challenges that she now calls the Wahls Diet. She developed this diet after finding prescription medicines did not help reduce her own MS symptoms. Dr. Wahls applied her nutritional ideas to Parkinson's Disease during my radio show on April 18, 2012.

Each of our cells contains from 100 to 1000 mitochondria, the energy processing and storage facilities of the body. Mitochondria stimulate each cell to percolate the biochemistry of life. If the necessary chemistry is not functioning properly, hormones will be out of balance and the neurological system will scream bloody murder. When the chemical reactions required by the body are stifled, blood vessels are compromised, brains become demented, hearts weaken and neurons misfire. In the end, all health problems originate with dormant or harmful biochemical reactions.

Studies have confirmed the leading role played by poor nutrition in causing the symptoms of Parkinsons disease. A 2007 prospective Harvard study [10] tracked the dietary intake of 49,692 men and 81,676 women who were free of Parkinsons at the launch of the study or "baseline." Sixteen years later, 508 new cases of Parkinsons had been diagnosed. Prospective studies are very sophisticated designs because they asked study subjects about their dietary practices now rather than asking them what they ate 16 years ago. Most people do not remember much

---

[10] **Xiang Gao et al., 2007). Prospective study of dietary pattern and risk of Parkinson disease, American Journal of Clinical Nutrition, Vol. 86, No. 5, 1486-1494.**

© 2013 Parkinsons Recovery

about their diet 16 years ago. Please also note that the sample size of this study was huge - over 130,000 subjects. They then tracked study subjects over a long period of time.

Dietary practices that were significantly less likely to be associated with Parkinsons were:

- high intake of fruit, vegetables, whole grains, nuts, fish and poultry

- low intake of saturated fats (e.g.: cream, red meat, pork)

- moderate intake of alcohol

Eat food in its natural state – otherwise known as raw – and the bio activity as well as the cellular structure remains intact. Cooked food degrades the integrity of enzymes and nutrients needed to sustain life. Thirty percent of the vitamin content of food is lost within two minutes of cooking it. This is why some people with Parkinson's symptoms decide to convert to a 100% raw food diet.

While in theory it sounds like a smart choice, a diet composed of 100% raw food can create problems if good bacteria and fiber in the digestive system are insufficient. Consuming all raw foods can pose formidable digestive problems under such circumstances. People with Parkinson's symptoms do not have sufficient enzymes in their digestive system to extract the minerals from raw foods as they pass through their digestive system. Larry Wilson (www.drlwilson.com) argues a combination of 80% cooked vegetables and meats with 20% raw foods works better for people with Parkinson's symptoms.

Larry Wilson also recommends that people with Parkinsons do not eat fruit which is a yin food. The body of persons with Parkinson's (and other diseases) is primarily Yin in content: cold and expanded. Healing occurs when the balance of the body is shifted to be more in balance. This requires a shift to eating foods with more yang content (hot and contracted). Eating a greater proportion of cooked foods relative to raw foods fulfills this need.

The initial diet should be composed of 70% to 80% cooked foods including vegetables, meats and some sardines. Larger fish such as tuna are too polluted with toxins, especially mercury. As the digestive system comes back on line, the proportion of raw foods that is consumed can be increased gradually. The ideal combination of raw versus cooked foods is likely to shift over time as the digestive system comes back on line and the necessary enzymes become more readily available to extract the minerals needed by the body to function.

Laurie Mischley, ND specializes in treating persons with Parkinsons. She also does not believe that the disease is necessarily progressive or irreversible. The rule of thumb she recommends is very straightforward: Avoid eating foods that do not look healthy. This includes donuts, potato chips, pasta, soda, candy, fast food, ice cream, etc. She explains that one of the greatest gifts you can give yourself is to reduce your intake of dead foods. Food that is good for your body has vibrant colors and carries high energy. I highly recommend her 2009 book, *Natural Therapies for Parkinsons Disease*.

Naturopath doctor John Briggs, ND from Clatskanie, Oregon offered the following brilliant analogy during my radio show with him on April 16, 2009 that clearly illustrates the critical importance of nourishment.

> *"The body has to have the correct kind of fuel. If you put the wrong kind of fuel in, you can't expect good function. You have to make sure you are rested. You have to have good water in the system. You have to get oxygen to the system.*
>
> *The body is like an automobile. If you fail on the maintenance, your vehicle is going to fail you. When I look at Parkinsons, I have to find out what failed and on what level.*
>
> *As a physician, when people bring the vehicle in to me to kick the tires and check the dip stick, I have to start finding out what are they doing from a physical standpoint that might be predisposing them to disease such as Parkinsons. I have to start looking at:*
>
> *What are they putting in their body?*
>
> *One of my mentors - Dr. Christopher, had a saying that I love:*
>
> *"Live Foods for Live Bodies"*
>
> *If you want to eat the dead foods, you know what you can expect. I like to advise people to eat at least 50% of their nutritional intake as raw fruits and vegetables. We will have higher enzyme content and those enzymes are responsible for the appropriate function of our body.*
>
> *As we age one of the things we start seeing is lower and lower enzyme levels throughout our system. In fact, it has been shown that after about the age of 30, we all start declining in all areas, mainly because of enzyme damage. Of course, if we are not eating foods that are rich in enzymes, then we are going to be speeding that along that much faster. You figure that if you are eating the dead foods, the enzymes that you have must work that much harder.*
>
> *We are born with a large enzyme account. When we are young we have a lot of enzyme potential going for us. As we get older, we keep signing these checks on the enzymes and eventually we become bankrupt. That is when we see a lot of these diseases show up.*

© 2013 Parkinsons Recovery

There are various things that can be done to help with enzyme function. You have maybe heard of Wobenzym out of Germany. This is an enzyme system. There is one called Vitalzym by World Nutrition which helps the body restore normal function."

John Briggs writes that both products are "excellent in breaking down fibrin and re-establishing circulation as well as cellular function". If you are interested in learning more about either product line, I suggest you contact Dr. John at 503-728-4732. He sells the Vitalzym through his office and ships it all over the world. I think it is smart to order it from a naturopath like John Briggs, ND because you get the additional advantage of having a knowledgeable professional who is available to answer all of your questions about enzyme products. You can connect to Dr. Brigg's newsletter by visiting http://drjohnscorner.blogspot.com

What evidence is there that eating raw foods instead of processed, cooked foods gives marked relief from the symptoms of chronic diseases like Parkinsons? Here is what Dorit has to say which, in my book of common sense, is an insightful perspective.

"You need to try it for yourself. It is only when you try it. I do not mean try it with all of this dread and fear.

> *'I cannot stand this. I miss my burger.'*

If you do it that way you will not see the results. Try it with an open heart, an open mind and an open body. The evidence lies within your own experience.

Do not go according to what someone else tells you. Just because you see somebody else healing and you do the exact same thing that they did and you do not heal - it does not mean there is something wrong with you. That is their path and their soul's journey. Your soul's journey is different.

Their mindset is different from your mindset. You are not ready for it. It is ok not to be ready because that is your soul's journey. Accept it. Acceptance is what we need. Acceptance creates self love. You cannot jump from acceptance and rigidity and self love. Self love is where all healing lies. "

Your body needs live food in order to heal. Most foods sold at the supermarket and served in restaurants are "dead" foods. When we eat dead food, there is no chance our cells will have the nourishment to rejuvenate.

MAKE EATING RAW FOODS A HABIT?
I asked nutritional author Dorit how a person accustomed to eating meat and french fries can motivate themselves to change a long standing habit of eating "dead," processed food.

© **2013 Parkinsons Recovery**

"You cannot eat raw foods if you are not willing to become raw yourself. In other words, you cannot change a habit overnight by changing one aspect of a habit. With a habit, everything supports it which means you will have to change everything in your life to support your new habit.

It means you are going to have to give up your meat and potato friends and meet raw food friends or vegan friends. It means you are going to have to find new tools and ways of being in the world. You cannot live in your comfort zone anymore. If you run towards fear you are going to run away from it. You confront all your fears. You see that there are gifts in them. You make friends with them. That is how they get released. You have to magnify that which you fear.

You have to become totally willing to give up everything for the truth of who you are. Either you do that or you live with what you wish to live with. It is about acceptance. If you wish to eat meat and potatoes, then accept that your life will reflect that and be ok with that. But it is not enough to change the food. You have to change everything around that supports that lifestyle.

To summarize, a habit is supported by everything else in your life. You build a whole structure around that habit. That is why it is so hard to give it up.

HEALTHY HABITS

What are the three most important habits that people with Parkinsons need to have when it comes down to what they put into on onto their body? Dorit recommends the following:

1. Never take a bath or shower without putting on massage oil before (or after the shower) using warm sesame, coconut or organic mustard oil.

2. Add hemp oil to your diet.

3. Change the salt you use to Hawaiian sea salt or Portuguese sea salt or Celtic sea salt. The white salt most people use is actually creating illness in the body.

Nutritional Counselor and pharmacist Randy Mentzer offers his own recommendation on diet.

"You should avoid any foods that cause inflammation. You should avoid fats that are at room temperature (margarine, fats found in meats). The liquid fatty acids like olive oil, fish oil flaxseed oil are fine because those are anti-inflammatory. Any fats that are solid at room temperature cause inflammation. Some of them cause a lot of inflammation. Some of them cause a little bit of inflammation. You should avoid anything that causes inflammation."

© 2013 Parkinsons Recovery

One of the most important decisions you can make is to never eat fried foods. Everyone has heard that the fatty acids in fish oils are important to good health. They nourish your myelin sheaths, the insulation that covers and protects the nerves. Few people know that there are different forms of fatty acids: Omega 3 and Omega 6. The relationship between the two should be one to one. When you eat fried foods, the Omega 6 fatty acids soar and this critical one to one is wacked.

There are also foods that are necessary to reduce the natural process of oxidation in the body that creates inflammation and accelerates aging. Anti-oxidant foods are a wise choice for anyone over the age of 21. Here is a list of foods that are at the top of the list for their antioxidant properties. If you like to indulge in eating any of the following foods – allow yourself the pleasure of eating them anytime the urge arises (unless your doctor recommends otherwise): blackberries, walnuts, strawberries, artichokes, cranberries, raspberries, pecans, blueberries, cloves, grape juice, unsweetened baking chocolate and sour cherries.

What does naturopath doctor John Briggs, ND suggest when it comes to nutrition?

> *"Your body has to have healthy fats. We have to have a certain amount of ... healthy saturated fats in our diet... Fifty percent of the weight of your brain is fat. It is necessary for your nervous system.*
>
> *We have changed the levels of what is acceptable in the human body so much that we are now using drugs to lower our cholesterol levels to such a low level that we are actually inviting disease. It concerns me greatly when I see somebody with a cholesterol count under 140. How are we going to maintain the insulation of your nerves?"*

Research conclusively shows that calorie restrictions reduce the progression of Parkinsons. Eating less protects neurons against oxidative and metabolic assaults and, better yet, stimulates the grown of new neurons. Eating fewer calories increases brain-derived neurotropic factor (BDNF) which enhances learning and memory.

It is difficult for most people to deny themselves the pleasure of eating delicious foods, but if you are serious about getting well, consider this as an option. An advantage of calorie restriction diets is that they save you a lot of money on your food bill every month. You should, however, consult with your doctor before restricting your calorie intake.

AYURVEDA

Principles of Ayurveda medicine are the following:

- Build a healthy metabolic system

© **2013 Parkinsons Recovery**

- Attain good digestion

- Maintain proper excretion

Do this and you will attain vitality, balance and wellness. Ayurveda more specifically focuses on diet, exercise, yoga, meditation, and massage. The guiding philosophy is that the body, mind, and spirit together need to be addressed for health to ensue.

One of the Pioneers of Recovery, Nathan Zakheim, attributes his full recovery from Parkinsons to Ayurveda medicine. He was given a pouch of herbs to take by a doctor in India who treats people with the symptoms of Parkinsons.

Nathan explains,

> "I was supposed to take Ginger Juice, so I got a coffee grinder and I used that for grinding ginger and squeezing it through a cloth."

Nutrition and diet played a leading role in his recovery:

> "I was very strict with the diet he [the doctor] gave me. I was not allowed to eat any potatoes, tomatoes, okra, eggplant and stuff like that. ...So I just basically ate mung beans, rice, vegetables, beans and spices. I ate that for two years.
>
> The effect was good. I began to show symptoms of improvement very, very soon after taking the medications."

Return to balance and harmony was critical to Nathan's work in art restoration. When he works on multi-million dollar oil canvasses that have been painted by the masters, it is important that he have a steady hand and rock solid centeredness. Now that he has recovered, Nathan has returned to doing the work he loves and is handsomely rewarded for - the work of art restoration.

A commitment to embrace Ayurveda principles entails a significant shift in eating habits for most people. You must avoid all foods that contain yeast which means breads and pastas. You also cannot eat refined sugar products, vinegar, fried foods, aged cheese, peanuts, canned products, bottled juices and junk food. And of course, results are not immediate. You must stick with this strict diet for some time before results are seen.

I have heard several excellent recommendations for a reputable company that sells high quality Ayurvedic herbs – Banyan Botanical Herbs which is based in Albuquerque, New Mexico.

© 2013 Parkinsons Recovery

MACROBIOTICS

A macrobiotic diet is an ominous term for a set of straightforward ideas which have been adopted by people for thousands of years to reverse illness and sustain health. The approach can vary considerably, but generally involves

- Eating more whole grains, beans and fresh vegetables.

- Choosing organic foods.

- Increasing the variety of foods that are eaten.

- Varying the methods used to cook them.

- Selecting smaller quantities of food.

- Establishing a regular routine for eating meals.

- Chewing each bite more thoroughly.

- Maintaining a positive outlook.

Consider the merits of this approach. Is it effective to eat live foods? Yes indeed! Eat live foods and we feel more alive. Eat dead food and we feel lifeless.

Does it make sense to eat less food more frequently? Yes indeed. Just ask your body whether it prefers to digest little amounts of fresh food more frequently or if it prefers to digest a belly full of food once every day. Your body will not hesitate to demonstrate that it is much easier to digest smaller quantities of food more frequently.

Is it smart to eat a variety of organic foods? Yes indeed. Our bodies need a variety of vitamins and minerals to function. Eating a rich variety of foods makes it more probable we will be giving our body all the fuel that it needs to maintain peak performance throughout the day.

What then is the best diet for persons with Parkinsons? There is no one "best diet." It all depends! As noted, experts disagree on the ideal diet for Parkinsons. Of course, taking certain medications complicates the question of how much protein to eat. I believe the ideal approach is to listen to your body and adopt an individualized nutritional program that is perfect for you and your body.

For example, you may have insufficient flora in your intestines to digest live, raw foods. If you try a totally raw food diet, you may be miserable. I have heard reports of cases where people stuck to a raw food diet for six months and were miserable to entire time. Instead of listening to their body they were listening to an "expert."

The flora in the intestines might be depleted. In this case, it would not matter what food you eat. Dog food would do just as much good as organic food. A chronic intestinal infection may be gobbling up all the good flora that is required to assimilate foods rich in vitamins and minerals.

I believe it is a mistake to be rigid about following any "expert's" diet. It may well be that you need to follow Dr. Wilson's protocol and eat cooked foods for a year and can then begin eating more raw foods over time – or Dr. Wahl's diet with its primary emphasis on raw foods. Each doctor has a compelling argument for why their diets should help people with Parkinson's symptoms, but their approaches are diametrically opposed to one another.

At a minimum, it makes sense to eat organic foods that are not genetically modified. It is ideal to eat food grown by people who live locally. Just because a product says it is organic does not mean, unfortunately, that it is free of pesticides and toxins or that it is rich in vitamins and minerals.

The key is to become sensitive to how your body reacts after you eat certain foods. If you have more energy and feel great after eating, the food you just ate is the perfect food for your body at this time. If you feel lousy after eating, you just crammed food into your body that is bad for it.

It may well make more sense to begin eliminating certain foods in your diet (like sugar). Think of it this way. If you put a poor grade of gas in your car, it will not run well. Our bodies are no different than an automobile. Many people treat their automobiles better than they treat their bodies.

You may well experience dramatic improvements in your energy level when you stop eating certain foods. It is not so much a question of eating the right foods, but avoiding foods that you are allergic to. Many people are allergic to foods they eat every day. They have become so accustomed to feeling lousy that they do not realize the reason is tied to foods they assume their body can tolerate. This assumption is often proved to be dead wrong.

In summary - what is the best diet to help reverse the symptoms of Parkinson's? It all depends on the factors that are causing your symptoms in the first place. Solve that mystery and you are 90% down the road to recovery.

NOURISH YOUR BRAIN

Some people believe that they have the symptoms of Parkinsons because the cells that produce dopamine in their body have died and can never be rejuvenated. Baloney I say.

© 2013 Parkinsons Recovery

The science of cell regeneration is compelling. New cells are born every day in our bodies. The science of neural plasticity is well established in the scientific literature. I am not making this up! Do an internet search. Go to the library. The evidence is compelling.

Neural networks get obstructed in everybody for lots of screwy reasons. As noted, pathogens, bacteria, viruses and fungi get in the way to create road blocks that obstruct the neural communication pathways. Trauma tenses up tissues to create obstructions. Toxins muck up neural pathways to be sure.

There is clearly a lot we can do to clear the neural signaling misfires: toxin cleanses, trauma releases, critter removals. There is also something we can do for ourselves every day that makes a huge difference.

We can challenge our minds with a puzzle or a problem that we have not seen before. Thinking about problems we have not solved before challenges neural networks to construct new pathways. People I interview tell me one of the keys to feeling better is to embrace a new challenge or solve a new problem each and every day.

Our body has a special ability to rejuvenate neural networks. This does not happen when we sit on a sofa all day long, eat potato chips and watch the soaps on TV. A little effort on our part is required.

The more often we take on new challenges and solve new problems the more success we will have with creating new neurons and new neural pathways. We will gradually feel better over time. This is true for everyone, but it is especially important for people with Parkinsons.

MINDWORK

People with Parkinsons can be trapped into a vicious cycle of escalating symptoms. Here is how the process unfolds.

Symptoms tend to creep up gradually. Little signs pop up here and there - a twitch here or a muscle cramp there. Signs are ignored or dismissed as being minor annoyances. Symptoms gradually become more persistent.

A search is launched for therapies that have the potential to provide relief. The search for relief in itself is stressful. Stress from the search inflames symptoms further. A diagnosis is made which hammers away at the idea that recovery is no longer possible.

The person begins to believe that recovery will never be possible. Since our thoughts affect our health, the next step is obvious. Other more troubling symptoms emerge. Movement becomes more challenging. Exercise becomes painful. Movement becomes more limited. Without physical exercise symptoms are destined to get worse.

Everyday tasks become much more challenging. Hope of recovery begins to hang on a very thin thread. The person is no longer able to exercise or even lift a finger for that matter. How can this vicious cycle be reversed?

My answer is simple. If you can't exercise your body, you can always exercise your mind. Why not build new neural networks without lifting a finger?

Simply put, you do not have to exercise your body to get the benefits of exercise. Research suggests that you can actually get two thirds of the benefits of physical exercise by exercising your mind without lifting a finger.

Isn't that a cool idea? I think so.

We can exercise our mind through memory exercises and guided visualizations. This results in the creation of new neural networks. Memory exercises facilitate the body's ability to make dopamine. As the symptoms subside, physical exercise becomes a viable option.

Presto. You are on the road to recovery.

I call this approach to recovery "Mindwork." Memory exercises and guided visualizations are posted on the Parkinsons Recovery member website. I ask everyone who participates in the Mindwork exercises to track their symptoms so we can all get an idea of how the recovery process unfolds when the mind is used as a form of exercise.

The good news is that Mindwork is fun, non-intrusive and safe. Oh, I should provide a disclaimer. The only side effect – and there is one side effect – is improved health on some level.

VIBRATION THERAPY

The practice of using vibrations to offer relief from the symptoms of Parkinsons is 120 years old. In the 1890's Jean Charcot, MD, one of the pioneering medical neurologists who was the first to associate the name "Parkinson's disease" with the neurological symptoms we see today, invented a novel way to vibrate the bodies of his Parkinson's patients. Why did he do this?

Jean Charcot's vibration therapy invention emerged from a most curious observation he made about the patients who came to see him. Patients who rode in carriages and trains were much more functional on average than those who came on foot or by others means. Charcot deduced that the vibration experienced by patients who traveled by carriage or train was the "difference that made the difference". The more a person vibrated the muscles and tissues of their body, the less severe was their symptoms.

© **2013 Parkinsons Recovery**

Charcot did not just propose vibration therapy as a theory. He actually constructed a vibration chair that he used to treat his patients with (reportedly) considerable success.

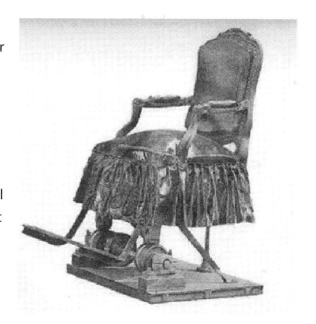

The invention was crude by all accounts. Charcot's patients sat in the vibrating chair while a nursing assistant jiggled the chair mechanically with a handle. Or, the assistant monitored a small steam engine that jostled the chair. The assistant was present throughout the therapy session to insure that the vibration was not too extreme for the patient to tolerate or too gentle to produce the intended effect.

Charcot died in 1893. Vibration therapy as a treatment for Parkinson's was abandoned by Charcot's students. I have no idea what happened to his chair. A medical student of Charcot modified Charcot's chair into a head helmet that vibrated the brain. There is no evidence on the success of the head helmet, though there are anecdotal indications it may have done some harm to patients.

Vibration therapy has now returned to the forefront in the 21st century as a companion to sound therapy in the form of Vibration Therapy. The cushions and lounges of 2011 vibrate to the binaural beats (or holosync) that beam into the right and left sides of your brain. No assistant need be present. The patient can turn down (or up) the degree of vibration by turning down (or up) the sound volume.

Charcot's enthusiasm over vibration therapy has been revived by neurologist Christopher Goetz, director of the movement disorder program at Rush University Medical Center in Chicago, who is completing a 2011 study to evaluate the effectiveness of the SMART Lounge for 20 Parkinson's patient study volunteers. We will have a much clearer idea on its effectiveness soon.

The company who makes the SMART Lounge is donating a SMART Lounge for use by study volunteers in their homes. Rush Medical Center is conducting the evaluations. I will disseminate Dr. Goetz's results when they have been compiled and released.

Parkinsons Recovery was literally one of the first organizations to acquire a SMART Lounge [http://www.vibrationtherapy.org]. The feedback we are hearing about people who have tried it is very encouraging. We actually started with the dinosaur model. The technology has been advanced light years ahead in just six months. We have just purchased the next generation of the SMART Lounge for use by everyone who will be attending our Jump Start to Wellness Programs.

I interviewed Lee Bender on my radio show on August 13, 2009 who is the father of Ed Bender, the creator of this new product. Lee has Parkinsons. He has benefited greatly from relaxing on the SMART Lounge every other day for 30 minutes.

Our own experience at Parkinsons Recovery with the Smart Lounge is that the combined effect of binaural sound and vibration forms new neural connections between the brain and the body. Movement becomes more agile and effortless.

You lie down on the lounge. You put the headphones on. You turn on the CD player. You wear dark glasses to block out the light. Then, you rock and roll for 30 minutes. The tissues of your body vibrate to the beat of the binaural sounds. It is very trippy and quite fun.

The acoustic CDs that are used in conjunction with the SMART Lounge build on groundbreaking research that tracks impulses in the brain with sounds. The brain reacts differently depending on the sounds that enter into the right and left ears. When there is a juxtaposition of the sounds that enter into each ear at the same time, new neural networks are born. By listening to music you can thus create new neural networks.

Feedback I hear from users is that people have more energy, are less stressed and have better balance. Lounge therapy appears to be safe, nonintrusive and totally enjoyable. Some people have described the experience as an awesome "head trip".

I am excited about the prospects for Vibration Therapy for the following reason. What therapies offer hope to people who have become totally debilitated from damage to their neurological system? If a person cannot exercise or eat healthy food or even visit a therapist from one specialty or another, what hope can they ever have that recovery is possible? Since they can still lie down on a bed or sit in a chair, they can always give Vibration Therapy a trial run.

SOUND THERAPY

Sound therapy has persisted through thousands of years because it helps people feel better. Sounds that are transmitted to the physical body induce physiological and emotional changes at the cellular level. If you do not feel like exercising or fixing yourself a yummy, nutritious meal, listen instead to music that warms the seat of your soul and the wings of your spirit. Sound medicine comes with a guarantee. It is also free to use and available anytime.

Sound conveys a spectrum of vibrations on a physical level. Vibrations are a concrete source of energy that nourishes our life force. When the full spectrum of frequencies our body needs for nourishment is present, we will be healthy and happy. When the frequencies our body needs to function are absent, we will be off balance, sick and ill. The delicate combination of hormones is disrupted. A wide variety of health problems emerge. We may be unable to properly talk, walk, swallow, eat, digest, think, breathe, see, hear or all of the above.

The argument I am making here is simple, but profound. If you are experiencing the symptoms of Parkinsons, your body is missing one or more frequencies it needs to be properly nourished. What does this mean precisely? Consider the example of a vitamin D3 deficiency.

It is well known from the research that people with Parkinson's have significant vitamin D3 deficiencies. People who know this take vitamin D3 and begin to feel better. Vitamin D3 has a very specific frequency, as do all vitamins and minerals our body needs.

Since a deficiency is present, you can choose to take a vitamin D3 supplement or you can expose the tissues of your body to the sound frequency that is specifically associated with vitamin D3. I admit this must seem outrageous to you. You are likely wondering:

> *How in the world can a person compensate for a vitamin D3 deficiency without taking a vitamin D3 supplement or getting sunshine?*

The answer I have for you to consider is just this. When you take vitamin D3 (or any vitamin or mineral for that matter), you are exposing your body to the very specific frequency of vitamin D3 itself. It is not so much the D3 itself that matters. It is the frequency that cuts the mustard here.

This means that music (or sound) is medicine. When we give our bodies a healthy infusion of the frequencies that are missing, our bodies are able to heal themselves. In Europe, doctors actually prescribe Music Medicine CDs for various illnesses including Parkinson's. You have to have a prescription to get the CD. And get this: The Parkinson's Music Medicine CD that is prescribed in Europe by doctors is as expensive (or more expensive) as any prescription medicine in pill or liquid form.

A number of people from the Parkinsons Recovery community have volunteered to participate in a Music Medicine study that was conducted by Dr. Suzanne Jonas who is an educator, Vibroacoustic Therapist and a pioneer in the field of Sound Therapy. Her findings showed that listening to the Parkinsons CD resulted in welcome relief from a variety of symptoms. You can order the Parkinson's CD (there are several to choose from) by visiting her website at http://www.innerharmonyhealthcenter.com/music.html. People who have been using it tell me it has been helping them get relief from their symptoms.

Dr. Jonas has also created a wide range of music medicine CDs that offer frequencies needed to provide relief from many different chronic conditions including addictions, anger, depression, dementia, jet lag, anxiety, stress, insomnia, fatigue and many others.

One of her most recent creations is entitled Resonance which assists people in maintaining a healthy connection with the earth during the current active solar cycle. Solar flares disrupt the neurological signaling mechanism in the body and are one reason many young people are experiencing neurological symptoms. This particular CD contains the Schumann resonances that are used to facilitate the reentry of astronauts to earth from space travel.

It is also possible to activate essential frequencies by a short chant that elicits the full range of frequencies needed by the brain needs to function. Howard Shifke repeats the following brain chant as fast as he possibly can for five continuous minutes:

ling yow chee chee chee – joe ling bah
ling yow chee chee chee – joe ar ar sih sih
NOTE: sih sounds like sit without the "t"

Howard reports that he feels a special vibration in his head after several minutes so he knows its effect is powerful. Why not give it a try and see what happens for you?

FOOT WHISPERING

Most people with neurological symptoms hold near and dear to their heart that the focus of attention should be directed to their head. The direct pathway to the head and all other organs in the body is through your feet not your skull. Foot Whisperer Randy Eady helps people with Parkinsons get sustained relief from their symptoms by stimulating acupuncture points on their feet. People who walk through one of his foot gardens or wear his specially configured sole insets report great results. Randy has been a hugely popular presenter at the Parkinsons Recovery Summits because his work has been so effective in helping people reverse their symptoms.

REJUVENATE CELLULAR ENERGY

Why do cells degenerate over time and die? A primary reason for low cellular energy is a lack of oxygen. What is the solution? It does not take a rocket scientist to reason that better breathing will rejuvenate your energy.

Perhaps you doubt such a simple, free solution? How could a natural therapy like deep breathing lead to a rejuvenation of your stamina and energy? Do not take my word for it. Try out this natural remedy for yourself. When you have low energy, devote several minutes to

© 2013 Parkinsons Recovery

breathing deeply and continuously – in and out – for several minutes. You will see after several minutes I am not making this up!

When you have several minutes to observe people in a public place – like a restaurant or sports stadium – notice how most people breathe. Shallow breaths are the norm. Infrequent breathing is common.

Observe your own breathing more mindfully. When I take this challenge, I become aware I do not breathe often for several minutes at a time.

One medical doctor who is serious about the effects of oxygen deprivation as a factor which has caused many illnesses is Frank Schallenberger from Carson City, Nevada. He has been administering Ozone Therapy (Major Auto Hemotherapy) to his patients for over twenty years. This procedure involves extracting your blood through an IV. He then infuses your blood with Ozone (which has an extra oxygen molecule). Ozone is denoted as O_3 rather than oxygen which everyone knows as O_2. The ozonated mixture of blood and saline is then re-infused into the body.

Is this a permanent solution? Obviously not. Does it offer a quick infusion of new energy? Obviously yes. This is a great way to kick start your body if you are running low on oil.

I also believe an oxygenated body is better able to eliminate bacterial infections that are hiding out along your neural networks and clogging up the intricate signaling system used by the body that makes effortless movement possible.

GROUNDING

Life in the 21st century has created a profound disconnection with the earth. We wear shoes made of plastic and rubber that insulate us from the nurturing energy of mother earth. The earth has an abundant supply of neutralizing electrons. When we walk barefoot or directly connect to the earth through other means, inflammation is neutralized. Free radicals are reduced. More energy will result. Better sleep is a welcome side effect.

Could something as simple as walking in the grass without shoes really help give relief from Parkinson's symptoms? You will only know if you experiment. Grounding was an invaluable strategy for the US team that has been successful in winning the Tour de France recently. Word on the street has it that team members purposefully did grounding exercises every evening they raced. This gave them the extra boost of energy needed to exceed the limits of their physical abilities and beyond.

© 2013 Parkinsons Recovery

The profound possibilities that grounding offers to our health is previewed in Earthing: The Most Important Health Discovery Ever? If one reason for your symptoms is electrical short circuiting, I can assure you that the simple exercise of grounding will help tremendously.

THE LAKOTA WAY

I had the pleasure recently of meeting Brian High Horse, a descendent of the Lakota Indiana leader High Horse from the 1800's. We are connected because my great uncle took a famous photo of his grandfather High Horse.

I explained to Brian that I worked with persons who had been diagnosed with Parkinsons. My question was: how did the American Indians treat the symptoms of Parkinsons? How did they feel better?

> *"Pardon?" Brian said.*

I gave a brief list of the symptoms for Parkinsons, but that was not the source of his confusion.

> *"You ask a strange question. No Lakota ever had such symptoms."*

Not willing to give up, I asked,

> *"So, how did the Lakota stay healthy?"*

> *"Simple. Sweat Lodges. Prayer. Vision quests."*

Feel the balance in his answer? The earthliness? The groundedness? Seems as though a sweat lodge or a vision quest just might help balance out your hormones, eh?

SUNLIGHT

Many people believe that exposure to sun is unwise because it may give you cancer or other horrendous diseases. I believe exposure to sunlight is essential to good health and wellness. No doubt you can overdo it and become sun burned. You can also under do it and become deficient in vitamin D3. Most people under do it.

When you have too little exposure to sunshine, it is imperative to take a vitamin D3 supplement. Note that it is vitamin D3 (not just vitamin D) that is produced by sunshine. Vitamin D3 is one of the foundation vitamins that make it possible for the body to maintain a balance of hormones.

Life on earth would not be possible without the sun. Doesn't it make perfect sense that as one of the living beings on earth (along with butterflies and fireflies and coyotes), we should make a special point of exposing our bodies to the sun? This therapy is not available every day, but

© 2013 Parkinsons Recovery

when it is available, it is free for the taking. Take it when it is available and your body will thank you.

EXERCISE

The news is unequivocal. Exercise helps you feel better. Study after study reveals the same result. Move your body every day and you will have relief from your symptoms. Move any way it feels good to you. Move as often as you can.

David Heydrick, MD is a Maryland neurologist with Parkinson's symptoms who says the most important therapy for him has been exercise. He confesses that when he exercises he does not have to be so careful about his diet. Why? Exercise cleanses the body of the bad stuff that is so tempting to eat (like sugar and processed foods). Now that is not a bad incentive to exercise, eh?

Exercise also helps the body to process, release and even tolerate toxins. Judy Cameron, Ph.D., University of Pittsburgh, reported stunning results from a fascinating study which divided monkeys into two groups – those who exercised every day for three months (the runners) and those who watched (the watchers). At the end of the three months the monkeys in both groups were injected with the toxin MPTP that induces Parkinson's symptoms. May we all send out a prayer of gratitude to the monkeys who endured this abuse.

Runners showed little evidence they had even been injected with MPTP. They were able to make normal use of their arm on the side where they were injected. Watchers on the other hand were not able to use their arm on the side where they were injected.

Subsequent brain scans showed that dopamine production had been decimated in the brains of the watchers. There was little evidence of lesions or destruction in the brains of the exercisers. Dopamine production remained normal. Exercise somehow changes how the brain functions and at the same time protects it against damage from toxins.

Toxins are highly correlated with exercise. If you exercise infrequently, toxins will inevitably cumulate in your body. The more frequently you exercise, the less likely toxins will be obstructing the ability of your body to maintain the hormonal balance needed for optimal functioning.

Lisa Schulman, Ph.D., from the University of Maryland, argues that exercise is more effective than taking most medications. Exercise increases growth factors which are needed by the body to manufacture dopamine naturally.

© 2013 Parkinsons Recovery

John Coleman, ND, has fully recovered from Parkinsons. John also exercises daily. He believes exercise is so important that he has illustrations of his personal exercise routine in his book at http://www.parkinsonsrecovery.com/startliving.

Michael Zigmond, MD a neurobiologist at the University of Pittsburgh, even goes so far as to suggest that exercise in itself has the potential to arrest the progression of Parkinsons. He theorizes that exercise stimulates the production of neuron protective chemicals in the body.

Who could ask for a better remedy? Exercise is the natural way to balance hormones in your body. Of course you do have to do something yourself to make this happen. But this is as it should be. Healing always must come from us.

Affinity for Exercise

Some people love to exercise. Other people hate to exercise. I talked with one woman last week who loves to exercise - so much so that her physical therapist has limited her exercise routine to 90 minutes. She gets significant relief from her symptoms.

Other people have never exercised in their life and are proud of it. Making a practice of moving every day is an annoyance. Too bad for them since exercise clearly has a profound impact on how you feel.

The solution for anyone who has never enjoyed exercise is to find a way of moving that is motivated from a place deep inside them. When you find a way of moving every day that works for you your body will let you know:

"Yes. This is what I need. Do it today. Do it every day."

What exercise is the right exercise for you? Remember what you loved doing as a child.

- Did you enjoy swimming when you were little? Then swim now.

- Did you love to play marbles? Then play marbles now.

- Did you love to play hide and seek? Then play hide and seek with your dog Fido now. (My apologies if your dog is not named Fido).

You get the point.

I have always been a runner, so I run frequently. I get high when I run. Running always makes me feel better. It is the natural remedy that works for me.

© 2013 Parkinsons Recovery

Some people with Parkinsons tell me running on a treadmill is their exercise of choice. Running itself is clearly not the best form of exercise for many people.

If any one of us (you or your husband or your wife or me) is told that we must exercise in a specific way using a specific routine for 60 minutes a day, we will not do it for very long if we do not like doing it. Period.

I will stick to a routine I do not like for a week – maybe – but that is probably being optimistic. Perhaps you are good for a month. Maybe you are more disciplined than I and will last four months.

Eventually, we all abandon any type of exercise if it does not give us intrinsic joy and genuine satisfaction. The desire to move must, again, be motivated by a place from deep inside us.

Another problem can surface if we exercise because we are told we must do it to feel better - not because we want to exercise to feel better. Isn't that just what I am telling you now? I suppose this recommendation is sure to backfire now, eh?

If the exercise is forced, we are likely at some point to stretch and challenge our muscles incorrectly. Tissues can be torn. Serious injuries can be the consequence. Injuries do not happen when exercising is done mindfully.

Of course, if you are injured you cannot exercise. Is not this the perfect outcome for anyone who has always hated to exercise? The steps are simple to follow:

1. Force yourself to exercise in a way that is not right for you.

2. Injure yourself.

3. Stop exercising.

4. Feel worse.

5. Conclude it is your body's fault for not working correctly.

If the question you ask yourself repeatedly when you exercise is:

> *"How much longer do I have to endure this torture?"*

Stop. Consider the possibility there is another form of exercise that is a better way of exercising.

You may very well have expected a different answer to your question about exercise. Perhaps you were looking for an answer like this from me:

© **2013 Parkinsons Recovery**

"Everyone with Parkinsons should do "Professor Bob's Zippy 2 Hour daily workout for Parkinsons." (Just to be clear in case anyone is wondering - this program does not exist.)

This is not the response I can give you because I do not believe that any single exercise program – even Professor Bob's Zippy program – is right for everyone. Any particular type of exercise will always work for some people, but it will never work for all people. Far from it.

What is important is to move.

- Move.

- Move.

- Move every day.

The more you move the better you will feel. The benefits are multifaceted. Muscles get stronger even for a 90 year old. The heart improves its function. Muscles get bigger. Movement gets easier. Falls are prevented. Mood improves. Depression is cut off at the pass. Weight is controlled.

Are you exercising hard enough to achieve the maximum benefits? Use the talking rule. If you can carry on a conversation with someone on a cell phone you are not exercising rigorously enough.   Rev it up a notch.

Everyone - people who are healthy and people who are not - should move the equivalent of 5 miles each day (weekends included). Total up each of your separate movements throughout the day to reach your goal.

For example: Let's say a walk from your bedroom to the kitchen in the morning is .005 miles. A walk from your car to the store at 9 am is .02 miles. And so forth. By the end of the day, the sum total of all such movements should total 5 miles.

There are many, many ways to move your body: Pilates, Tia-chi, yoga, swimming, daily walks -- the list is endless. If you do not move every day, your body will eventually go on strike. Symptoms will flare.

Have you noticed that there is redundancy in my writing here? This is just what exercise is all about, going through the same routine over and over, day after day. So get with it.

There is a way of exercising somewhere out there in the universe that is perfect for you. Make it a high priority to discover it.

© 2013 Parkinsons Recovery

There are also physical therapists that are specifically trained to help persons with Parkinsons. They assess your strengths and weaknesses and recommend specific exercises.

Good options surround you. Explore the options. Try them out. An exercise routine is not working for you if you are not doing it regularly and loving it. Find another. Try it out. Keep experimenting until you find a way of moving every day that gives you joy.

Your body will thank you. And you will thank yourself.

FORCED EXERCISE

Jay Alberts, Ph.D. from the Center for Neurological Restoration at the Cleveland Clinic at Cleveland Ohio, has seen exciting benefits to "forced exercise". Excerpts from my interview with Jay Alberts on April 23, 2009 follow:

> *"In 2003 I rode a tandem bicycle across the state of Iowa with a Parkinson's patient...She made a statement after we rode that week. She said,*

>> *'For this week, it didn't feel like I had Parkinsons.'*

> *We were really encouraged by that. We started thinking about what might be happening here with Parkinsons and exercise. We followed that up in 2005. I rode a tandem bike with Dave Heydrick, MD. He has had deep brain stimulation for Parkinsons. He turned his stimulators off that day when we did a 50 mile ride. About 15 miles into the ride we were stopping to have a doughnut - to fuel up as we were peddling across Iowa. He looked at me and said,*

>> *'Where did my tremor go?'*

> *I said,*

>> *'I don't know. Let's hop back on the bike and see if we can keep it away.'*

> *About 4 hours later he was still asymptomatic following the tandem bike riding.*

> *It was after that that I realized we really needed to follow this up and do some more systematic studies. That is when we recently conducted a preliminary clinical trial to compare the effects of "voluntary exercise" to what we are calling "forced exercise".*

> *"Forced exercise" is essentially assisting or forcing the Parkinson's patient to peddle faster than they can on their own. One of the things with Parkinson's disease is that patients have this poverty of movement or slowness of movement.*

Essentially, patients who ride the tandem bicycle typically peddle only 50 to 55 revolutions per minute. When they rode the tandem with me, I tended to peddle around 85 revolutions per minute. The idea was that maybe we are overdriving to some degree the central nervous system. That is changing brain function that allows them to have better or greater improvements in their motor function.

We have followed these field observations up with this preliminary clinical trial. Our data are very encouraging here with respect to the positive effects of "forced exercise" on motor function compared to "voluntary exercise."

The tandem bike used in the study was a two seat bike. A healthy adult trainer known as the "captain" sits on the front seat. The person with Parkinson's symptoms – known as the "stoker" sits on the back seat. The bike was stationary in the experiment to insure the safety of the research volunteers. In the pilot experiment, the captain:

"...controlled the rate of peddling and made sure that the Parkinsons patient continued to peddle between 80-90 revolutions per minute, three times a week, essentially 40 minutes per session. There was a little bit of a warm up period before the main exercise and a little bit of a cool down period following the main exercise. This was an eight week intervention.

We were pleased with the clinical outcomes. The UPDRS (Unified Parkinsons Disease Rating Scale) estimates motor functions or symptoms of Parkinsons. What we found after eight weeks of "forced exercise" was that Parkinson's patients experienced about a 35% decrease in their clinical scores. If you look at the data, that is equivalent to what you see in some studies looking at unilateral or even bilateral Deep Brain Stimulation.

The other encouraging aspect of this to us is that if you think about this type of intervention - what is happening- you are exercising the lower extremities but we are seeing an improvement in the upper extremities in function. To us, that was pointing to some kind of a change in the brain or central nervous system function.

We did access upper extremity function in our recent study. The biomechanical measures used to assess function were consistent with our earlier in the field observations. We saw a general relief of symptoms.

Ironically enough, the items in the UPDRS that showed the smallest change were actually gait and postural stability. It is important to note that in terms of assessing gait and postural stability, the UPDRS is not a real precise tool. We are following those measures up with more precise biomechanical measures to look and see if maybe we have

© **2013 Parkinsons Recovery**

changed the lower extremity function as well. In general we actually found that tremor was quite responsive to "forced exercise" as well as akinesia and bradykinesia.

Some clinics are evaluating the use of treadmills which replicate forced exercise. There is a safety issue with treadmills, so the clinics are looking at systems where part of your body weight is supported by some type of overhead harness. A small proportion of subjects (estimated at 15%) are able to increase their heart rate before falling.

The tandem bike is a little safer if you are trying to increase exertion by 30%.

> *"Once patients started to feel some of the benefits, they did not want to miss. We did not have a difficult time recruiting subjects. After they finished the study, they all wanted to re-enroll."*

> *It may not be just aerobic exercise. It may be the rate at which you exercise that is the critical factor in terms of leading to global improvements in motor function.*

> *We are looking to see how "forced exercise" changes blood flow and patterns of activity in the brain relative to the administration of medication. Our preliminary data look very favorable in the sense that it appears "forced exercise" is having a very similar effect on brain function as is the administration of l-dopa.*

> *Many who are on medication are a passive recipient in terms of how well the medication works. They have very little control over that. Either it is working well today or it is not working well. Patients with Deep Brain Stimulation Surgery - though they weren't in the study - say the same thing. Their function is dependent on something else - how well the stimulation is working or how well their meds are working.*

> *All of the patients in our forced exercise study said they really felt with this type of intervention they were an active participant in the treatment and fight against the disease. That was a secondary benefit - a warm and fuzzy feeling we had here - that we were empowering these individuals to really treat or fight the disease on their own in addition to medication."*

In collaboration with the <u>Lou Ruvo Center for Brain Health in Las Vegas,</u> the Cleveland Clinic is currently conducting a follow-up study to evaluate the effects of forced exercise for persons currently experiencing the symptoms of Parkinson's disease. Dr. Alberts reported that preliminary findings reveal that forced exercise had a positive impact on olfaction (or the ability to smell). MRI scans also show that forced exercise increases brain activity in the basal ganglia.

Forced exercises nourish the plasticity of the brain. Effects are wide ranging.

© 2013 Parkinsons Recovery

- *It reorganizes the intricate function of existing neural networks.*

- *It protects neurons from premature death.*

- *It regenerates neural synapses.*

- *It grows new nerves.*

The research is conclusive: Effects of forced exercise are wide ranging.

Nan Little has been helping hospitals in the Seattle area set up in house forced exercise clinics. She is a true expert on how to find the equipment you will need. Contact Nan Little for more information.

There is another twist to forced exercise. Studies show that the forced exercise of a handicapped appendage increases its functionality. Are you having more difficulty with one side of your body or one arm or one leg? Consider setting up exercises (with the assistance of a physical therapist) where you force yourself to exercise the appendage of your body that is the most problematic.

Tai Chi

Research evidence clearly demonstrates that Tai Chi helps to prevent falls. Steven Wolf, Ph.D. from Emory University has developed of program that reveals positive benefits of tai chi for persons who have difficulty walking. One of his award winning studies selected a group of 300 study volunteers who were "transitioning to frailty." Wolf observed a 40% reduction in falls by study participants. Study participants in general became less dependent on walkers and wheelchairs over the course of the 48 month study. Results of Wolf's study have been replicated in other studies as well.

Author and tai chi master Arieh Breslow reports the positive experience with one of his students Danny who had been diagnosed 10 years ago:

> *"Danny was able to reduce his level of medicine through Tai Chi and diet. He felt that when he did tai chi on a regular basis, it was the same as taking his Parkinsons medication. He had to take the medicine but he was able to keep the dosage on a fairly low level.*
>
> *He is still doing great. He went to a Parkinson's conference with his wife recently. They sat down in the circle. He had already had Parkinsons for eight or ten years at that time. They asked them —*
>
> *'Which one of you has Parkinsons?'*

© 2013 Parkinsons Recovery

There are some signs but you really have to knows he has Parkinsons to pick it up.

My own personal experience with people that have Parkinsons ... is that Tai Chi can definitely improve balance and walking and feeling more confident about yourself."

Arieh Breslow explains that tai chi is a Chinese martial art that is very useful for promoting balance and stability. People with mobility problems have weaker legs. Tai Chi develops strong legs. With Tai Chi you develop better balance and stronger legs. Stance is emphasized - how long, how wide, how much you should sink.

"We do the movements very slowly. It takes a few seconds to shift all the weight from one leg to 70% on the front leg and 30% in the back leg. We then step again with the opposite leg forward with 70% on the front and 30% on the back leg. We do it very slowly. The knees are bent.

The second important part is being able to sink into what we call the hip joints...teaching people to bring their hips so they are level with the ground. The sitting bone is level on both sides. The waste and pelvis area provides a cradle for the spine to be upright.

We sit into the hip joints which allow the lower back and coccyx to be more level. The whole pelvis becomes more parallel to the ground so it does not cause the spine or upper torso to lean in any direction.

The body finds its own internal organization. You have the cradle of the pelvis that sits parallel with the ground. The spine does not lean forward or backward.

When we find that balance point where the body is perfectly integrated ... we actually use gravity to make our bodies stronger. When we sink into our legs with the gravity we are also at the same time lifting the head above the spine and opening the whole spine so the whole energy of the body can move freely between the brain, the head and the rest of the body all the way down into the legs."

Arieh Breslow explains that the effects of tai chi are cumulative. You have to keep the exercise up and work with it every day.

Tai Chi can also be adjusted to each person's circumstances. It is possible to do tai chi even if you are in a wheel chair or use a walker. All of the tai chi movements and exercises can be adapted to meet the needs of the individual. Listen to my radio program interview with Arieh Breslow on August 6, 2009 to learn more about Tai Chi and how it has helped people with Parkinsons. Arieh Breslow has created a number of very powerful DVD's and books for people with Parkinsons which are of enormous help for those on the Road to Recovery.

© 2013 Parkinsons Recovery

QiGong

Zhineng, Wisdom Healing, or Chi-lel Qigong involves a carefully constructed combination of stimuli including slow movements, meditations, sound therapy and color visualizations. It has successfully reversed the symptoms of some individuals with Parkinson's symptoms including Bianca Molle who has assumed leadership as a coach, helping others reverse their own symptoms (www.mettamorphix.com).

Bianca explains:

> "Most who come to this practice, come with the intent of physical healing. Many receive that and so much more: equanimity, confidence, joy, and a general sense of expanded well-being."

Through the Chi Center in San Francisco Master Mingtong Gu has exposed a wide range of individuals with Parkinsons (including Bianca) to QiGong. Master Gu summaries its benefits:

> "Qigong connects the mind and the body to awaken mental clarity, to improve body balance and movement, and to sustain daily activities – functions that can be greatly impacted by Parkinson's."

The chi Center (www.chicenter.com) offers a variety of opportunities to learn QiGong using a beautifully produced collection of teaching resources that include DVDs and on line courses. They have made learning QiGong accessible to persons who live in any country the world. As with many natural therapies, QiGong has no adverse side effects.

YOGA

Perhaps you are someone who believes yoga is only for people in their twenties who have bodies that can twist in every which direction like a rubber band. Perhaps you have dismissed yoga as a potential therapy because it would surely be too physically demanding. These limiting and untrue thoughts – and they are just that – inhibit you from experiencing an activity that has been the source of endless joy and relief for a surprising number of people who currently experience Parkinson's symptoms.

While many people think yoga is reserved for athletic types, a dedicated group of individuals with Parkinson's practice yoga at least once every week at Northwest Hospital in Seattle, Washington. Participants report feeling more physically fit, less stiff and rigid, more flexible overall, better balanced and centered, stronger and less likely to stumble, fall and freeze.

You are probably thinking this extensive list of benefits must surely be exaggerated. Benefits listed above are documented by the testimonials of a dozen guests on my radio show

© 2013 Parkinsons Recovery

December 21, 2011 who talked about the amazing benefits they derived from attending yoga classes at Northwest Hospital. Some people even reported that attending regular yoga classes had transformed their lives. Listen to this radio show and you will understand why I do not hesitate to state these claims. You certainly cannot expect these outcomes from taking medications or supplements!

You may now be thinking – right. I bet these people lost their life savings paying for these classes. No my friends. The Yoga classes are free.

DANCE

Why should dance be considered a useful therapy for persons currently experiencing the symptoms of Parkinson's? Professional Dancer Pamela Quinn offers a succinct and eloquent perspective on this question during my radio show September 30, 2010.

> *Dance involves strength. It involves alignment. It involves balance. It involves music. It involves memory and learning combinations. It is a social form so it brings people together. There are a lot of characteristics of dance that make it particularly suited toward Parkinson's.*

Pamela offered a fascinating observation about the complexity of dances. She finds that the more complex the movement, the easier it is for her to do. Why is that? She believes different neural networks are required to help her body move in a complex way. When involved in simple movements such as walking or turning, there is an impairment not found with the complex movement. So if you are seriously considering dance as a outlet for fun and as a natural therapy to facilitate your recovery, experiment with dances that involve more complex movements.

A recent study found that the symptoms of people who danced the tango were significantly reduced. The tango is particularly well suited for two reasons. There is a repetitive sense of rhythm and your weight is held low to the ground.

TANGO AND SALSA DANCING

Tango is certainly not the only or even best dance option. Try Salsa dancing! Morry Krispijn, owner of a professional dance company in the Netherlands, tells me that persons with Parkinson's symptoms are markedly better at dancing the Salsa than persons who do not experience the symptoms. Isn't that fascinating? If you are not having enough fun this year, one smart option to consider is to learn how to dance the Salsa. This would be a marvelous activity to explore for a support group!

Mordechay Krispign from a Dutch Dance Company, Salsaventura (www.salsaventura.nl) has produced a marvelous DVD for persons with Parkinson's symptoms which is now available in English. Learn how to Salsa by watching his remarkable DVD in your bedroom. Form a dance group yourself and create your own class using his DVD as the teacher. Morry Krispign talked about the creation and success with his new Salsa DVD for Parkinsons on my radio show January 4, 2012.

Any form of dance can be beneficial because it involves exercise in combination with music which by itself facilitates effortless movement. This is the magical combination that fires new neural networks and clears obstructions in the neural networks that happen to be blocked.

What type of dancing did you enjoy when you were a child – square dancing perhaps? Then square dance now. Just do it as Pamela Quinn would say! Whoever said that recovery has to be painful? The best recovery options are fun.

DANCE FOR PD

The Mark Morris Dance Company in Brooklyn, New York has developed an entire training program for dance instructors who wish to teach dance to persons with Parkinson's symptoms. I love their philosophy and approach which is explained by Program Manager David Leventhal during my radio show on October 19, 2011.

Classes are taught by professional dancers. When you attend a DanceforPD (www.danceforpd.org) session, you are exposed to exactly the same training a professional dancer receives. Why? Dancers have to practice certain skills sets over and over before they become habituated. David explains that persons who currently experience neurological challenges too must practice motor skills over and over before the movements become effortless. Dancers and individuals with Parkinson's thus both benefit from learning the same skill sets in the same way – through repetition and consistent practice.

No one in the class is treated as handicapped or disabled. Accommodations are of course made for persons who currently have mobility challenges, but no one in the class is treated any differently than is given in a class of dancers who are professionals. People report loving the DanceforPD classes and experience an improvement in symptoms. Yea!

The purpose of classes is to have fun, learn a new skill and receive the awesome benefits that accrue to the neurological system from movement. With David's assistance, dance groups for Parkinsons led by professional dancers are forming across the United States. Contact David if you are interested in seeing a Dance for PD group form in your own community if one does not currently exist.

© **2013 Parkinsons Recovery**

GigerMD

Physical Therapist Ed Gray has been using a new technology invented by Swiss inventor Adrian Giger known as the GigerMD. The person lies on their back and peddles a bike upside down. Ed is currently the only physical therapist who uses the GigerMD in the USA, but all reports are that he is having wonderful results. Ed discussed his experience with the GigerMD on my radio show October 3, 2012 and will demonstrate it at the 2013 Parkinsons Recovery Summit in Santa Fe.

Meditation

Norman Fischer writes extensively about meditation and travels throughout the world teaching people how to meditate. During my radio show that aired September 24, 2009, Norman explained what meditation is all about:

> "In meditation you use the feeling of the breath in the belly and the feeling of the sensations of the body as a container in which thought can arise if it wants to arise. Instead of getting hooked on the thought or letting the thought push us around we let it go by coming back to the breath, coming back to the body.
>
> The goal is not to make the mind free of thought. The goal rather is to allow thoughts to come and go without getting hooked into them. That is a subtle difference, but it is really important. If you think you are supposed to have no thoughts, you are going to be frustrated.
>
> So, what we want to do then is find a way to let thoughts come and go, not getting hooked in old patterns and old routines which we can do most easily on the cushion, although as we all know, it is not easy there either. We want to then be able to extend this into our daily lives, little by little by little.
>
> We are always breathing. There are people who have to some extent compromised breathing. But we are all breathing to some extent with whatever degree of freedom we can manage. Paying attention to the breathing and to the sensations of the body regardless of the posture is the point.
>
> One does not need to sit in a lotus position in order to meditate. The most important factors for the posture and the body in meditation are the ability to have the spine lengthened, somehow sitting up straight and lengthening the spine. You can do the same thing laying down which opens the spine and opens the heart area. That is the first thing.
>
> Partly connected to this is that the breathing is conscious and full and open.

© 2013 Parkinsons Recovery

- *This can certainly be done sitting in a chair.*

- *It can be done lying down.*

- *It can also be done with walking meditation. You can do it when you are walking very slowly.*

The fundamental meditation that I always come back to and that I think is the most valuable is the practice of just sitting in the present moment with the sensations of the body and with the breath. Just being present with whatever is there, with whatever pleasant or unpleasant sensations, with whatever thoughts, with whatever feelings may arise, staying with the feeling of the body and the feeling of the breath to create a container for whatever else arises.

Although it is very counterintuitive, one would think – now how is that going to help me? The fact of the matter is – that is the most helpful thing – the willingness to actually be present, without hating what you are feeling or trying to make it stay there always – just to be present and allow something to come. Allow something to go. That is the most powerful and the most fundamental of all meditations.

There are people who have spinal issues. They may not be able to lengthen the spine. But they can do that as much as it is comfortable for them and then, pay attention to the breathing.

In a way – you do not even have the disease. You have a set of sensations in the body. The disease is a convenient label that is put on top of that so that doctors can know what to call something and can know how to treat it.

We wind up identifying ourselves with that label and with that disease as if that is ourselves. Actually, it is really a succession of various sensations in the body. That is what it is. That is what we have to cope with.

It is really terrible in a beauty and health obsessed society like the one we live in. It is very difficult to feel you are not in the swim of that. There is something different about you or something wrong with you. The isolation and loneliness of that is really one of the most painful aspects of chronic illness."

You can find extensive explanations about meditation on Norman Fischer's website at http://www.everydayzen.org. His mission is to bring the practice of meditation to all people, all nations and all religions. You will find a wealth of resources on his website that explain everything you need to know about how to meditate if you would like to start a daily practice.

Many people with Parkinsons tell me meditation helps them tremendously. Why not give it a spin? There are so many different forms – surely you can find one that meets your needs.

Do you not have enough time in the day to take out 20-30 minutes to meditation? Here is what Norman has to say about this excuse:

> "Meditation saves you time. You don't have time not to meditate. What one is busy with when one is not meditating is all the messes and mix ups that occur because we are not mindful.

Norman explains that the following statement is closer to the truth:

> 'I am busy. I do not have time to meditate because I am cleaning up the mess when I dropped my coffee all over the floor which I would not have done if I had meditated.'

> If you analyze your day, you are putting out fires, many of which would not have started in the beginning if you were more mindful".

Research published in Movement Disorders shows that guided imagery reduces tremors. That is why I post a new meditation on the Parkinsons Recovery member website every week day.

HYPNOTHERAPY

Hypnosis is similar to meditation in many respects. Research reveals that the brain waves of a person who meditates are similar in pattern and form to the brain waves of a person who is hypnotized. We all move in and out of a hypnotic (or meditative) state throughout the day. The simple act of day dreaming is a hypnotic state.

Hypnosis (or day dreaming or meditating) induces a profound sense of relaxation. The internal voice of judgment and criticism is silenced. Ability to focus and manifest is enhanced. The conscious mind goes on vacation. The internal dialogue which plays the same tired record over and over is silenced.

If left unchecked, an endless babble of thoughts that do not serve our best and highest good will continue to grease the hamster wheel in our heads. Left unchecked this hamster wheel will spin out of control. Our bodies rebel. Symptoms flare.

When we cycle thoughts over and over that are not in our best and highest good with criticisms and judgments that are untrue, we perpetually suspend ourselves in a state of fear. Ability of the body to maintain a steady state of balance and harmony is compromised.

The idea behind hypnotherapy is to shut down the hamster wheel, to quiet the mind and induce a relaxed state. It is in a relaxed state that it is possible to remove all of the knee jerk responses we have used since childhood to perpetuate fear. The process of activation becomes so automatic that we have to deactivate the hamster wheel and silence our overactive minds first.

Hypnotherapists facilitate a dialogue with your subconscious mind to remove the internal triggers that are causing the fear reflex to activate. Perhaps more importantly, it is helpful to learn how to do self-hypnosis so that you can remain in a state of safety and calmness throughout the day.

Are your symptoms in your face all the time? If so, you are in fear and may not know it. Learn how to maintain a steady state of calmness and watch those symptoms vanish. It can be very magical indeed. Better yet – this is something you can do for yourself. No outside intervention is required or necessary.

Hypnotherapist Steve Frison teaches his patients how to hypnotize themselves. Contact Steve to obtain guidance on how you can learn how to shift into a hypnotic state when you want relief from whatever symptoms you may be experiencing in the moment.

Mindfulness

Moment to moment we have a choice about how we perceive the marvelous world that cuddles and embraces us. We can fixate on pain and on body parts that are flying in every which direction imaginable. Or, we can focus our attention on the details of our surroundings – the sound of the birds (or the heater) or the color of the tiles on the floor or the texture of the wood that holds up the ceiling or the smell of a pet in the room or the sound of breathing. When attention is directed toward the wonders of the world, other issues fade away from consciousness. As Darlene Cohen so beautifully says, this is one guaranteed way to turn suffering inside out.

I concluded that becoming more mindful is the key to reducing stress, so I invented a year long series of weekly mindfulness challenges specifically created to help persons with Parkinson's reduce their stress level. I tried each challenge out myself before releasing it. Some of the challenges are truly engaging but have been very useful to me as well as others. For more information about how to reduce stress through an engaging mindfulness visit www.stress.parkinsonsrecovery.com

© 2013 Parkinsons Recovery

Music

Wendy Magee, Ph.D., International Fellow in Music Therapy at the Royal Hospital for Neuro-disability in West Hill, London, England explains that music regenerates and rejuvenates the pathways in the body that sense perception.

> *"Music acts in global pathways all over the brain. What this means is that when somebody has damage to one particular part of the brain as in a scenario involved with language production ... music can sometimes skirt around this by finding alternative routes.*
>
> *Listening to music, singing music and playing music is something that lights up other areas of the brain. The brain finds new routes to actually access functions that may be damaged."*

Listening to a systematic beat or a regular musical pulse can have a significant impact on a person's ability to walk. Wendy Magee, PH.D. explains:

> *"Hearing a pulse can affect somebody's gait pattern. The person hears the sound. Before the sound actually gets processed at some higher level within the brain - it cuts across straight in to the sensory motor pathways and can have a direct effect on somebody's walking pattern and gait pattern."*

One of the most exciting findings from research on music therapy has been to track improvements of people with gait problems - whether they walk too fast, take too many steps or walk too slowly. Wendy Magee, Ph.D. elaborates:

> *"What we know is that the use of pulse and the careful planned use of music where you are particularly focusing on the manipulation of pulse is that people improve the length of their leg gait, their walking pattern. It also can improve speed and regularity of the walking pattern. Somebody can actually manage their walking so much better and of course reduce the risk of falls.*
>
> *Some of the most interesting research results have looked at a home program after people have experienced auditory stimulation in a clinical setting. They have gone away with their tapes that have been made specifically for them at a pace with which they can walk. They practiced at home.*
>
> *Follow up studies looked at how that person is walking six weeks later without any musical stimulation. What has been shown is a significant improvement in how people walk weeks after having the initial training and even outside of the music condition."*

How does a music therapist help a person with gait challenges? Wendy Magee, Ph.D. says:

> *"The first part is meeting the person and assessing what their problems are. As we know, somebody with Parkinson's disease is likely to be having problems particularly with their gait and their walking pattern. They may be having problems with their speech and their voice production. They may be having problems with their facial expressions or maybe having difficulty with their fine motor control and their finger and hand movements."*

The music therapist evaluates the person's ability to walk without any auditory stimulation. They assess how fast they walk over a certain distance. They evaluate the gait pattern. The therapist then starts the individual off at one particular tempo.

If that tempo is not too fast or slow, the therapist incrementally increases the tempo, making sure the person can manage the upward adjustment in the beat. The music is then gradually withdrawn so that the person can walk confidently without the assistance of music.

Wendy Magee, Ph.D. says music is a mega vitamin for the brain. It is a natural and safe form of nourishment for our body and soul.

> *"Particularly if conventional treatment isn't doing the right thing or you don't feel you are getting very far with those, as an adjunct to those … think about trying music therapy."*

Hear more about the value of music as a mega vitamin and healthy nourishment for the brain by listening to my radio program with Wendy Magee, Ph.D. on June 25, 2009.

Heather MacTavish uses drumming and singing to help herself and groups with mobility challenges. She expresses the value of music beautifully in her new book, *Songs, Science and Spirit: Musical keys to open special doors of ability*.

> *"Music and song take me away from worry and regret, bringing me back to happier remembrances and feelings. My body remembers and responds to what my emotions perceive. I need to feel this on a sub-conscious level"* [11] *(p. 155).*

She also uses song to jump start her movements:

> *"When I am low on dopamine, I often drag my right leg. It is as if I am pulling a lead weight along with me. I have found that my movements can be jump-started if I do not*

---

[11] **Heather MacTavish with Zubin Balsara (2009). Songs, Science and Spirit: Musical keys to open special doors of ability. Provident Publishing, Tiburan, California, p. 155**

focus on the movement itself, but use the emotions evoked by rousing songs to galvanize me to action."

The more difficult the initiation of movement is, the more I sing. I basically spend my life as if I were in the shower.[12] (p. 161)"

Here are some of the songs that Heather sings during her day:

- *Ain't She Sweet*

- *When the Red, Red Robin Comes Bob, Bob Bobbin Along*

- *I'm Walking*

- *These Boots are Made for Walking*

DRUMMING

Do you like the title of this section of my book? I do. Are you surprised that drumming helps to relieve the symptoms of Parkinsons?

I am not. I must make a confession before I tell you more. I have been a drummer since I was in elementary school. Much of my time in high school was spent playing in bands and orchestras. I still love to drum on anything - chairs, tables, walls and of course drums of all sizes and shapes.

Some people say drumming relieves the symptoms of Parkinsons so I drum at Jump Start to Wellness events. The purpose of drumming is to have fun and feel better. Drumming fulfills both aspirations effortlessly. Everyone becomes young again.

The drum is a powerful force in healing. It:

- Releases stress

- Energizes the spirit

- Heals troubling emotions

- Releases anger

- Creates euphoria

It is hard to beat this list, eh? The body's ability to heal is boundless. Drumming is a fundamental way to support this ability.

---

[12] Ibid. p. 161

© 2013 Parkinsons Recovery

Connie Tomaino has found that listening to drumming gives people with Parkinson's better control over their movements and helps to improve their gait in stressful situations. Connie Tomaino, DA, MT-BC, uses drumming in her work with persons with Parkinsons. Here is her report:

> *"I once worked with a young person with Parkinson's disease who had trouble initiating movement. I explored different rhythm patterns with him. We then made a cassette of different kinds of African drumming that he seemed to find very stimulating and helped him get moving."*

> *"Anytime he had to walk across a street, whereas in the past he may freeze, he would put on his headphones and listen to African rhythms to get to the other side without freezing in the middle of rush hour traffic."*

> http://www.remo.com/portal/pages/health_rhythms/library_article9.html

There is a marked tendency for persons with Parkinsons to be hyper-vigilant. Mental activity is usually turned up to the top notch. Hyper-vigilance is a good trait. It is one reason why people with Parkinsons succeed in whatever they choose to do. Hyper-vigilance also takes a heavy toll on the human body which has a foundational need for rest and relaxation.

The body was not designed to pump out adrenaline 24-7 without registering loud complaints. You know the story. People who are always working and never playing have health problems.

People who are hyper-vigilant also have a much greater chance of having no alfa brainwaves. Zero. Drumming helps to jump start this deficiency by inducing alfa brainwaves at 8-12 cycles per second.

The alfa state is that delicious, relaxed place that ever so gently nudges the body into a state of pure relaxation, the place where dopamine is manufactured. The hyper-vigilant person has difficulty producing dopamine because they rarely experience this state.

I suspect that what happens in transcendental meditation is similar to what happens with drumming. Twenty minutes (or so) of a 30 minute transcendental meditation are spent floating in the alfa state.

Stress and trauma are embodied by a disconnection from the earth. One good way to survive stressful circumstances and trauma (especially when we are young) is to disassociate from ourselves and from our surroundings. We yank our roots up from the earth and let them flop about in thin air.

© 2013 Parkinsons Recovery

- *Drumming helps to connect you back to the earth. Drumming calls you back to the embrace of mother earth where it is safe and exciting to be alive.*

- *Drumming helps you accept everything and everyone - including ourselves - just as you are.*

- *Drumming invites the body to relax and unwind.*

Results happen when you start. You do not have to wait weeks or months for the "therapy" to take effect. Pretty neat, eh?

Testimonials tell us that drumming helps people with Parkinsons. We have no formal research to indicate that it helps but I say why even bother.

Why not give it a try and find a drum this week? You can often find great drums at garage sales for a few dollars.

- It certainly cannot hurt you.

- It is bound to be fun.

- You may laugh while doing it.

- When you have fun and laugh ...

You give yourself the best dose of dopamine that exists. It is all natural and entirely free.

So be honest with me here. Do you think this is a silly idea? If you do, please take this opportunity to laugh at me. That will do you some good for sure!

As for myself, I am on the lookout for drums at garage sales. Euphoria is calling me.

You do not have to just listen to drumming. You can drum yourself. Drumming is stress free and fun by design.

- *No musical ability is necessary.*

- *No talent is required.*

- *No sense of rhythm is necessary.*

- *No musical training is a prerequisite.*

The only requirement is to have a body. Everyone meets this requirement. Right? The only agenda is to have fun. Everyone is qualified to participate.

Any type of drum will do. Bongos, bass drums, snare drums without the snare, tympani, hand drums, African drums - you name it. If it sounds like a drum it is a drum no matter what it looks like or how it is made.

You can drum alone or in groups. If you drum with others, someone in the group can volunteer to maintain a steady beat – often like the beat of a human heart. Everyone else in the group then beats away on their drum to their hearts content with whatever beat calls to them.

Some people make simple beats that are meditative. Others are show offs. It is not the beat per se that matters. Whatever way you drum is the right way for you. The room rocks.

Let no one convince you otherwise. You may be one who does not like to "keep the beat." Good for you. Go for it.

When we are in groups it is fun to sit around in a circle and drum together. Even if you are not drumming yourself, it is healing to feel the thump of the airwaves. The thumps crawl under your skin and sit on the lap of your soul.

What you get in return for having fun by just sitting in the group is euphoria. What other remedy for Parkinsons can beat that? You also receive the welcome benefit of dopamine. Who could use a little more dopamine today?

Heather MacTavish has written a book which provides step by step instructions on how to lead drumming groups. Are you bored with what your support group is doing these days? I suggest you purchase her book and get started having more fun. Purchase her new book *Songs, Science and Spirit*, nominate a leader from the group and start drumming during your get togethers. It is fun. It opens up chakras. It helps balance and center the body.

ART Therapy

Several Parkinsons art therapy groups have emerged out of Australia that have had remarkable success. The good news is spreading to other countries as new groups are popping up across the globe. Most of the participants in art therapy groups have had no prior experience as artists. Novices receive just as much benefit from creating art as the professional artists who have Parkinson's symptoms.

Art therapy offers far more punch to recovery than you could imagine if you have not experienced it firsthand. I have aired several marvelous interviews with pioneers of art therapy for Parkinsons who facilitate art groups for persons with Parkinson's symptoms. Anne Atkin (whose radio show aired January 11, 2012) writes:

> *"You know Robert, when I look back about four years ago to how I was doing as a person with Parkinson's I can't believe how much both the group and myself have developed. I*

have found it all to have been a most amazing journey and one that I would not have missed for the world. I have changed so much as a person and developed skills that I never thought I would have."

Nancy Tingey (whose radio aired <u>April 25, 2012</u>) created a *Painting for Parkinsons* group in Canberra Australia. Nancy reports the quality of the work that is produced by people who have never painted before is stunning.

"I started Painting for Parkinsons when my husband (diagnosed with Parkinsons 25 years ago and still going) was made president of the local Parkinson's support group. We have 12 or so participants (people with Parkinson's and their carers) in the group, five facilitators and half a dozen volunteer helpers and we have a great time. The work the participants do is magic."

Jesse Lyle previewed her experience with facilitating art therapy for persons at the <u>2011 Parkinsons Recovery Summit</u>. To watch a <u>video</u> of her in action facilitating art therapy at the Summit, visit the Parkinsons Recovery Blog post on April 4, 2011.

COLOR THERAPY

Our life force is sustained by energy that vibrates on many different frequencies. A rich complement of frequencies that capture the full range of the color spectrum is necessary for the body to maintain balance and wellness.

Frequencies vibrate through portals known as chakras. Chakras in the lower part of the body vibrate at lower frequencies than chakras at the upper part of the body. The body remains healthy as long as all of the chakras are nurtured with frequencies that are needed to maintain an adequate flow of energy through the body.

We need an infusion of the full rainbow of colors to be healthy. Next time you see a rainbow notice how the colors are sorted in the order of their frequency: Red (which corresponds to the first chakra at the bottom of the body's trunk), then orange (which corresponds to the second chakra which is a few inches below the belly button) then yellow (which corresponds to the third chakra which is just below the rib cage), then green or blue (which correspond to the fourth heart chakra and fifth throat chakra). As you gaze at the colors of the rainbow observe the colors that correspond to the frequencies that are running through each chakra, respectively from the lower part of the body to the upper part of the body. The order is not random.

© 2013 Parkinsons Recovery

According to quantum physics we are all frozen light at the level of subatomic reality. Think of yourself as a "light being." When we absorb all that we have experienced fully and completely with all of our feelings and sensations, we exude the full rainbow of colors through our biological prism. Some experiences, especially those that are frightening or traumatic, are unresolved. They linger as unfinished business within the crevices of our cells. Our minds fail to digest what we have experienced. The flow of our life energy is constricted. This nurtures a biological resistance of sorts, a resistance which is manifested through the distortions of light that are emitted from our bodies. As a "light being" we emit a segmented rainbow of colors.

Blockages in the flow of energy distort the flow of energy and lead to illness of one type or another. Energy flow is obstructed by physical injury, emotional disturbances, stress and traumas. No one in a body escapes traumas in one form or another that distort, mute or silence the flow of energy through the chakras.

The explanation is certainly intuitively plausible to everyone. When we are stressed, we feel sick. When we are traumatized, we get sick. Traumas and stress distort, freeze and/or alter the specific vibrations that are critical to all health and wellness.

Frequency distortions manifest in the body as discomfort or pain. Some people feel the impact of traumas and stress in their body as a lump or growth that needs to be removed. Others feel them as a hole that needs to be filled.

When the complete rainbow of frequencies do not flow freely through the chakras, our life force is depleted. Other physical manifestations result. Some fall in the category of chronic illness. Symptoms that happen to be associated with a diagnosis of Parkinson's disease offer a rich preview of the consequences when energy is not flowing through one, several or all of the chakras.

How can we revitalize our life force? First, any blockages need to be removed and cleared. Second, specific vibrations that are distorted, missing or muted need to be reactivated.

A variety of approaches are available to reintroduce the frequencies needed by the body to function. One safe, nonintrusive and engaging approach is color therapy.

Arlene Arnold uses complements of colors to remove blockages and reactivate vibrations that have been blocked or distorted. Color complements are positioned opposite one another on the color wheel.

Introduction of the right combination of colors jump starts the energy that is not vibrating just as you might jump start the engine of a car. Listen to my radio show with Arlene on February

16, 2011 to hear a rich explanation and illustration of how she uses color therapy to move energy through the body.

Arlene first asks a client where they feel discomfort in their body. If, for example, their knee is hurting, she has you bring to consciousness red (which is connected to the knee) and green (which is its color complement). Arlene then helps her clients shift the blocked energy (which in this case is causing pain in the knee) using a breathing technique combined with a visualization of specific colors (in this example - red and green). She also works in pairs of colors to shift the vibrations that are stuck or distorted.

You may be thinking - how can such a simplistic approach really help me find relief from my symptoms? My spin on this criticism is simple. Simple therapies are the ones that provide the biggest bang. Want to feel better? Breath. Drink more water. Move. Hang out with your friends. You will feel 50% better (if not 90% better). Everything I just listed is simple and free.

Don't some colors feel good to you? Healing is all about embracing the full spectrum of frequencies. Each color is tied to a specific frequency. You can use colors to shift the frequencies that need adjustment or revitalize the frequencies that are dormant. Arlene offers an inexpensive course on the internet where you can learn how to use colors to heal yourself. Visit her website for more information http://www.thepowerofcolor.com

Still not convinced? Does color therapy still appear too simplistic and implausible as a viable therapy for you? Check out this 2 minute You Tube video that shows a dramatic improvement in a man's dyskinesia when he simply looks at a blue colored sheet or wears blue tinted glasses. The shift is remarkable. You don't need to put colored lenses on to see the immediate results in this video.

http://www.youtube.com/watch?v=OrcO2oRv75I

Why not experiment with color therapy as a way to get back into the natural, healthy flow of life? Wear glasses with different colors and see which ones help. No harm can be done. The only possible outcome is improved health on some level.

OPTOMETRY

What do glasses, prisms and color have to do with Parkinson's disease? Dr. Janet Kohtz, a Neuro Optometrist, has found that glasses and neuro-rehabilitation therapy can help reverse the symptoms of Parkinsons Disease. During my radio show interview with her January 18, 2012, Dr. Kohtz reported that her patients had been able to adjust their posture, balance and gait. They even freed themselves from walkers after being fitted with glasses specifically configured to address their current limitations. Glasses with prisms extend the range of sight which is

© 2013 Parkinsons Recovery

restricted in many persons with Parkinson's symptoms. Use of certain colors in glasses can also be extremely useful.

In my opinion, optometry therapy (while unknown to many) is a viable option especially for persons who are currently having difficulty walking. If you cannot move with ease, exercise in any form is problematic. If you cannot exercise, the chances of reversing your symptoms are poor.

What if being fitted with special prescription glasses facilitates the ease with which you can walk, run and play? Is it possible that by simply wearing classes the opportunity for regular exercise can become immediately available? Dr. Kohtz has convinced me that the answer to these questions is yes. Isn't that exciting news?

The best news of all is that you do not have to wait to see if optometry therapy can help! Once you put on the glasses which have been prescribed, you will know! For further information about how neuro-rehabilitation therapy can help reverse Parkinson's symptoms, visit Dr. Kohtz's website at www.optometrists.org/Riverside.

PHYSICAL THERAPY

Kevin Lockette is a physical therapist from Hawaii who has produced a dynamite DVD for people with the symptoms of Parkinsons called Move It. His groundbreaking DVD contains marvelous strategies that can help anyone whose mobility is currently challenged to get back on track.

Kevin was my guest on my radio show June 10, 2010. The following is an excerpt from my interview with Kevin who emphasized the importance of posture.

POSTURE

"Posture plays a very important role. I really focus on the postural muscles and try to keep people upright as much as possible. My experience has been that the stronger your postural muscles are (hip extensors, upper back muscles) the less likely that freezing episodes will happen.

A lot of times it is when your center of gravity gets so far advanced in front of you that it triggers a lot of the freezing. If I can help people train their postural muscles, then they can avoid a lot of the issues with freezing.

My experience has been – once the posture starts going down – a typical posture you might see with Parkinsons is:

- *Your knees are bent*

© 2013 Parkinsons Recovery

- *Your hips are bent*

- *Your shoulders are rounded and forward*

That posture feeds into the Parkinsons symptoms. A lot of times this posture will trigger the freezing or difficulty with walking which is known as a festinating gait or shuffling type of gait. You are basically trying to keep up with your center of gravity. If you stop you may fall.

One very young patient who has Parkinsons would get going and literally run into the wall (or some structure that was stable) to right herself because she could not stop. If you can keep your center of gravity and have your postural muscles strong you will have that tool to hopefully avoid the episodes.

BALANCE AND MOBILITY

Physical therapist Cynthia Gibson-Horn has invented a novel method for improving balance and mobility using the strategic placement of weights on the torso. She calls her invention Balance-Based Torso-Weighting (BBTW). The BBTW method assesses the directional instabilities which are causing difficulties with being able to walk and maintain good balance. These assessments often detect a twisting of the torso which is why the placement of weights has proved beneficial. Once the weights are placed strategically on the person's torso, Cynthia has been successful in providing improvements in people with Parkinson's symptoms who have difficulties with balance and mobility. Cynthia explains the BBTW method during my radio show April 4, 2012. For more information, visit: www.motiontherapeutics.com

Physical Therapist Lisa Brown recommends people stay as active as possible:

"I think the most important thing would be to stay as mobile as you possibly can and engage in activities that are something you enjoy. One thing that can be hard is that if I give you a specific exercise program but you are not interested in it – you are not going to keep up with it. Find activities that you enjoy, whether it is a walking group or going to a local gym or a yoga class or a Pilates class or some type of a community facility where you can go to for exercises."

HERBS

Herbalist Andrew Bentley, one of the Pioneers of Recovery, discusses the specific use of herbs that have provided relief from the symptoms of his clients who have Parkinsons.

"There are certain things that are fundamentally helpful with getting the nervous system to repair itself. One of the things I use in that capacity is an herb called Bacopa. Bacopa comes to us from the traditional medicine of India. As such it has a very long

© 2013 Parkinsons Recovery

documented history of use for helping the nervous system repair itself. That can sometimes help. There are a few other herbs that help along those same lines that help with actually physically repairing the tissue in the nervous system. There are others ones that help to change the chemistry of the nervous system.

A good example of that is Barley Malt Extract. It is a particular extract prepared from barley malt that contains a substance called Hordenine which has a very strong effect on the dopamine pathways in the brain. If someone were taking dopamine or Levodopa I probably would not use that herb. It might increase the amount of those or decrease the clearance of those substances because then you start seeing things which are not really the goal. It depends on a lot of things but definitely the presenting symptoms are a very big factor in choosing which herbs to choose.

There are some other things that may help on a more symptomatic level or help more with the peripheral nervous system. For example, Oat Straw extract helps to calm the tremors that most people have. Valerian can also be helpful in that capacity sometimes.

There are several different categories of herbs that help with different functions and different structures in the body and in the nervous system. In each of those categories there are many different herbs that might be helpful depending on the particular individual.

As far as rigidity goes, one of my favorite things for that is an herb called Artemisia or sometimes it is called wormwood. That is a herb that helps the mechanism by which the nerve impulses are transmitted in the body. It is very good for rigidity of all sorts including what sometimes accompanies Parkinsons."

Andrew Bentley

One of the issues many people with Parkinson's symptoms confront is an exhausted adrenal system. Adrenals are the small organs located on top of the kidneys which secret hormones such as adrenaline. When a person sets the engine of their body in overdrive most of the time, their adrenals will eventually become exhausted. One herb which is used to sooth the adrenals is licorice root which you can readily find in a tea.

I hear encouraging reports from people who have been taking the herb Mucuna. Some people use Mucuna as their primary treatment. Others use Mucuna in conjunction with Parkinson's medications under the close supervision of their doctor. The word "on the street" is that Mucuna seems to help traditional medications last longer and reduce the dose that is needed to relieve symptoms.

Mucuna is an Ayurvedic herb that is also known as velvet bean or cowhage. It is a natural herb that grows over 15 meters in length. Mucuna bears white, lavender or purple flowers with pods that hang in long, dangling clusters. The seeds are shiny black or brown in color. Mucuna is found primarily in tropical regions of the world.

Mucuna seeds contain high concentrations of levodopa which is a direct precursor of the neurotransmitter dopamine. People who have Parkinsons are deficient in dopamine relative to the other neurotransmitters. Dopamine does not cross the blood-brain barrier and therefore cannot be used directly as a treatment. However, levodopa does gain access to the brain where it is converted to dopamine.

I have a warning for those of you who are motivated to search for more information about Mucuna on the internet. Mucuna is also an aphrodisiac. It is widely promoted on sexual enhancement websites. Dopamine has a profound influence on sexual function, mood and movement. It increases libido in both men and women because of its dopamine inducing properties.

Mucuna has been used for generations as a remedy for Parkinsons in Ayurvedic Indian medicine. In large amounts it has been shown to be as effective as pure Levodopa in the treatment of Parkinson's disease. Mucuna also has antioxidant properties which are helpful in repairing damage to neural tissues.

Herbalist Andrew Bentley does not prescribe Mucuna to his patients. Why? He has been unable to identify a reliable source for Mucuna. Herbs that grow naturally in the wild have the most potency. Andrew harvests most of the herbs he prescribes himself or he obtains them from sources that he knows harvest the herbs in the wild. When grown commercially, the herbs just don't cut the cake and Andrew never considers using them.

I receive frequent questions from people asking about a reliable source of Mucuna. Several people have told me that they received Mucuna from a source that was working for a year or so, but when receiving a new batch in the mail, the Mucuna had literally no effect. It was like swallowing a sugar tablet.

Andrew explained to me this is very common. Commercial sources of Mucuna (and other herbs) are usually unreliable. Some people I have interviewed made it a hobby to grow and harvest Mucuna in their backyards.

Needless to say, Mucuna is not a "cure" nor should it be used without the close supervision of a doctor. The good news is that it is an entirely natural alternative to traditional medications and offers hope that symptoms can be relieved.

UPSIDE AND DOWN SIDE OF MUCUNA

There is an upside and a downside to taking Mucuna to treat the symptoms of Parkinsons.

THE UPSIDE

Mucuna bean (or Mucuna Pruriens) is derived from a plant that grows in tropical climates. The Mucuna herb has been used for generations in India and other eastern countries to treat Parkinsons with varying success. Mucuna is by no means a new revelation.

People use Mucuna in part because it does not have the side effects of prescription medications. Several volunteers from the Portland Parkinsons Energy Project who do not take prescribed medications for Parkinsons have been pleased with the results they get from taking Mucuna. Other people have been able to reduce the dose of their prescribed medications or even wean themselves off medications altogether.

Research on the effectiveness on Mucuna is encouraging, but everyone responds differently of course. No changes in the dosage of prescription medications should of course be made without consulting with your doctor first. Even though it is not a prescription medication, it is just as important to consult with your doctor before taking any natural herb supplement like Mucuna. It may be natural, but it is still a medicine.

THE DOWNSIDE

It is clear from talking with other health professionals that Mucuna is not a cure nor does it provide relief for everyone. After all, if Mucuna were a panacea everyone with Parkinsons would be taking it and no one today would be suffering from its symptoms.

Many people think of Parkinsons simplistically as a deficiency of dopamine. In fact, the "disease" is described by most health care providers as such. The truth of the matter is that reasons for the symptoms of Parkinsons are far, far more complicated than this.

Symptoms of Parkinsons are aggravated by an imbalance of over 39 different neurotransmitters. When you take Mucuna (or any dopamine supplement for that matter) you are making a decision to focus on only a tiny fraction of the problem.

The body is making fine adjustments to the production and distribution of hormones continuously, second by second, minute by minute. Consider the maze of complicated adjustments your body makes to produce and distribute the other 38 neurotransmitters when you take any dopamine lookalike.

Ingesting a single synthetic hormone once a day creates an instant imbalance. The body is challenged with the task of re-balancing all the other 38 hormones that must be continuously

© 2013 Parkinsons Recovery

manufactured and distributed to the tissues. The "adjustment" that comes from taking a dopamine supplement is crude.

Mucuna is taken once or twice a day. The body produces and distributes hormones continuously each and every second of the day. Do the math. The difference is mind-boggling. If the choice is between the body and Mucuna I am betting on the body any day of the week.

A second challenge you will encounter if you decide to take Mucuna - and keep in mind this may be a good choice for you - is that you are giving your body the signal it does not need to produce dopamine on its own. Think like your body and you will understand the long term consequences of what happens when you take a dopamine producing supplement like Mucuna.

Here is the decision sequence: Your body is busy with the work of adjusting and balancing hormones which, after all, is one of its important jobs. Mucuna mysteriously appears in the digestive system. There is suddenly and unexpectedly an external intrusion into the body. The body begins to ponder:

> *"Who is in charge here?"*

A critical function of the body is suddenly and unexpectedly being handled by someone else. The mind then says to itself:

> *"If someone else is doing my job, why should I bother?"*

Isn't this just what you do when someone else begins doing the job you thought was your responsibility?

A reason that cells in the substantia nigra die is because dopamine is being supplied by an external source. Cells that produce dopamine are no longer needed. You either use it or lose it. In this case you lose it. The body eventually surrenders responsibility for producing dopamine.

John Coleman, ND points out that most of the Mucuna bean that is packaged and sold in the marketplace is not actually "natural." It is processed. The Mucuna pill capsules are manufactured and refined, purified and converted to powder.

John Coleman has also observed in his clinic that Mucuna can induce the "same adverse effects as synthetic levodopa if consumed in large quantities over a long period. Coleman has a different recommendation for his clients. He suggests you hydrate your body by taking a natural homeopathic remedy called the Aquas (www.aquas4life.com). The body has an easier time producing and balancing hormones when the cells are adequately hydrated.

Mucuna may provide welcome relief in the short term. But if it is used as a lifetime remedy your body's intricate system for monitoring hormones will be short circuited. Sensitivity of the monitoring system is degraded and the system itself is eventually disabled.

Your body gradually gives up its charge at birth to maintain health and wellness. You eventually begin to feel lousy. Your health deteriorates.

Why not give your body a chance to do its work whenever possible? Wait. Be patient. Acknowledge to yourself that you will not necessarily feel good every day. Accept the reality that some days you will likely feel lousy. Helping the body re-remember how to balance hormones is not an easy task but the rewards are worth it.

Fava Beans

Many foods help to provide relief from the symptoms of Parkinsons, but fava beans are of particular interest. They are a staple throughout much of the world, especially in the Mediterranean, though fava beans are not well accepted in the western world.

Fava beans grow in pods much like green beans and are a food that has been around for thousands of years. The bean pods are clearly most effective when they are very young and green, even before a string like fiber forms along the pod.

You can eat the beans after steaming them or boiling them in water. Of course, you can add the seasonings like sea salt, butter or herbs. The best effect comes from eating fava beans that are green and fresh. Some people like eating the shells. Or, you can grind them up, add them to other foods or beverages or take them like a pill.

The resident expert on fava beans in my book of experts is Aunt Bean from Tennessee who I interviewed on my radio show February 4, 2010. She says that fava bean sprouts are the best way to get l-dopa supplementation. Here is her method of sprouting fava beans:

> *You just soak the beans overnight (about a 1/2 Cup in a bowl). In the morning drain & rinse them well. Drain them well and cover with a paper towel to keep light out. Rinse and drain well 3 times a day until they start to sprout. It only takes about 3 days. Then rinse well and let them stand in water about 15 minutes to soften the skins.*

> *Drain & remove the skins. Rinse well again. Then put into a steamer (beans not in water) & steam covered for 6 minutes after the water starts boiling good. Remove from steam. Rinse with cold water. Dry. Put on a plate or cookie sheet in a single layer to freeze. Then after about 45 minutes put in a plastic freezer zip lock and freeze until needed.*

> *Experiment with eating 2 or 3 every couple of hours or/ just in the in between times when you are not taking meds...everyone is so different & so are the doses of meds &*

time schedules and activity levels...you will have to find your own dose amount and how often to take them. Always start with a small amount as with any medicine...They are medicine...just a natural whole food medicine for us.

Also, remember to have a G6 PD blood test done to make sure you are ok to take them (having the right enzymes necessary, or they can hurt you!) Also, ask your physician if you are on any MAOI's. Fava bean supplementing can cause a quick and dangerous rise in blood pressure when mixed with these drugs. Let your doctor know, so they can work with you and be aware of your experimenting!

Goya Favas usually sprout well. If you wish to cook dry fava beans: Soak them overnight to hydrate them. Then rinse well in the morning and put in clean water and cook until tender. After they are cooked, they taste great stir fried with garlic & onion.

Alternatively, you can boil or steam them till they are tender. Add them to salads. The longer they are cooked, the less dopamine enhancing value they will have. Here is how Aunt Bean prepares them:

I have found that picking the immature pods at about 2 1/2 inches is the best for us. They have a great buttery taste and no strings. We steam them for about 6 minutes, then freeze them on cookie sheets for about 15 minutes, then place them in freezer bags and return them to the freezer. My friend enjoys them the right from the freezer...2-4 pods with her Sinemet dose.

Bean chips & cookies were made by putting large favas (past the stage of eating the pod) through a Champion Juicer, which takes out all the indigestible fiber and using that juice to make tasty l-dopa treats. We keep our "treats" frozen and use them to ward off symptoms. They are great also for car trips, just to carry along if needed. The possibilities are endless.

Fava bean pods have a tough outer skin so it takes time, focus and commitment to harvest the little green beans which look a lot like limas. They are bitter in taste and have an aftertaste, two characteristics which are not appealing to people who love their sweets.

Favas are as popular in the Mediterranean as grits are in the South (of the US). People in the Mediterranean do not eat grits. People from the South do not eat fava beans, unless they have the symptoms of Parkinsons.

Beans of the fava plant contain levodopa, the medicine contained in the Parkinsons medication known as Sinemet. The leaves, stems and pods of the fava plant also contain levodopa. I am told some people juice the entire plant.

Aunt Bean cuts the tips of the leaves of Fava Beans she grows on her farm in Tennessee and places them in alcohol for 6 weeks to make a tincture. When she begins to shake, she places a drop of her tincture under her tongue. Presto. Her tremor vanishes.

Her tincture is not for sale – at least not yet! You can contact Sandra through her blog and learn from her about how you too can grow fava beans in your own backyard:

http://www.favabeans.parkinsonsrecovery.com

I have talked with a number of people who grow and harvest their own fava beans in their backyards. It is a fun and engaging hobby which has a much appreciated side effect: relief from symptoms when they harvest and eat their own beans.

ESSENTIAL OILS

Have you considered using essential oils? They are a yummy application of aromatherapy that helps you cozy up to the sweetness and purity of your much underappreciated life force. You can apply them yourself or ask a spouse, partner or friend to help.

Essential oils are a pleasure to experience. Pleasure is the signal your body needs to make more hormones like dopamine, serotonin and melatonin. It doesn't get better than that. You get the double benefit of pleasure and more dopamine.

Allergic reactions and side effects from using essential oils are rare. Their use is generally reported to be safe because they are a product that is derived from nature. Check with your doctor or nutritional counselor before using them to make sure that there will be no adverse interaction with any medications or supplements you currently take.

Essential oils provide nourishment to the body. It doesn't matter if you can smell them or not. The will have an effect whether your olfactory organs are up and running or if they are on vacation this week.

Why are essential oils effective? There is certainly a long and complicated explanation of the chemical reactions that subdue the symptoms for each oil. I suppose could write a series of books about the value of each essential oil, but that would be a silly waste of time.

Why? Essential oils help people with Parkinsons. Will they help you? Who knows, but why not give them a trial run?

They are relatively inexpensive, noninvasive and a joy to use. The symptoms of Parkinsons are not likely to clear with a single application of essential oils but people do report immediate, though temporary relief.

© 2013 Parkinsons Recovery

Which oils should you use? It depends on your symptoms! Jean Oswald, RN in Pioneers of Recovery discusses her own challenge with insomnia:

> "There are many causes of insomnia as well, so there are many options in essential oils: Lavender comes to mind of course, but so does Roman Chamomile and Valerian.
>
> There is a new essential oil blend that Young Living made last year combining Ruta, from the rainforest in Ecuador, with Valerian and Lavender and they call it RutaVaLa[13]. This oil has helped me fall asleep better than any other and I sleep soundly! Sometimes I use that Citrus Blend called Peace & Calming or the Lavender for a long time and find that I need to make a switch. I have a variety of oils to choose from".

Jean Oswald discusses a variety of options for specific symptoms in Pioneers of Recovery. Jean Oswald offers consultations. You can reach her at 1-585-872-6242; e-mail: jean@compassionateconsulting.net

Gary Young from Young Living Essential Oils invented a new technique in 2008 that is specifically helpful to people with neurological challenges he calls Neuroauricular (pronounced nor- i- cu- lar) or NAT. A technique that uses six essential oils, NAT has been used with great success with persons who have the symptoms of Parkinsons.

NAT uses 6 oils and can easily be applied by a lay person. One man's wife reported to Jean that she "has her husband back" after doing the NAT technique for about 2 and a half months. Her husband has Parkinson's symptoms. Aroma therapist and nurse Jean Oswald also talks about which essential oils can be used to treat Parkinsons symptoms on my radio show which aired September 17, 2009.

More detailed experiences with essential oils are reported next by Joachim, Eleanor and Leslie. Although there are vast differences in the type of essential oils used by each individual, they all are experiencing wonderful benefits.

JOACHIM'S PROTOCOL

> 1. Valor - left foot and left side of body from head to hip.
>
> Take 4 drops of each oil for neck and feet – start on the right side –always three times
>
> 2. Frankincense
>
> 3. Cedarwood

---

[13] **RutaVaLa promotes relaxation of the body and mind. It helps ease tension and relieve stress. The blend helps overcome negative feelings while encouraging a positive attitude and comfort.**

4. *Vetiver*

5. *Sandalwood*

6. *Melissa –for oxygen*

7. *Geranium*

8. *Peppermint*

ELEANOR'S STORY

"*I've been diagnosed as having Parkinson's disease. This is a very scary thing to happen when one has always been extremely healthy and independent.*

I began looking for alternative health methods to augment the traditional medicine. I tried many things -- too numerous to recite! Then along came Young Living Essential Oils, and they have made a tremendous difference to me. I say, "Young Living allows me to live again"!

In May of 1999, my two sisters came from northern Maine to central Massachusetts. They did Raindrop Technique on me for each of the four days they were here. They started me on the following supplements:

The Cleansing Trio (Comfortone, I.C.P., Megazyme – now called Essentialzyme), Sulfurzyme, and Thyromin, then more slowly we added VitaGreen, Master Hers, Chelex, and Be Fit. I also began with Power Meal and Body Balance.

The initial oils I used were: Valor, vitex, frankincense, lavender, along with the Raindrop oils. Since that time I've added: Helichrysum, Brain Power, geranium, M-Grain, Roman Chamomile, 3 Wise Men, Magnify Your Purpose, Release, Idaho Tansy, Joy, Harmony, Clarity, bergamot, tangerine, orange, lemon -- whatever I think may help with my liver, nerve regeneration, etc. It seems during some periods of time, I intuitively use some combinations, at other times other oils.

I put the oils on the bottom of my feet, on my brainstem (back of neck), behind my ears, on my temples. I inhale the oils from the bottle, diffuse them in my home with Young Living's diffuser, I spray our bed with floral waters and I add lemon/grapefruit to my drinking water. I love them all -- and buy as many as I can afford each month.

I also do weekly sessions of deep muscle massage, reflexology, and the Young Living oils. My therapist is now a firm believer in the power of these oils, which definitely complement her work.

© 2013 Parkinsons Recovery

A few of the differences that I see since last May when I began are: my energy level has improved so much (before I had none); my arm tremors are a bit quieter, but sometimes still there; I have hope again!"

LESLIE'S REPORT

I have received requests to elaborate on what my father-in-law (who has Parkinsons) is doing for his health regimen.....

He uses the whole Essential 7 kit each for various reasons mainly for the nutritional value ... his body has been depleted of nutrition for so long that he needs help to get the value from his food and water.

He has been using Frankincense to help with building his immune system and to help with depression ......this is being very effective.

Thieves to build his immune system... and this is helping to stop the aching in his mouth from rotting teeth... he really needs to get the rest of them pulled out ......he can't use the Thieves inside his mouth because it is too hot for him ...so he uses it on the outside of his cheek and gets fantastic results ..no more pain... within a few seconds.

M-Grain for headaches and helps him with aches and pains ... he gets really tired and sore from shaking all the time.

> *RC helps him with breathing and he just likes the smell of it!!*

> *Acceptance helps him to come to a place where it is ok just to be him!*

There are many other oils he uses too and this would get too long to describe each one so here is a list:

- *Sage*
- *Clarity*
- *Valor*
- *Marjoram*

He has just started to use the Vitex so I have not yet seen a marked change in his shaking but there are so many things that effect persons with Parkinsons that we are very patient and we know that he did not get Parkinsons overnight and we do not expect a miracle cure ....any relief is a miracle in itself!

Dad has never had a winter (in the 8 years I have known him) where he was not very sick with the flu or depression......until this year he has had one cold and it was not too severe ...he is not suffering with his chronic depression (which he has had for 20 years) and I would say he is happy to be on the planet!! The Essential Oils have been the best thing that has ever happened to Dad!!

BACH FLOWER ESSENCES

The following is an explanation from Allan who found using Bach Flower essences offered him relief from the symptoms of Parkinsons.

"For those who might have questions, the Bach flower essences affect the emotions only with no guarantee that physical healing will result. It was Edward Bach's genius to notice that one's emotional disposition has a lot to do with the course of physical healing."

"This was observed when two people would have the same disease or two returning British soldiers would come back from WW I with the same type of injury. One would heal easily and rapidly; the other would have a difficult time in the healing of the same problem! Bach took his research into the emotional dimension of his patients to try to help those who had difficulty in healing. I am grateful to him."

AQUAS

Naturopath John Coleman, ND recommends that his Parkinsons patients take Aquas, a homeopathic remedy originally developed to reverse the problem of dehydration for marathon runners. John Carlin, a bicyclist who was diagnosed with Parkinsons in 2003, has a simple though eloquent explanation of how the Aquas work.

"The Aquas are a formula that helps get the water out of your gut into your system faster and then from your system to your cells faster. It also has a detoxifying effect. The only thing I can say is that I have seen the results in person.

It was meant to be a hydrator for shall we say well people, marathoners...It is a homeopathic hydration therapy of sorts. It doesn't cross with any of your meds. I am taking three.

My neurologist said I do not know what you are doing, but keep doing it because it is helping you on a daily basis."

I began taking the *Aquas* myself three years ago and also experienced positive results. Since there was no direct source of Aquas in the western hemisphere I collaborated with Leonie Hibbert, a developer of the Aquas, to establish a website at http://www.Aquas4life.com in

© 2013 Parkinsons Recovery

2007 so people living in the west could obtain them. The Aquas are approved by Australia's *Therapeutic Goods Administration*, the Australian equivalent of the *FDA* in the US. John continues to tell me that the *Aquas* made a huge difference to his own recovery and continue to make a difference to the recovery of his patients.

OIL MASSAGE

What follows are author and nutritional Counselor Dorit's suggestions for oil massage conveyed to me during my radio show June 3, 2010.

> *"Oil massage is very calming to the mind and nurturing to the heart and strengthening to the bones and nerves. This should be done on a daily basis right after you have your bath. This is another way you can apply food which is in the form of sesame or almond oil. It is great for people with Parkinsons. You can supply it into your body without having to eat and digest it. If your system is off that day make yourself a massage with oils.*
>
> *Everybody should have an oil massage on a regular basis every day after taking a shower, including those who are experiencing the symptoms of Parkinsons. You should definitely make this a part of your treatment. This is one of the ways to get those foods into your body.*
>
> *The oil should always be applied warm though. They should be left on for some time for proper absorption, just like the food needs to stay inside your digestive system for proper absorption. The skin is our largest organ. The skin will take it in. Afterwards when you apply the oil you can always take a shower or steam bath to remove the excess oil if you want. Keep it on for at least 15 -30 minutes. To make this easier, try a powder like calamus to absorb the excess oil, then rub off the power if you wish to. You can use sesame oil, coconut oil, mustard oil.*
>
> ***Sesame oil*** *is specific for removing toxins from the body. If you find that you are very stimulated and you are very frantic, sesame oil is very grounding and nurturing to the mind. It can also be applied to the head, to the hair, the back or the feet in order to calm the nerves as well, particularly in the evening before going to bed. Again, this can all be left on for at least 15 minutes. If you do not wish to keep it on, then wash it off in a warm shower. For all people suffering from pain and anxiety regular sesame oil massage is a must. It is much better than actually eating it in your foods.*
>
> ***Coconut oil***. *You have probably heard a lot of nonsense about coconut oil not being great for us, but it is not true. Raw coconut oil is cooling and calming to the mind and especially to the nerves and the skin. There is a certain herb called Brahmi also known as gotu kola that can be prepared with coconut oil as well, then applied to the head, hair,*

© 2013 Parkinsons Recovery

and the sensory openings like the ear drums and the nostrils as well as used as a general massage oil.

Mustard oil. *You have to be careful with mustard oil. It must be organic mustard oil. It can actually be toxic if it is not organic. It is very warming and stimulating and improves circulation. It particularly helps clear the channels of the lungs and the head. It is excellent for mental dullness and depression and used a lot in India for these conditions. It can be used as a general massage oil or massage to cover regions like the lungs especially in the winter time. For those of you who say:*

> *'I am trying to eat these raw foods but I am just too cold'*

This is what you do instead. Warm the oils. Use them on your skin. You eat the food raw inside of you."

PRESCRIPTION DRUGS

How many side effects do you experience because you are taking a particular drug? Of course there is no sure way to sort this all out. You can however get some hints about what might be happening. How? Get the pharmacy information sheet on the drug you take. Read the side effects. Are you experiencing any of the side effects that are listed?

Guess what. Some of your symptoms may be directly caused by the drug you take. For some people, the side effects of the drug (or drugs) they take can be worse than the symptoms of Parkinsons itself.

Parkinson's drugs can clearly help people in the short term. Some people have told me that prescription medications literally saved their lives. The sad news is that the research literature is clear on one point. The effects of most Parkinson's drugs begin to wear off after several years or less. A stronger and stronger dose of the drug has to be taken in order to have symptom relief.

There are consequences to taking higher doses. As you take more of the drug each day, you add more chemicals and substances to your body that need to be eliminated. The kidneys become challenged. The liver is taxed. The volume of chemicals and toxins in the body eventually become so great they cannot all be eliminated.

Chinese medicine describes the symptoms of Parkinsons of stiffness, tremors, freezing and numbness in the limbs as a liver-wind condition. There is a depletion of Yin (the feminine energy that invites us to receive and be nourished) juxtaposed to an overabundance of Yang energy (the masculine energy that takes action and makes things happen in the world). Persons

© 2013 Parkinsons Recovery

currently experiencing the symptoms of Parkinsons are often movers and shakers of the world who find it extremely challenging to chill out and receive from others.

From a Chinese medicine mindset, Parkinson's symptoms imply that the liver is compromised. Some people with Parkinson's prefer to pursue natural therapies because they anticipate prescription medicines will further degrade the function of their liver.

Toxins accumulate in the cells of the body, more and more each day. The cells can no longer eliminate all of the waste that is deposited.

-        *More and more cells die.*

-        *Fewer and fewer cells are born.*

-        *You feel worse.*

-        *And worse.*

-        *Unhealthy cells eventually outnumber the healthy cells.*

You find yourself saying to your friends.

>   *Perhaps my time on earth is about to end."*

You get totally frustrated. A bold decision is made.

>   *"I am going to stop taking my drugs today. Cold turkey is the only way. It works for alcoholics. It will surely work for me."*

A courageous decision? To be sure. Smart? The only gentle way to say this is - No. The decision to go cold turkey is actually very stupid.

Most drugs for any disease (including Parkinsons) have a strong addictive character to them. You cannot just stop taking the drug one day and expect to feel better the next. You will likely pay serious consequences if you stop taking a prescribed drug.

You can experience very painful withdrawal symptoms. For some people the withdrawal symptoms are similar to what a drug addict experiences. People who stop taking their drugs all at once can wind up having to take a stronger dose later. In the end nothing is accomplished other than having to experience discomfort, pain and frustration.

If you do decide to reduce the dose of any drugs you are taking, do so only in close collaboration with your medical doctor. A program to reduce dosage will take a very long time - months and sometimes years.

© 2013 Parkinsons Recovery

You can reduce the dosage very slowly if you give your body the nutrition it needs and if your body is adequately hydrated. Good luck with whatever you decide.

The most encouraging news I have heard in response to this question comes from John Coleman, ND. Here is John's answer to the question "Has anyone improved enough to discontinue Sinemet?" in his own words.

> "*I chose not to take any western medication during my journey. There were a number of reasons for that, mainly around the way doctors treated me. But that was my choice, and I'm glad of it.*"

> "*However, all my clients who have recovered were taking western medication (Sinemet, Madopar, and/or others) until they got better. The first was taking around 1500 mg of levodopa per day, and gradually weaned himself of it over two years. Another was on Sinemet 100/25 three times daily and reduced that to 0 over about 18 months. Another was on Madopar and went cold turkey (I don't advise that) after three years or so and has stayed well. Others have started on high medication and reduced to very low doses while they still work towards recovery.*"

> "*I saw a client this week who just gave up Sinemet in January because he didn't like the way it made him feel. He is a little stiffer without it, but feels better in himself and has more energy to work towards wellness. He is improving in health steadily.*"

At Parkinsons Recovery we are hearing more and more stories from people who have successfully reduced the dose of the medications they have been taking under the close supervision of their doctor. If you are interested in learning how the dose of a prescription medication can be reduced, be sure and listen to my radio program that features Compounding Pharmacist Randy Mentzer who explains how he helps people reduce the dose of their prescription medications. My radio show interview with Randy aired on March 11, 2010.

Researchers are working on identifying medicines that can switch on (or off) genes that are responsible for sustaining symptoms. Some are enthusiastic about the proposition that Parkinson's symptoms are caused by the accumulation or proteins in the brain. This accumulation, according to their theory, is due to an inactive DJ1 gene. These researchers hope to show in clinical studies that taking a prescription drug known as phenylbutyrate (which has been in use for 30 years and is currently a very expensive medication) will switch on the DJ1 gene and thus reduce the accumulation of proteins in the brain.

© 2013 Parkinsons Recovery

NEURO-LINGUISTIC PROGRAMMING

Carl Buchheit is one of the international leaders in the Neuro-Linguistic Programming movement and one of the Pioneers of Recovery. Below are excerpts from my interview with Carl where he explains what NLP does for people, how it is done and what success he has had with individuals who have the symptoms of Parkinsons.

'NLP is a respective and eloquent change format, a human format, a self discovery format for assisting people to fully respect the experience that they have created for themselves and that they are having, especially when that experience seems to be just about impossible to appreciate or respect.

Properly done what we want to do is to bring the person into a very deep rapport with themselves, with their own creative force, with the larger creative forces that they participate in terms of their own internal world, their identity and their family as well.

We never seek to overcome or defeat anything that is going on within us or within anyone else. All we do is to respect the intended positive that is behind it all, to include it with respect, allow it to transform so that it is producing the experience the person truly wants. Doing NLP change work is a process of coming into deep, deep respect for oneself and for all of the intentions that operate inside us humans though conflicting as they may be.

What we typically find and pay attention to – which we always do when we are dealing with any kind of change working with the NLP model - is as preposterous as this question might sound:

> *'What are the intended positive outcomes of the symptoms, of the illness?'*

We pre-suppose that all experience, all behavior (Parkinsons included) - however difficult - is prompted by some kind of intended positive outcome. Now the question is what version is this, where and when? When people are in such distress with the symptoms it is really difficult to imagine that there could be anything positive trying to happen as I am sure everyone can easily imagine.

What we usually do is ask this first question when we are doing NLP change:

> *'What would you like?'*

That can take two hours to answer obviously or it can take two days. Then we ask:

> *'What will having that do for you?'*

© 2013 Parkinsons Recovery

> *'Is there anything you might lose that you value when you have the outcome that you like?'*
>
> *I have had some experience with people who have shifted their symptoms quite a bit and several other people not at all. So I have a mixed report. I would probably put it at half I am sorry to say or slightly less than half. Maybe 45 to 55 or something like that.*
>
> *The belief system that I have very often found sitting underneath the symptoms of Parkinsons ...is a commitment to or an entanglement with or an apparently unstoppable focus on not having choice about movement. It is opposite of the metaphor of paralysis.*
>
> *The metaphor that we find in Parkinsons is something along the lines of:*
>
> > *'I will never stop moving and you can't make me stop."*

NEUROFEEDBACK

There are two distinct approaches to Neurofeedback, a therapy that is painless and nonintrusive. The first involves training the brain. The second involves resetting the brain's beta band.

TRAINING THE BRAIN

Angela (who was a guest on my radio show October 28, 2010) describes her experience with training her brain to activate new neural pathways:

> *During the first session an EEG (electroencephalogram) was done to determine those parts of my brain that had abnormal brainwave patterns. My dorsolateral prefrontal cortex was deficient in theta wave output. Subsequent sessions (one hour each) involved application of a single electrode at the position on my head corresponding to the dorsolateral prefrontal cortex. I was provided with headphones to listen to the sound of surf while my eyes were closed.*
>
> *Whenever my brain produced Theta waves I could hear the surf; when no theta waves were being produced all I heard was static. At first, I struggled to hear the surf, but later just let my brain do all the work of figuring it out.*

BRAIN RESETS

Resetting the brain involves an innovative approach refined by Jaclyn Gisburne, Ph.D. from Rocky Mountain NeuroAdvantage For a rich and fascinating explanation of her approach, listen to my radio show which aired December 30, 2009. Videos that demonstrate Brain Resets are posted on the Parkinsons Recovery Blog. To watch the videos, visit the Parkinsons Recovery blog [http://www.blog.parkinsonsrecovery.com] and click on the "Neurofeedback" category.

© 2013 Parkinsons Recovery

Here is the approach in a nutshell. Four electrodes are attached to the patient's head. A reading is then taken of the parameters present in the brain. This initial analysis sets the baseline parameters. Once the parameters have been established the patient watches a video game. If their brain shifts outside the parameters that have been set the video game stops. If it is within the established parameters, the video game keeps running. Points are tallied when the video game runs. The brain figures out how to keep the video game running in no time flat.

With Parkinson's, the frequency bands of the brain have become deregulated. Her resets encourage the brain to do what it normally does but with greater flexibility and without the deregulation present. Hard wiring of the brain is reset in a fashion similar to resetting your computer by turning it off and on. You stop doing the deregulated activity and begin doing what the brain is hard wired to do naturally.

When Dr. Gisburne and her colleagues work with persons who currently exhibit the symptoms of Parkinson's, most symptoms are pretty well mitigated. Some symptoms vanish. Tremors stop. Patients regain their strength. Normal sleep patterns return.

Dr. Gisburne has found that everyone with Parkinson's she has treated has had a significant trauma in their life that is related to their symptoms. She says when then the trauma is addressed the person heals.

I like her innovative approach for many reasons. Her approach is noninvasive, safe and effective. You can't beat that combination.

Biophoton therapy

The body emits light in the form of biophotons that contain dense packets of information that hold our history from the moment of conception and the life histories of our ancestors. The intensity of the light that we emit is very dim. It is analogous to seeing the light of a candle twenty miles away, an image that is not possible to see using the human eye or most magnifying devices.

The invention of fiber optics in the 1990's changed everything. This invention made it possible to detect the light that is emitted by the body. When the light does not flow in a straight line it is distorted. This signifies an imbalance somewhere in the body.

Johan Boswinkel, a guest on my radio show September 26, 2012 has invented a neurofeedback device he named the Chiren that tracks all such distortions. His new invention identifies distortions in the light emitted by the body. The person's own light is corrected for these distortions and fed back into the body. This resets the body's ability to recognize problems.

A reason the body does not heal from a chronic illness is that the imbalances that cause the symptoms are not recognized. The body has isolated the problem and placed it in an isolation container of sorts. This is why so many conditions like Parkinsons become chronic and resist reversal.

If the body does not recognize a problem there will be no response to correct it. The body knows precisely what to do to correct an imbalance. It will not take action however when the imbalance (whether an infection or toxin) is not recognized.

Once the body's signaling system has been reset, the body quickly recognizes infections as well as toxins and gets busy releasing them from the body naturally. Light therapy reactivates the body's magical ability to heal itself. There is no diagnosis of a condition. As a neurofeedback device, this approach simply resets the body's natural ability to come back into balance. For more information visit www.biontology.com

ELECTRO-STIMULATION

One factor that impedes recovery from most illnesses is oxidative stress. It becomes problematic at the cellular level when you find yourself stressed and strung out day after day. If oxidative stress settles in for the long run, circulation is inevitably compromised.

One fundamental approach for enhancing circulation throughout the body and reducing oxidative stress at the cellular level is to stimulate the nerve endings with a low level of electrical impulses. Donald Rhodes, MD, has invented an approach using low level electro-stimulation for accomplishing this.

What happens when you stimulate nerve endings in the feet and hands with a very low level frequency? Chemicals are released known as Neuropeptides that stimulate circulation throughout the body. Neuropeptides are small protein-like molecules used by neurons to communicate with each other.

Do you happen to have digestive issues? It is likely that your Neuropeptide reserve is on empty. Do you have pain in your feet or hands? Your nerve endings are probably not receiving the circulation necessary for renewal and regeneration. Are your feet or hands usually cold? You need to heat them up to get better circulation. Moreover, you body probably needs a "fill up" of Neuropeptides.

Dr. Rhodes has developed a machine he has named Vecttor (http://www.vecttor.com) that he tells me is currently being evaluated by the FDA and is approved for use in Europe. Once approved for use in the US a doctor's prescription will be required to use it. Vecttor's wires are attached to the feet and hands. A low level of current stimulates the body's natural production of Neuropeptides.

The stimulation improves circulation which in turn helps to reduce the cellular damage caused by oxidative stress. The basic idea is to get more oxygen to the nerves through better circulation so that the nerves begin communicating more efficiently. Although we have little evidence for persons with Parkinson's symptoms the approach is intriguing because it is natural and has no side effects.

To get the complete details on this new treatment option listen to my radio show with Donald Rhodes which aired on July 20, 2011. The Vecttor machine itself costs in the vicinity of $4,000. While the cost is high, the logic and theory of the therapeutic approach is certainly plausible.

Other less expensive approaches will also facilitate circulation such as acupuncture and acupressure. If you have pain in your hands or feet, see what happens when you shake your hands or feet. Does the temperature rise? Are your hands or feet warmer? If so, circulation may be a key issue for you. Any methods to enhance circulation will help. Knowing that poor circulation is an issue for you will help you find ways to enhance it. Many options are free and always available:

- *Deep breathing*

- *Stimulation of acupuncture meridians*

- *Exercise*

ACUPUNCTURE

Research has shown that acupuncture helps to reverse Parkinson's symptoms, particularly those associated with an impairment of movement. Ease of movement is facilitated when energetic pathways of the various meridians in the body are cleared.

Acupuncturists focus on one point in particular to treat tremors. They call this point on LV3. It is located on the foot's dorsum between the first and second metatarsal bones. Treatment on LV3 addresses liver issues, a factor other researchers have found can be a cause of symptoms for many persons with Parkinsons. While acupuncturists use needles, you can also find relief using self administered acupressure which is a fancy way of saying you can press on the point with your own fingers. You can either find the point on your foot to press or be open to comprehensive foot massages from massage therapists or family members. A foot massage will certainly tap into LV3 even if you have no idea where it is located!

Chinese Scalp Acupuncture (CSA) is a unique therapy that targets specific areas on the scalp to treat Parkinson's symptoms as well as other chronic conditions. It stimulates the cortical area of the brain. By stimulating targeted acupuncture points on the scalp, CSA communicates with the endocrine and neurological systems of the body. Chinese Scalp Acupuncture (CSA) is a noninvasive form of acupuncture, existent in its current form for about one hundred years, that has been shown effective for neurological disorders. Peter Doyle, an acupuncturist who practices Chinese Scalp Acupuncture in New York City, reports encouraging results when working with persons with Parkinsons during my radio show September 12, 2012.

PROCESS WORK

Process work is uniquely suited to making conscious the reasons why a person with the symptoms of Parkinsons might unconsciously not want to heal. It is one (among other) approaches for helping a person transform their unconscious "no – I do not wish to feel better" to a conscious "yes – I am healing myself now."

Psychologist Steven Fenwick, Ph.D. in Pioneers of Recovery describes the rich meaning that is conveyed by symptoms and the various forms process work can take.

> "Symptoms aren't just bad things. Of course on one level they are negative. It's horrible to have a chronic symptom like Parkinsons that you have to deal with. Nobody likes to have those kinds of things happen.
>
> On another level we can look at them as being meaningful in our lives. They have a message to tell us something about ourselves and the way our souls are trying to grow and develop in this life.
>
> As you look at the underlying meaning and purpose of the symptoms, what are they trying to tell you? It is like it has a gift for you. Even though you may hate the symptoms - we all hate symptoms - but even though we hate them and we want them to go away and we do everything we can to make them go away (which is good) we also want to look at what the meaning is.
>
> What is it trying to tell you about your life?
>
> What is it trying to tell you about your life's purpose and meaning?
>
> And as you unfold that and get more in touch with that and express it more in your life, often times the symptoms do get better.
>
> To be whole, you need to let a little of everything in your life that needs to be expressed. Sometimes if those things aren't expressed and are alive, then they come up as dreams

© 2013 Parkinsons Recovery

or they come up as symptoms or they come up as relationship problems or various things in our life.

We try to find what is right for each person. We view people as "process." A process is always changing, moving and unfolding.

It is like a river. So, it's kind of like following the current of a river. The rivers current can take you to different places.

- *Sometimes it takes you into working with movement.*

- *Sometimes it takes you into working with dreams.*

- *Sometimes it takes you into working with visualizing things or doing artwork.*

- *Sometime it takes you into role playing – how to express this in your life with various people.*

There are a lot of different methods that we use. Sometimes we just sit and talk about what's going on."

ENERGY HEALING

Energy healing is perhaps the oldest medical specialty of all. You will find references to energy healing in many of the ancient writings.

Many subspecialties of energy healing have popped up over the past ten years including Reiki, Therapeutic Touch, Breathwork, Pathwork, Zero Balancing, Zen Massage and others. I have experienced them all. I would have never dreamed I would be seeking energy work a decade ago, but today I do not know I could function without it! Each of these therapies has offered me rich insights into who I am, why I am here and where I am going with my life. And, each therapy helped me release stress and trauma that had been trapped deep within the fabric and constitution of my cells.

All forms of energy healing focus on balancing and charging the human energy field. Energy practitioners realign the light and biophotons that stream through the meridians in the body which have been distorted from trauma and stress.

The energy work Deborah Russell is multidimensional and involves a wide range of modalities including energy work, Reiki, craniosacral therapy, medical intuition and intuitive counseling. Visit Zero Point Healers for a more detailed explanation.

© 2013 Parkinsons Recovery

Karl Robb (www.asoftvoice.com) found that Reiki was so helpful to him in offering relief from his symptoms that he and his wife became Reiki practitioners who now provide treatments to others. Karl provided a fascinating discussion of his experience with Reiki on my radio show that aired on March 20, 2012.

For a perspective on a unique form of energy healing called CHORD Therapy. Listen to my radio show with Roni Angel, Ph.D. on August 27, 2009. She is the inventor of CHORD therapy which she now uses in her own private practice. She explains her nonconventional approach in detail during the interview. Roni Angel, Ph.D. has used CHORD therapy successfully on people with chronic illness now for several decades.

WHAT THERAPIES DO NOT HELP

Here is John Coleman's perspective on this question:

> "There were a lot. In general, any form of body work that was firm or hard. Deep tissue massage, sports massage - those sorts of massages – created extra pain. Vigorous therapies like chiropractic and other manipulative therapies also tended to increase my symptoms and create pain."

> "Excessive intake of nutritional supplements tended to have no effect or make me nauseous or simply be a waste of money. I had to be very careful about homeopathic remedies because the normal approach in selecting potencies and frequencies seemed to aggravate me where a very gentle, a very cautious approached worked."

> "Many counseling modalities helped. Psychiatry did not. I am sure there are good psychiatrists out there, but I saw four and none of them helped me at all. Antidepressant therapy did not work."

> "I choose not to take pharmaceuticals, but other forms of herbal, vitamin homeopathic remedies for depression, but I realized I actually was not depressed. I was certainly anxious, but the antidepressant therapies were just no good for me."

> "I needed to be active and proactive in my approach. In general, anything that was too hard, too vigorous, too enthusiastic didn't work, and gentle, cautious, loving therapies worked."

POWER OF THE MIND

Gord Summer exposed me to the power of the mind to reverse the symptoms of Parkinson's at the First Parkinsons Recovery Summit in Vancouver. Gord uses the power of his mind to shift the energy from his "good" side (which exhibits no tremoring) to his "bad" side (where a tremor is evident). The shift takes seconds. The result?

He calms his tremoring to stillness. Preview four videos where Gord demonstrates his ability to calm his tremors using the power of the mind by visiting the Parkinsons Recovery Blog (www.blog.parkinsonsrecovery) and clicking on the category to the left entitled "Power of the Mind." Gord presented workshops on the Power of the Mind at the 2012 Summit in Cincinnati and the 2013 Summit in Santa Fe. The most compelling evidence that demonstrates the power of the mind is to watch a person like Gord with Parkinson's symptoms calm his own tremors.

Research has also demonstrated compelling results for the power of the mind to facilitate unbelievable outcomes. Italian researcher Fabrizio Benedetti gave subjects saline treatments in lieu of their Parkinson's medications. Tremors and stiffness were reduced as documented by brain scans. Other studies generated similar results. University of British Columbia researchers demonstrated using PET scans that the stores of dopamine in the brain increased when subjects given placebos were told they were being given dopamine.

Use the power of your mind to get any result you want. Isn't that cool? No medications are necessary or needed!

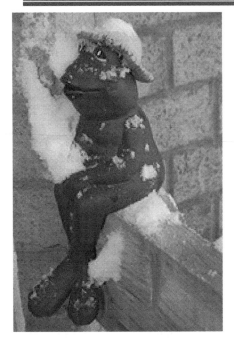

HOW TO DECIDE WHICH THERAPIES TO TRY

Photo by <u>Peter Thompson</u>

There exist so many options ... so many products ... so many supplements ... so many people offering one remedy or another.

- *Where do I turn?*

- *Who do I see?*

- *What precisely do I need to do for myself to feel better?*

It would cost a fortune to purchase all of the supplements on the market that are presumed to help the symptoms of Parkinsons. Worse, your body can not tolerate an overload of too many supplements, herbs or drugs. Taking too many supplements or doing too many therapies may turn out to do more harm than good.

The challenge of determining the essential food your body needs is specific to you and your body. Your body may need more magnesium and calcium. My body may need more protein, vitamin C and vitamin B12. How in the world does anyone figure out what their own body needs?

An option is always to request medical tests. Medical tests are expensive. They are also relevant only to the time and day when they are administered and they are specific to a particular question. For example, is there a depletion or overabundance of magnesium in the body?

© 2013 Parkinsons Recovery

The nutritional needs of your body are also shifting continuously as a function of what you eat. Having an array of tests every week is cost prohibitive. I might also add it is very unpleasant to be poked with a needle.

A decision needs to be made of one type or another. No one can afford to take everything that is suggested by one person or another and your body would not like it if you did.

Do I personally know the answer to this question? No. Does anyone know the answer to this question? Yes. So who is it? I know. I know. You are now thinking to yourself - "Can't this guy get to the point?"

I have four suggestions for you to consider. The first involves getting information from Bioenergetic Testing which can be done by a naturopath doctor. The second involves asking your body for the answer through muscle testing. The third involves a self constructed argument of the two sides of the question. The fourth involves voice profiling. An explanation of each approach follows.

BIOENERGETIC TESTING

I will first explain how a naturopath doctor approaches illness. Then I will explain how Bioenergetic testing is done by a naturopath.

A naturopath investigates the root causes of sickness. They do not treat symptom with temporary bandages. When you seek assistance from a medical doctor because you have a headache, you will most likely be offered a prescription for a drug or herb. With a little luck the treatment works and your headache is temporarily relieved.

Tomorrow is another day. The root cause of the headache is not addressed or considered.

In contrast, naturopath doctors ask the question: Why is this person sick? Why is this person having these symptoms? Symptoms simply relate to something that is presently out of balance in the body. The body is telling us:

> *"Something is not right here. I need to be fixed."*

The pain, the discomfort, the impairment of function sets off an alarm.

Not all naturopaths use Bioenergetic Testing but I personally believe that they are a key diagnostic tool of the future. Naturopath doctor <u>Ivy Faber, ND</u> has been using Bioenergetic testing for 20 years and has been getting unbelievable results with her patients.

Bioenergetic Testing does not generate a diagnosis of an illness like Parkinsons. Naturopaths like <u>Ivy Faber</u> use bioenergetic testing because it targets the root causes of the imbalances. The

© 2013 Parkinsons Recovery

intent of the test is not to diagnose and treat a disease which is how medical doctors approach illness. Here is what Ivy Faber has to say about Bioenergetic Testing:

> "What I like about Bioenergetic Testing is that it looks at toxicity on a cellular level. It doesn't matter if it is not in the blood. We see many people who have great blood tests. Everything is normal. They have gone through every test, yet they are sick. This test looks at things from a cellular standpoint...Other testing may not show it.
>
> We can identify toxicity. We can identify allergies. We can identify hormonal imbalances. We can identify nutritional imbalances. This test has the ability to test for 18,000 different scenarios. It is a great way to get information and have guidance as to what is going to work.
>
> It is a frequency generated program. Basically, everything in the program is in there via the frequency that it relates to. Let's say, parasites. Every parasite exudes or releases a certain energy which enters our body if we come in contact with it. If you have a frequency for that parasite, the body is going to say -
>
> 'Yes. I got that'.
>
> Also, in another way, when there is a deficiency, another part of the test is utilized where it says:
>
> 'Oh - I need that. I am deficient here.'

Ivy Faber, ND has been using this test for many years as her only diagnostic tool. She summarizes the potential contribution of the test quite succinctly:

> 'You will get the biggest bang for your buck with this test."

I personally began using Bioenergetic Testing ten years ago after my dermatologist at the University of Kentucky was unable to provide any relief from a persistent rash. I was astounded at the specifics of the report which Ivy Faber generated for me from the test.

I received a very detailed report about organs in my body that were compromised, names of toxins that had invaded my tissues, names of bacteria and viruses that were having a party at the expense of my health, the location of infected teeth that were causing a systemic infection, the source of hormonal imbalances and information about other systems in my body that were compromised. The test generates very specific results because it uses frequencies to detect the source of the imbalances.

If you do not take action to correct the imbalances, the test gives you a rich idea of the illnesses you can soon expect to confront. My reaction after seeing the results of my first test ten years

© 2013 Parkinsons Recovery

ago was to wonder why I was still alive. I like using the test for myself because no matter what the results reveal, I can always take action to put all of my systems back into balance.

Nothing is "progressive" or "degenerative." The body just needs a little loving care and attention to come back into balance. We just have to start paying a little closer attention to what our bodies are telling us.

Ask Your Body

Your body knows the answer to what action you should take. Look in the mirror, the answer is literally staring you in the face.

OK, you are probably thinking great. How do I get my body to tell me the answer by looking at myself in the mirror? The answer is by muscle testing.

There are a variety of methods that can be used to ask your body what it needs through muscle testing. We show, demonstrate and practice several methods in Jump Start to Wellness.

Here is the method I personally use to muscle test myself. Touch the thumb and index finger of your non-dominant hand. This makes a natural ring. Do the same thing with the thumb and index finger on your dominant hand, but this time interlock the two rings. Let the other fingers on both hands flop around as they might wish.

Now experiment with pulling the two rings apart through the weakest point which is where the thumbs and fingers meet. Experiment at first to get a sense of how this feels. Try to make it difficult to separate the two rings.

To get started you will want to ask a question that has an obvious answer. I might say: "My name is Robert." I then see if I can pull the interlocked rings through at their weakest point where the thumb and fingers meet. Go ahead and try this using your own name now.

I know the answer to this question since I know that my name is Robert. My body will signal the "yes" answer to me with a strong response, so I will not be able to easily pull my fingers through the interlocked rings I have formed.

Alternatively, when I say "My name is Sally" my body will respond with a weak response. My muscles become flabby and weak. I can easily pull the two rings apart. There is little or no resistance.

Sometimes when I begin muscle testing myself I will say "My name is Robert" and I can pull the rings I have formed apart. Is my body saying my name is not Robert? Did my mother lie to me when she told me my name was Robert?

© 2013 Parkinsons Recovery

What is wrong if my body is giving a weak response to a "yes" question? In this case my body is not hydrated adequately. I only need to drink a glass of water, wait a few minutes and try again. You can always count on getting good answers from your body as long as it is adequately hydrated.

There are other ways to muscle test yourself. A second popular method requires the assistance of another person. Hold your arm out straight from your body so that it is parallel with the ground. You then make a true statement. In my case I might say "My name is Robert." Now ask your friend to try and push your arm down. If the statement is true, your arm will remain firm and your friend will find pushing your arm down extremely difficult. Many people are surprised at their own strength.

If the statement is false (in my case I might say "My name is Sally"), your friend will easily be able to push your arm down. The body always gives a valid answer.

There is a third method I use when I am out in public - the sway test. I do this in public because no one will ever realize what I am doing. The interlocking ring test is a little weird to do in public.

I am standing up in a grocery store looking at ice creams. I pose the True/False statement. Do I need to buy this dessert? For the strong or true response, I sway forward. For the weak or false response I sway backward. If I am determined to buy the dessert regardless of what my body needs, I do not muscle test myself. I already know the answer I want to hear and I know the answer my body will give me. I already know sugar is not good for my body.

No one method is better than another. They all work beautifully. Choosing a method is more a question of personal preference and convenience. I recorded a Muscle Testing CD which gives explicit instructions of four different methods you can use to muscle test that can all be done all by yourself. Your recovery will be expedited if you learn how to use a self-administered method of muscle testing you can use anytime, anywhere to address a long list of questions such as which supplements to purchase (if any), which practitioners to see (if any), which books to buy (if any), etc.

Regardless of the muscle testing method that you adopt, the basic procedure is the same. You ask your body whether you need a particular supplement, drug, food or therapy. It is a good idea to hold the substance in your hand if it is available. If not, just ask the question out loud.

Let me take a specific question by way of example. Let's say you are currently taking fermented Papaya and are wondering if this is really what your body needs. Ask the question: "Does my body need fermented papaya?" You can muscle test with the ring test or the arm test.

© 2013 Parkinsons Recovery

Using the ring test place the papaya in your lap and muscle test using interlocking rings. Using the arm test with the help of a friend to help, place the papaya in one hand and hold the other arm level to the ground. Ask your friend to try and push your arm down after asking the question "Does my body need fermented papaya?"

The psychic Lenore from New York City who I interviewed on my radio program muscle tests by lifting up a chair at home or a water jug at the grocery store. The possibilities of how to muscle test are endless!

If the answer is yes (i.e. it is difficult to push your arm down or unlock the rings in your fingers) follow up by asking more questions that can help you figure out how much to take and how often. You should also test whether the addition of other specific foods, supplements, herbs and/or therapies with papaya are good or bad for your body.

The miracle of this method is that your body gives you the correct answer every time. You just have to ask what your body needs.

Muscle testing is a simple procedure. It is accurate. It costs nothing. It is simple to do. You can do it anywhere. You can do it by yourself. You can do it with a friend.

Why wouldn't you want to muscle test to find out what your body needs every time? Oops, I do not have time to answer that question. The dessert I bought at the store is calling me. I did not have time to ask my body whether it needed the dessert before I bought it. After all, muscle testing takes 10 seconds and I am a busy man.

All of us confront the challenge of making decisions moment by moment. Do we make an appointment with the neurologist this week? Do we visit Parkinsons Recovery to get information? Do we take a vacation from our symptoms and have a piece of chocolate cake?

There is no way around it. Life is all about decision making moment to moment.

How do you go about making the big decisions in your life? How do you go about deciding which therapies or treatments to pursue? There are so many choices. There is so little time. Money is a challenge for most.

LISTEN TO YOURSELF ARGUE THE TWO SIDES

Here is an awesome suggestion offered by Hans from Holland. Hans uses a strategy of fleshing out the arguments on each side to make big decisions. The example he shared with us involved making a decision about whether he needed to start taking prescription medications for Parkinsons. Here how Hans' system works:

On the First Day:

Take the position:

> "Yes, I need to take medications now."

Everyone you talk with this day, listen to yourself giving all the reasons and arguments why it will be a great idea for you to start taking medications. No criticism is allowed. All discussion throughout the day with anyone you talk with is about the advantages of taking medications.

On the Second Day:

Reverse the position. Devote the entire day talking about the negatives with your friends and loved ones. (This is not your only work this day. It just focuses the discussions you have with your friends). Everything that comes out of your mouth is about the negatives.

> "No, I should not take medications now."

Talk about all the reasons why it will be a stupid idea to start taking medications.

On the Third Day:

Talk only about the positives. Listen to yourself as you talk with others. Is your body excited? Are you excited? Are you losing energy? Are you gaining energy? How does it feel? Do you speak with confidence and enthusiasm? Listen to yourself.

On the Fourth Day:

Talk only about the negatives. Listen to yourself as you talk with others. Is your body excited? Are you excited? Are you losing energy? Are you gaining energy? How does it feel? Do you speak with confidence and enthusiasm? Listen to yourself.

You can do the routine for two more days, or it may be clear by now. Your body may have given you a clear signal about which decision is best for you now.

Hans' method of alternating positions helps you listen to the wisdom of your own body. Your body knows what is best. The idea is to just listen to your own babble. If you are confronting a tough decision, give Hans' decision making method a spin. It works for him like a charm.

VOCAL PROFILING

Did you know that any and all imbalances in the body are revealed in a 30 second profile of your voice? Sharry Edwards from Sound Health in Albany, Ohio has developed a sophisticated diagnostic tool that uses a profile of your voice to determine the source of the imbalance that is

© 2013 Parkinsons Recovery

causing your symptoms. After recording your voice and analyzing the profile in a computer program, she is able to determine the sources of imbalances.

Is your problem toxins? The program shows if this is the cause and reveals which toxin is the culprit. Is your problem bacterial infections? If so, the analysis reveals the specific bacteria that are creating the problem. Is your problem the inability of your body to assimilate folic acid or L-dopa or vitamin B-12? All is revealed. All of our secrets are buried in the nuances of our voice.

Voice profiling makes it possible to see where the link is broken in the complex chain of metabolic sequences to cause one or another neurological symptom. I believe Sharry Edward's research is at the cutting edge of where medicine is headed in the future. I also believe doctors will soon be using frequencies to diagnose and treat disease.

Perhaps you are thinking it would be a waste of money to get a voice profile? That is no excuse! Sharry offers free monthly sessions she calls "Happy Hour" where you can call in and volunteer to have your voice analysis analyzed by her. Click on Sound Health practitioners to see a current listing of Sound Health professionals who offer vocal profiling services in your locality.

Sharry Edwards is passionate about training individuals who currently experience the symptoms of Parkinsons to learn vocal profiling. The idea is that once you learn how to take voice profiles on yourself, you can do them every week or so. Everything in the body shifts as you enter the road to recovery. With regular assessments you can determine the nature of the imbalance that is present now and take appropriate corrective action. You do not have to pay someone else. To learn more about the vocal profiling training courses that are offered every month in Ohio visit Sound Health Training Options.

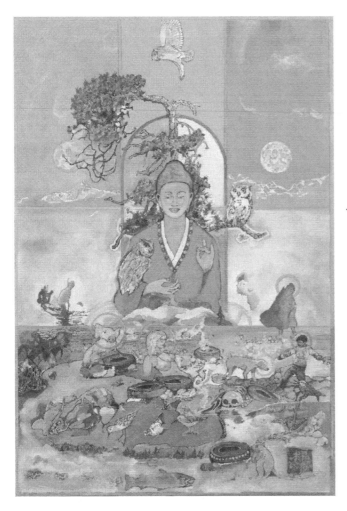

Medicine Buddha (2003) Michael Sawyer

THERAPIES FOR SPECIFIC SYMPTOMS

DYSKINESIA

Dyskinesia is a jerky, dance-like movement of the arms and/or head which typically occurs after several years of treatment with L-DOPA or levodopa. The surgical procedure known as deep Brain Stimulation (DBP) is sometimes recommended when the "on" periods of the medications begin to shorten.

There is an alternative to DBS that also increases the length of time that levodopa is effective (the "on" periods). Citicoline is a nutrient for brain health that has been shown to be effective in reducing the dose of levodopa that is needed by as much as 30-50%. Citicoline is a natural substance derived from soy and egg yolks that is available as an over-the-counter supplement in health food stores. It has few side effects and costs less than most prescription medications. The dosage of levodopa usually has to be adjusted when Citicoline is taken, so it is important to consult with your doctor if you want to pursue this alternative. Find more information about this alternative in *Natural Therapies for Parkinsons Disease.*

© **2013 Parkinsons Recovery**

Pamela Quinn has observed that Michael J Fox is brilliant in how he moves his body. He is continually shifting his body in all directions as he talks. He follows the way his body wants to move rather than resist and face the possibility of freezing up.

Pamela Quinn has also found that applying pressure can be helpful. For example, if you have a lot of dyskinesia or tremor in your head, ask a friend to press on the two sides of your head with their hands. If they apply pressure with a little force, your body will relax and your head tremor will subside.

TREMORS

A wide variety of supplements have been suggested to me for the treatment of tremors. One in particular stands at the top of the list magnesium. Magnesium helps to reduce tremors and facilitates natural detoxing of heavy metals and other harmful substances. I rub magnesium lotion on my body and spray oil under my arm pits every day from Ancient Minerals: www.ancient-minerals.com

The herb Ashwagandha has been identified in research as a useful remedy for tremors, freezing and muscle pain. Rosemary tea is a natural treatment that facilitates the brain body communication, easing mobility challenge which can arise from time to time.

Professor Dancer Pamela Quinn uses some counter intuitive approaches to control her own tremor:

> I take charge of the tremor. I shake the tremor. I don't let the tremor shake me. I do it. That way I am manipulating it. I am taking control of it. There is this sort of psychological benefit as well as a physical one.

> Then, when I release my arm the muscles are relaxed for a bit. The tremor won't go away totally. It will come back. Then I do that again.

> If I am in a social situation where I do not want to look like a crazy person shaking my body around - I will put my hand under my leg. When my tremor starts up I shift position. I will put my hand on my hip or behind my back. If my tremor starts up I will shift it again. I will even sit on my hands.

> As soon as my body enters a physical behavior that I don't want I interrupt it and I shift to another mode. That is a way of saying

> "No. I am not going there."

People report that use of herbs such as Barley Malt Extract, Rhodiola Rosea Mucuna and Fava Beans offer them relief from tremors. Whether any of these herbs can actually help you depends on the level of dopamine in your body and whether or not the dopamine that is present is actually being absorbed. Herbs are just as much a medicine as Sinemet. It is important to consult with your doctor when supplementing prescription medicines with herbs.

LACK OF ARM SWING

For some people, one or both arms stop swinging when they walk. Ask yourself the question – why does one of my arms (or both arms) not swing like they used to? Your body is always protecting you in one way or another. If you force your arm to swing, you may experience freezing or tremoring on an opposite leg.

Experiment on yourself. What happens when you swing your arm? What other parts of your body are affected? Instead of viewing the lack of arm swing as an impediment, it may well be the case that this is your body's way of protecting you against a fall or freezing.

Professor Matt Ford, Ph.D. explains that you get better at what you practice. If you practice swinging your arms, you will eventually have a better arm swing. If you try and think about coordinating your arm swing with you steps, you will probably succeed in the short run. No one however can sustain their focus on the mechanics of walking. It is an automatic process that cannot be mechanized.

Focus helps in the short run but in the long run it flops. What is the alternative? Matt Ford has the answer: Walk to the beat of music you like to hear. The arm swing becomes more natural when it is matched to rhythmic beats.

What music is best? Music you like to hear and music that has a strong beat. Professor Ford suggests that everyone listen to music as often as possible. It is an eloquent, simple solution to a perplexing problem.

Professional Dancer Pamela Quinn also offers a simple, yet effective solution to this problem which she explained during my radio show with her:

> "If you take a grocery bag that has some food in it or anything weighted and you swing that from front to back - that will help get that arm moving."

FROZEN SHOULDER

Angela Wensley has found that intramuscular stimulation (IMS) has been a very effective therapy that lengthens the muscles that have shortened due to misuse. Here is her explanation of IMS:

© 2013 Parkinsons Recovery

"IMS involves needling as in acupuncture but the needles are applied to the tendons instead of to fictional meridians. The benefits of IMS are immediate and last for at least several days. I see my physiotherapist weekly."

Johan Boswinkel finds that the root cause of frozen shoulder is a digestive system that is malfunctioning. Work on getting your digestion back on line and the frozen shoulder problem will resolve.

FOOT DRAGGING

As a soccer Mom, Pamela Quinn invented a solution to her foot dragging which works beautifully for her. She puts a soccer ball inside a plastic grocery bag and proceeds to kick the ball with her lazy leg. After helping the body to renew the neural pathways that are required to wake up a lazy leg, she puts the soccer ball aside and pretends she is kicking it. Try it if foot dragging is a problem. It works.

Howard Shifke had difficulty stepping onto the first step of his stairs. Initially, he held onto the stair rail and used his upper body strength to walk up the stairs. This distorted his posture and twisted his body. He then switched to a more calculated and docile approach. He held onto the rail and placed one foot on the next step. Then he placed his second foot on the same step. It took longer to walk up the stairs, but he did so without exerting upper body muscles or distorting his torso.

Howard found that less was more. Mobility challenges will totally exhaust you by the end of the day because muscles are continuously been challenged and flexed. Howard found a much better approach was to move slower and more mindfully. He never pushed his physical limits. He always walks slower than necessary. This way he was able to maintain a reserve of energy when it was most needed. Howard is symptom free today.

FALLS

Professional Dancer Pamela Quinn has a unique appreciation for the mechanics of movement. Here is her recommendation offered during my radio show for prevention of falls:

It is important to lead with your feet - to lead with your heels in particular as a way of preventing yourself from falling or tripping. In Parkinsons you tend to lead with your torso.

Sometimes I have people pretend they are on a fashion runway because it puts their chest up and their shoulders back and it makes their feet lead. If you are going backwards it is also very important for your feet to lead. The tendency with going backwards is for your upper back to go back. That can lead to a backward fall. You want to crouch forward and make your feet go back. Your body should always follow where your feet go.

FREEZING

Here are professional dancer Pamela Quinn's secrets to avoid freezing:

"There are different ways to take detours in your neurological pathways. One way is to take giant steps. Or, you are going to walk quietly. You can become a Marx Brother and bend your knees and take those big low steps. Anything that will take you out of your Parkinson's movement pattern and shift you into a different reality can be something that breaks through your problem and allows you to get going.

When I cross the street I either step over those white lines or on each one. I give myself a task which is related to visual cuing. Sometimes I use the visual cuing and the oral cuing together. If I have my IPOD, I sync up to music. I have all kinds of categories of music - so I am in a rhythm with my gait as I step over the cracks in the sidewalk.

One thing I did for years in walking is to place myself behind someone - not too close behind - and I sync my walk with theirs. I would take their rhythm. I would take their gait. It would help even out my gait. They would turn and I would find someone else to follow.

Just the other day there was a person walking with a pair of heels. I could hear: Click. Click. Click. Click. So, I put my walk right into her rhythm of the sound of her feet. Both visual and oral cues have helped me tremendously in working my body to move in as normal a way as possible."

Pamela also suggests that you attach masking tape on your hallway or floor. Increase the distance between each tape marker. The challenge is to step over the tape (not on the tape) as you walk. Your stride will increase because the distance between the tape markers increases. This will open up your stride and improve your gait.

Physical Therapist Kevin Lockette offers the following suggestion to address the perplexing challenge of freezing.

"I just read an attentional focus study that addressed teaching people strategies on how to move. There are basically two different ways to teach. They examined focusing on internal cues like your own legs or external cues which is something away from your body. In these studies, the external cues help people unfreeze and help people get out of it. For instance a lot of predictors that will trigger freezing are:

- *elevators*

- *escalators*

- *turning corners*

I train the people so that when they encounter those circumstances they can avoid freezing. One strategy is always to focus away from their body. For instance, if we are having a problem with freezing in an elevator and there is a lot going on –

- *You have anxiety.*

- *There are multiple elevators.*

- *Which one is going to open first?*

- *Can I get there before it shuts?*

- *How many people will be on the elevator?*

- *How long does it take for the elevator door to shut?*

All of these things can increase symptoms for people. If people have these strategies, the anxiety goes down. The external cuing is basically looking at the destination of where you want to go.

I always have people look past the threshold. If a threshold is the trigger of your freezing, I will have them focus not on their feet, not even on the threshold, but past the threshold – where they want to go on that elevator. I have them focus right on that spot and walk toward it. A lot of times it can be effective and they will not freeze.

A lot of times when people freeze both your legs are loaded. You are literally frozen. If you do not have a strategy you may try to move with both your legs loaded (which can throw you off balance) and sometimes fall. I will teach people to stop and try to take control. Basically, cautiously move.

One of the staples that I teach everybody is what I call the poor man's hula where if you are frozen, your weight shifts back and forth left to right like you are swinging your hips like a hula dancer. You can do this very subtly. You can do this maneuver in 3-5 seconds. You just shift to one side, shift to the other and then purposely take the first step towards a target away from your body. It pretty much works a majority of the time. Those types of strategies are helpful.

© 2013 Parkinsons Recovery

The whole idea is by shifting your weight you are going to off load the weight and now you can pick it up. The benefit of swaying is that now you are moving cautiously. Cautious movement will help get you out of freezing. The problem with freezing is that people don't have the strategies. They are operating on this automatic pilot that is not working. You turn off the automatic pilot especially during the freezing periods and then move consciously.

In most circumstances you can move out of it. The side to side weight shifting – the poor man's hula – forces you to turn off the faulty automatic pilot. You are grounding the steering wheel and driving your body yourself. You teach yourself to do that. You consciously are thinking about your movement. The weight shifts to one side. This off loads that leg and you can pick it up. Again, my experience has been if you can focus on where you want to step it seems to work better."

Howard Shifke (http://www.fightingparkinsonsdrugfree.com) invented a different way of solving the challenge of freezing that he faced. During the initial diagnostic assessment, his neurologist asked him to put his left arm out. To Howard's surprise, his right leg began to tremor. A similar result occurred when he put his right arm out – his left side began to tremor. While everyone knows that the right brain controls the left side of the body and the left brain controls the right, Howard speculated that he could rewire his circuits to avoid setting off undesirable tremors and freezing. When he learned to control the right side of his body with his right brain and the left side with his left brain, all would be well.

For example, Howard noticed that his left hand sometimes froze when he drove. Since he was accustomed to holding the steering wheel with his left hand and pushing on the gas pedal with his right foot, these episodes were genuinely problematic. He figured out by analyzing the electrical impulses in his body that the source of freezing in his left hand was caused by his right foot (which of course was on the gas pedal).

What was his solution? He started putting his left hand under his left thigh (to prevent his habit of holding the steering wheel with his left hand). When he holds the steering wheel of his car with his right hand he experiences no freezing episodes in his arms or legs. By stimulating the right side of his brain to move the right side of his body and stimulating the left side of his brain to move the left side of his body, all movement challenges were eventually resolved.

SLEEP DISORDERS AND INSOMNIA

Do you have problems sleeping at night? John Coleman, ND who once had Parkinsons himself and now helps others in his role as a naturopath doctor offers the following suggestions.

"Now this is a difficult challenge for those of us with Parkinson's disease symptoms. A poor sleep pattern can result from pain, restlessness, a neurotransmitter imbalance between serotonin and melatonin, adrenal stimulation, lack of exercise or lack of fresh air."

"It seems weird sometimes because we can - in fact we often do - feel really tired to the point of exhaustion. Yet we go to bed and cannot go to sleep or if we go to sleep, we wake frequently."

"Some of the things that can help are meditation before bed - say 10 minutes. There are some really good CD's to help that if we need that. Some of them can be played softly in the bedroom or some can be listened to through stereo headphones."

"Magnesium powder taken after dinner sometimes helps settle restlessness so that we go to sleep easier. Homeopathic magnesium phosphate or some other homeopathic remedies like coffea or chamomilla can help you sleep. Herbal mixtures like Passionflower, Hops, Jamaica Dogwood can help."

"One of the important aspects of this is to not become worried or anxious about the lack of sleep because that then sets up a negative feedback pattern. Our sleep pattern becomes even worse."

"We need to move around during the day as much as we can, particularly if we can get outside, that is good. Keep physically active. We need to get as much fresh air as we can. Make sure we do some stretches before bed to relax our muscles."

"Often we will sit all evening and then get up and go to bed. Our muscles have gotten quite tight and short so we can't get comfortable. If we do some stretching, some Pilates stretching, or yoga stretching or simple stretching before bed, that will often help our muscles relax better."

"It is also really important not to just turn off the television and go to bed. Television stimulates bursts of neurotransmitters in our brain that sets up sort of a chattery situation. If we just switch off the television and go to bed our mind is still chattery. It is important to have 10 minutes or so of quiet time, after we have switched off the television, before we go to bed and go to sleep."

I also would like to respond to this question using my own experience as a guide. I have attended seminars where doctors give step by step instructions that are supposed to help you sleep. You have probably heard the same recommendations: Go to sleep at the same time every night, don't watch TV before you sleep, eat (or drink) ... etc.

© 2013 Parkinsons Recovery

Speaking for myself, I cannot do these things before I sleep. The routine is too rigid for me. My life is too unstructured. If you have a similar response, you might want to investigate any one of the six strategies I have listed below. Surely one will be the winning ticket for you if you have problems with your sleep routine.

EAR PLUGS

It may sound silly, but many people are very sensitive to sounds. Spend a $1 at the dollar store. Buy some wax type ear plugs (like swimmers use). Put them in your ears before you sleep.

EXERCISE

When I exercise during the day, I am much more likely to get a good night's sleep. Sweat works wonders when it comes to rest.

WHITE NOISE

We turn on an air cleaner at night when we sleep. It is a soothing way to screen out extraneous noise that can put your hormonal system on alert. Noises that come from unknown places in the dark create fear in the body which is bound to keep you awake.

DARKEN THE BEDROOM

When we started closing the blinds in the bedroom at night, we discovered it is much easier to sleep. For years we looked out the windows at our beautiful view of the Puget Sound, but at the cost of restful sleep at night. Darkening the room promotes sound sleep.

HOLOSYNC

This is my personal favorite strategy for sleep, though it is the one recommendation that costs a little money. If I am ever unable to sleep, I pop on my holosync ear phones. I am out in two minutes.

ACUPRESSURE

Some people report that a brief acupressure treatment in the evening offers them a good night's sleep. Like acupuncture, acupressure activates meridians in the body using gentle pressure, but using your hands and fingers rather than needles. You can apply acupressure on yourself or ask your spouse to do it for you every evening. A few minutes can work miracles if you are having difficulty getting to sleep.

PROTEIN

Kristen Allott, ND, (www.dynamicpaths.com) argues that the body needs protein to maintain the right balance of hormones that are conducive to a restful night's sleep. She recommends that anyone who is having sleep challenges eat a little protein just before going to bed. Give it a trial run. I predict you will be pleased with the result.

EYE PROBLEMS

Are you having issues with your eyes? Perhaps dry eyes. Perhaps double vision. Perhaps jittery eyes. Perhaps cloudy eyes.

My uncle Gordon Ward developed advanced cataracts at age 65. A former college president of Sheridan College and Wyoming State Legislator, Gordon loved to play tennis, read books and write about history. Cataracts made it so difficult for him to read that Gordon reluctantly decided to have cataract surgery, one eye at a time. There was no other good option in the 1990's.

Cataract surgery on Gordon's right eye healed beautifully. Surgery on the left eye was a miserable flop. Gordon developed double vision and for all practical purposes was blind. He could not read. He could no longer play tennis. It was all a horrible mess.

My Aunt Betty said that the stress of cataract surgery caused Gordon to begin experiencing the symptoms of Parkinson's. He was diagnosed shortly after his botched surgery. Had Gordon been able to see, I believe he would still be playing tennis today. He died in the spring of 2009. Only later did we discover that Gordon had hepatitis C, not Parkinson's.

As part of my work to identify natural remedies, I am excited to report that I found a natural antioxidant eye drop that reverses cataracts and addresses other eye problems caused by inflammation. Had this antioxidant therapy been available to Gordon he could have reversed his failing eyesight without resorting to cataract surgery. Obviously, cataract surgery is a viable option for many people, but for my Uncle Gordon it was a disaster.

The discovery of an antioxidant remedy originated with the work of a Russian medical biophysicist Mark Babizhayev, Ph.D who made the simple, but profound observation that people who had no eye problems had sufficient levels of N-Acetyl-Carnosine in their eyes. People with cataracts and other eye problems had insufficient levels of N-Acetyl-Carnosine in their eyes.

Dr. Babizhayev took his research to the next level ten years ago by formulating eye drops that contained N-Acetyl-Carnosine which he called Can-C. He then began doing research to see if this antioxidant eye therapy worked.

Studies confirmed his hypothesis. Add the Can-C eye drops to the eyes and the eyes are able to heal naturally. Cataracts were reversed in about 95% of the cases. The Can-C eye drops resolve eye problems because they reduce the inflammation that is aggravating the problem in the first place. Isn't that totally cool?

© 2013 Parkinsons Recovery

I also want to make the obvious observation that our eyes are physically located next to the part of the brain that is responsible for manufacturing dopamine. I am wondering if healing eye problems might have an indirect, but positive impact on Parkinson's symptoms in general. The jury is still out on that one, but you never know...

You can find more information about Can-C eye drops and Dr. Babizhayev's research by visiting: http://www.cataracts.parkinsonsrecovery.com

I have aired two radio shows on the antioxidant Can-C eye drop therapy - an interview with company representative Jennifer Jones from Innovative Vision Products on February 11, 2010 and an interview with both Jennifer Jones and Dr. Babizhayev that aired April 1, 2010.

CAN-C PLUS. When I interviewed Dr. Babizhayev, he could not stop talking about his recent revelation concerning a dietary supplement that he formulated which bolsters the anti-inflammatory effects of Can-C eye drops. People who have advanced cataracts need extra support to reverse them, so he formulated a full spectrum antioxidant supplement that contains carnosine and an array of other antioxidants. This particular supplement gives people with advanced cataracts the extra boost that is necessary to reverse their cataracts.

Apparently, Can-C Plus does much more than to help reverse cataracts and address other eye complications that are caused by inflammation. Dr. Babizhayev's recent research shows that the Can-C Plus nutritional supplement reverses the increased aging effects of chronic illnesses at the DNA level. How can this be?

Can-C Plus lengthens telomeres which become shorter with natural aging and the cellular damage caused by all chronic illness. A telomere is a region of repetitive DNA at the end of a chromosome which protects the end of the chromosome from deterioration. His findings show that shortening of telomeres is not just stopped. Rather, it is reversed when Can-C Plus is used as a supplement. That is, the telomeres become longer!

Don't get me wrong here. Dr. Babizhayev has not done any research with Parkinson's patients, though I encouraged him to launch such a study. He makes no claims about what Can-C Plus can do for the symptoms of Parkinson's. But, I wonder if the Can-C Plus supplement might also provide sustained relief from the neurological damage caused by Parkinson's. If you are taking the Can-C Plus supplement, please let me know about your experience so I can document it. Discover more information about Can-C Plus at: http://www.cataracts.parkinsonsrecovery.com

DEPRESSION

This is a truly challenging illness. The feeling seems to be trapped in a vice grip that will not let go. It seems as though nothing can pull you out of the depths of despair. Absent is the motivation to do anything of any substance. Present is the thought that nothing you do makes a difference. Clearly, hormonal imbalances are taking their toll.

Depression can be so deep and penetrating that it is nearly impossible to take any action to reverse it without help. Even making an appointment with a health care provider takes up too much energy. The negative thought form that emerges is:

"It won't make any difference anyway, so why bother?"

Depression is a place of despair where all you can think about is going to sleep so you are not haunted by the black void of nothingness and immobility. Have I described the sorry state of depression adequately?

THE VICIOUS CYCLE OF DESPAIR

A marked tendency for individuals who currently have a diagnosis of Parkinson's disease is withdrawal from doing activities that are enjoyable and fun. When you spend less time hanging out with friends and doing activities that have been intrinsically fulfilling in the past, you are bound to get depressed. As you pass up opportunities to feel good, depression creeps in your life. It may sit undetected until your friends begin saying to you:

"What is wrong? You look depressed."

The cycle is self fulfilling. You do less and less. You feel worse and worse every day. Hope spirals into a downward freefall. When feeling sad, most people put on hold doing any and all of the things that you most enjoyed doing in the past.

Psychologist Roseanne Dobkin, Ph.D., recommends that when you are depressed, act according to your goals rather than your feelings. No one feels like doing anything when they are depressed. If you act according to your feelings, rest assured you will become more depressed. We can normally be guided by our feelings, but in the case of depression, Roseanne Dobkin explains that feelings are an unreliable guide. Depression is anything but a normal state.

Focus on the goal of feeling better. Certain actions must be taken even though you do not feel like taking them. Once the depression lifts you can return to the practice of trusting your feelings.

HOW TO BEAT DEPRESSION WITHOUT MEDICATIONS

The most straightforward and simplest solution to reversing depression is to eat protein at two hour intervals throughout the day. I picked up this valuable suggestion from Kristen Allott, ND, a naturopath doctor who specializes in treatment depression and anxiety through the right nutrition. You may be thinking – "This is too simple to work" – or I should admit that was my first reaction. Part of me said that simple is better, so I gave it a whirl.

© 2013 Parkinsons Recovery

Her method works. Yea! In the past I tended to become fatigued and slightly depressed around 2:00 in the afternoon. Once I began eating protein more regularly, the spells of depression lifted. Benefits of eating protein are less fatigue, improved sleep, better energy, fewer bouts of hunger and more muscle mass.

What foods contain protein? Certainly meat and fish fits have high protein. So do many vegetarian foods such as tofu, tempeh, lentils, whole beans, garden burgers, quinea, millet, oats, brown rice soy milk, nuts, seeds, cottage cheese and yogurt. Dr. Allott suggests that you start the day with protein with a Lizard Brain Treat which consists of ¼ cup of fruit juice and ¼ cup of nuts. For more information on how to combat depression by eating protein more regularly, visit Kristen Allott's website: http://www.dynamicpaths.com

If you are taking medications, be sure and consult with your doctor about the appropriate quantity of protein for your diet. Eating too much protein can undermine the efficacy of certain prescription medications that are used to treat the symptoms of Parkinson's.

FRESH THINKING COMBINED WITH INVIGORATING ACTIVITY

What safe, natural and nonintrusive therapies provide relief from depression that is frequently associated with a diagnosis of Parkinson's disease? Here is a short list of Roseanne Dobkin's suggestions for ways to combat depression without having to resort to medications (which of course may be necessary for some people).

1. Exercise every day. Exercise boosts your mood and decreases stress. It doesn't matter what you do for exercise – just get your body moving.

2. Increase the time you spend every day engaging in activities that are meaningful, rewarding and pleasurable. Do you enjoy playing bridge? Then play bridge often. Do you enjoy playing tennis? Then play tennis often. Do you enjoy hanging out with friends at the local coffee shop? Then visit the coffee shop often.

Test out new activities you have never tried and see what happens. Ever bowled? Why not give it a whirl? Why not join a book club or investment club or women's group or men's group.

Professor Dobkin explained during my radio show August 19, 2010 that when people are depressed they overestimate the extent of their limitations. Acknowledge that tendency. Everyone does it. Put thoughts of limitation on hold. Experiment. If an activity is no fun - drop it and try something else. If you cannot make yourself act, hire a coach that will gently nudge you into taking action.

3. Acknowledge negative thoughts and then pause them. Are these thoughts really as true as you think? With depression, thoughts are influenced by emotions more so than logic. We automatically accept all of our thoughts as true when in fact they are flat out silly or dead wrong. When we become depressed, negative thoughts are seldom as true as we think they are. They are also rarely accurate. Replace negative thinking with a more balanced view.

4. Treat every challenge as a problem solving opportunity.

> *You can't go to the party because you cannot drive? There is a solution to this problem. Find it and go to the party.*

> *You don't want to go out to dinner because you are having difficulty holding a fork? There is a solution to this problem. Solve the problem. Go out to dinner. Have some fun.*

Become more flexible. Make fewer demands on yourself. Depression is not a normal state of affairs. Act accordingly.

Elizabeth, a guest on my radio show, offered a lucid explanation of how she was able to function so beautifully despite having been diagnosed with Parkinson's two decades ago. Her trick was to carefully plan out each day so there was enough time to accomplish everything without rushing or stressing. She learned how to pace herself and move through each moment of her day with the grace of an angel.

5. Finally, Professor Dobkin recommends that if you are depressed, find a method of relaxation that works for you. There are many options including visualization, progressive muscle relaxation, deep breathing, meditation, self-hypnosis and others. You probably already have a method that works for you. Use it on the spot when you are stressed.

MUSIC

Professor Matt Ford, Ph.D. during my radio show on January 26, 2011 suggested that listening to music can provide welcome relief from sour moods. Play music around the house all the time as often as possible. Music helps you move with ease. Music helps with balance. Music has a powerful emotional impact. Music increases endorphins (which are the pain killers). Music enhances mood. You will move better, feel better and smile more often.

Depression can be very problematic if you happen to live in the northwest United States during winter time. What follows is my short list of strategies I have personally found to be useful for fighting off depression:

© 2013 Parkinsons Recovery

1. First, buy a seasonal affective disorder light. Use it every day. Drag yourself to the computer and order one online.

2. Second, purchase vitamin D3 and take it during the winter. Please note – this is D3, not a composite vitamin D supplement (which can include other forms of vitamin D).

3. Third, if there is sunlight, bask in it. You do not need to take D3 if you are able to get sufficient exposure to sunshine.

These are my simple suggestions because they work for me. You can pull these things off even in a state of deep depression. They will help pull you out of the darkness.

Take any or all of the steps above and you will see a gradual reawakening to the sweetness of life. If you are depressed and unable to act, get help. Asking for help is not a sign of weakness. It is a sign of strength and courage.

RIGIDITY

Physical Therapist Kevin Lockette from Hawaii suggests two exercises that will create more flexibility and reduce rigidity. He explains the problem resides in the lack of ability to rotate the hips freely. First, lie down on the floor or bed. Place both feet on the floor with your knees bent. Shift your legs to the left, then to the right. This simple exercise "oils" the hips joints.

Second, stand up. Pretend as though you are holding a golf club. Clasp your hands together and swing that imaginary golf club. When you do, you will feel the rotation in your hips. With each swing, the rotation becomes wider and easier. When the body is able to rotate at will, rigidity becomes less of a obstacle to effortless movement.

FACIAL RIGIDITY

Many people hold the mistaken belief that the source of the problem with facial rigidity – or social staring - is found in the facial muscles. As is the case with any localized issue in the body, the cause of the problem resides somewhere else. In the case of facial rigidity the problem is rooted in a spine which is rounded and hunched or a twisted pelvis. Body therapies help the problem of facial rigidity because they release the tension that is held and the misalignment that is found in the spine and pelvis.

Irene Pasternack explained in my radio show December 8, 2010 that when she helps you make little movements in your pelvis and shift how you balance on your sit bones, your sternum, chest and face are profoundly affected. It is easy to smile when the pelvis and spine are in alignment.

Feldenkrais™ removes the blockages and wakes up the neural pathways in the facial muscles. It is one therapy among others that offers the potential to reverse the embarrassing problem of facial rigidity that sends a misleading signal to others that you are uninterested in them and bored.

CONSTIPATION

Why should anyone be concerned about gut problems when "everyone" knows the challenge with Parkinsons involves a neural dysfunction? Function of the gut has a huge influence - I repeat huge - on the symptoms of Parkinsons. When the gut is working properly depression lifts, constipation is relieved and energy returns.

Let me be blunt. If your digestive system is not functioning properly, all of the money you spend on supplements and healthy food goes down the toilet.

The process is wicked. You spend money on supplements and healthy food. You pour the supplements and healthy food into your body each day like clockwork. The following day the supplements and healthy food from the day before come out the other end - unaltered. This happens over and over, day in and day out. Your body is not absorbing the nutrients.

There is a second reason to heal digestive issues such as constipation first if you have Parkinson's symptoms. People with neurological challenges are much more likely to have a store house of toxins such as heavy metals and pesticides that are trapped in cells throughout their body. If the digestive system is clogged up, these toxins cannot be eliminated.

To summarize:

You pour money down the toilet day in and day out.

1. *You do not feel any better.*

2. *You convince yourself it is impossible to feel better.*

3. *You stop doing the things that help you feel better.*

4. *End of story.*

The good news is that you can reverse this wicked cycle. Natural approaches for improving gut function are widely available. They fall into three categories.

1. *Increasing hydration in the body.*

2. *Maintaining a proper pH level in the stomach.*

3. *Improving overall function of the bowel.*

First let's consider the important role hydration which, as we age, becomes more and more problematic.

INCREASE HYDRATION IN THE BODY

If the body is not hydrated adequately, waste begins to accumulate in the cells. This is the underlying reason why many people feel sluggish and run out of energy by the afternoon. The solution is to hydrate your body.

John Coleman, ND recommends that people with Parkinsons take a homeopathic remedy for dehydration called the Aquas (www.aquas4life.com) This therapy involves taking a few drops of a unique combination of essential oils and Bach flower essences in the morning and the evening.

The mechanism in the body that signals thirst needs to be recalibrated as we age. I was totally unaware until last year that I had stopped drinking water. The tissues in my body had become chronically dehydrated. It is the type of problem that creeps up on you so slowly you do not even notice what is happening.

I have taken Aquas for about a year and have been amazed at their effectiveness. I now get thirsty when my body needs water. If I do not take the Aquas, I do not drink water because I am never thirsty. The Aquas have solved this problem for me. Discover more information about the Aquas homeopathic treatment by visiting http://www.aquas4life.com.

PH LEVELS

Everyone should maintain a pH level in the stomach of 2. The term "pH" is a measure of the acidity of a solution like a body fluid. The most acidic of liquids will have a pH as low as -5 (this is a negative five). The most alkaline of liquids have pH level of +14.

By way of comparison here is a sample of pH levels from selected foods: lemon juice pH = 2.4, coffee pH = 5.0, pure water pH = 7.0, tomato pH = 4.0, milk pH = 6.5.

A point of confusion for many people is to conclude that you need to eat more acidic foods in order to maintain the correct acidic content in your stomach. This is not true. Disease flourishes when the environment in the body is acidic.

A high proportion of the food you eat should contain a high alkaline content. Many doctors recommend that 60% of the foods should be alkaline. Others suggest 80% of the foods you eat should have a high alkaline content in cases of chronic conditions like Parkinsons.

© 2013 Parkinsons Recovery

Most people think of the acid-alkaline scale as linear: i.e., from 2 to 3 = 1 and from 2 to 4 = 2. It is not. Each individual pH unit is a factor of 10 more than the next higher or lower unit. An increase in pH from 2 to 3 represents a 10-fold change. An increase of 2 to 4 represents a one-hundred (10 × 10) fold change.

Shifting down from a pH level of 6 (which is very alkaline) to a pH level of 2 (which is more acidic) is thus not as easy as it might seem. Given the tricky nature of pH, is there any wonder that it is difficult to maintain the proper pH balance in the stomach?

The pH in the stomach needs to be low because acid is needed to break food down. Here is the key: If there is not sufficient acid in the stomach (i.e., the stomach is too alkaline), food does not break down. No. It crawls its way into your gut and - if you are squeamish do not read further - rots.

Please note that I said the pH level "in the stomach" should be around 2. The pH of other body fluids such as urine, saliva and blood vary considerably. For example, the pH of blood is 7.4. Secretions of the pancreas have a pH of 8.1.

In contrast, a fluid in the body that has a high acidic content in the body is plaque. Plaque's pH is low and will dissolve teeth if it is not removed.

How can you know if the pH level in your stomach is "2"? After all, having a pH lab test every day would be very expensive and time consuming.

There is an easy way to know. It costs nothing. It takes a second each day. Simply pay attention to the color of your bowel movements. OK. I know this is not exactly a sexy topic, but it is important to know.

If your poop is dark brown the pH level in your stomach is low enough. You are in good shape. If your poop is light brown, there is not enough hydrochloric acid in your system. That is to say, the pH level in your stomach is too high.

So if the color of the poop is too light corrective action is needed. What do you do? Take vitamin C and drink a lot of water.

Vitamin C is the body's antioxidant of choice. If we give our bodies enough vitamin C, our bodies are able to manufacture enough CoQ10.

There are many vitamin C products on the market, so be judicious in what you choose to purchase. I use a vitamin C product recommended by Randy Mentzer: Vital Mixed Ascorbates made by Pharmax which is loosely packed in a 9 ounce container. I mix it with water.

© **2013 Parkinsons Recovery**

How much vitamin C should you take? Your body will tell you the answer. Just ask it. Muscle test yourself. You will need to take more and more vitamin C until your poop turns to a dark brown color.

Most people are unaware that our natural biology calls for large quantities of vitamin C. You may be shocked at how much is needed for your body to come back into balance.

IMPROVE OVERALL FUNCTION OF THE BOWELS

You are now well hydrated and your pH level is good to go. Now it is time to focus on getting your bowels moving. Everyone needs one good bowel movement every day. Two to three movements are ideal.

Herbs that can facilitate bowel function are gentian, chamomile, fennel and St Mary's thistle. Which herb (or herbs) will do the best job for you? I must sound like a broken record, but just ask your body. Muscle test yourself. Your body knows the answer.

Your body may be having difficulty digesting animal fats. I have received several reports from persons currently experiencing debilitating constipation challenges who switched to a vegetarian diet. Their constipation difficulties were resolved within weeks of the change in diet.

HOME REMEDY

John Coleman, ND recommends a homemade cocktail for people suffering from digestive challenges including constipation. He suggests you take this cocktail in the morning and evening 1/2 hour before meals. You make this special cocktail yourself.

THE RECIPE:

> *12 ounces pure water*
>
> *1/2 - 1 teaspoon vitamin C powder*
>
> *1/2 teaspoon magnesium*
>
> *1 ml (eyedropper) zinc liquid*
>
> *Aqua drops (1 drop AM in morning; 1 drop PM in evening)*
>
> *1 drop selenium*

Once you get your digestive system back on line, nutrients from the healthy food you eat will be distributed to the cells that desperately need to be nourished.

© 2013 Parkinsons Recovery

As always, check out my ideas to improve your gut function with your doctor before you decide to do anything. Always treat anything I say as information that needs to be discussed and evaluated with your medical doctor.

- ♣ May your constipation resolve with each passing day.

- ♣ May your energy rebound as your gut function improves.

- ♣ Your body and your pocketbook will thank you.

MEMORY LOSS

People who have difficulty with their mental functioning often hold the belief the problem is centered in their brains. To be sure, this is the case for a very small proportion of persons. The root cause of memory problems for most people is much more likely to reside from a disruption in the healthy flora of their digestive system. The climate in their digestive track is too acidic. Good bacteria required for proper digestion vanish. Bad bacteria that disrupt the digestive process flourish. Without the presence of good bacteria in the digestive system, a person will see little benefit from eating organic, healthy food.

Find a doctor who is knowledgeable about the best probiotics to take (for your body) which can help your digestive system come back on line. When it does, celebrate a transformation in your cognitive functioning as your mind becomes sharp as a tack.

As another option, consider making your own probiotics. Sandor Katz has written a book titled Wild Fermentation which describes in detail how you can ferment foods in your kitchen and prepare your own probiotics. This is a fun, easy approach for helping your digestive system come back on line. You also get to prepare tasty fermented foods you love to eat.

PAIN

Do you really want to rush into a strategy to eliminate pain? On the one hand – you probably have a knee jerk answer – Duh. There is another answer to this question which is not as popular as the first. From a holistic perspective, pain is a sign you are making progress on your road to recovery. Pain gives you valuable information about the cause of an imbalance in your body. If you are interested in healing the cause of the pain, it is best to hang out with it for a while rather than numbing it with medications.

Nutritional counselor Dorit offered a fascinating perspective on pain during my radio show on June 3, 2010.

"It is normal to have pain. I see pain as weakness leaving the body. I do not see pain as something to be covered up. The question is - how can we assist the pain in leaving in a smoother manner in a way that would help us to release the reason behind the pain if there is a reason to release it at all. Sometimes we need to just acknowledge and be there for our own growth."

In some cases, pain is the body's distraction from feeling unpleasant emotions like guilt, abandonment, rage, deceit, sorrow or grief. Instead of fixating on the pain, drop down just underneath the pain and ask yourself:

"What lies beneath this pain of mine?

You may be surprised at the answer. Once the wounds of unpleasant feelings are released, the physical pain disappears as fast as a parrot from a magician's hand during a magic show.

For reasons that may surprise you, meditation can be a powerful antidote to pain. Radio programs I offer on the subject of meditation are typically the least popular. I suspect many people believe little benefit can be derived from sitting in a silly position doing nothing. Norman Fischer explains why meditation can be extremely beneficial for anyone who experiences chronic pain.

To be sure, sometimes there is relief from the pain as a result of the meditation practice. I suppose it is not impossible depending on the condition there could be some significant change in the physical condition.... Generally ...it is a matter of:

- *How do we live with what we have?*

- *How do we manage it?*

- *If there is pain, how do we have some happiness and some relief even in the middle of some discomfort?*

The first head is - you have a pain. [With Parkinsons it may be pain in the muscles or joints] That is one head. Putting a head on top of your head is when you say:

"Oh, I hate this pain."

"Why won't it go away?"

"What did I ever do to deserve this?"

"How come nobody else has this pain?"

All of that actually becomes in many ways more painful, or at least as painful as the original pain. The idea is this. Can you accept and be present with the pain and take away that second head that you put on top. If you then just have the original head, life becomes much more bearable and sometimes quite beautiful.

How can you get immediate relief from pain when it is literally driving you up the wall? Michelle Mill's mother suffered from the persistent pain. She has chronic fatigue syndrome. It is not Parkinsons, but some of the symptoms overlap.

With a mother who was unable to find relief from any remedy that was prescribed by health care practitioners, Michelle took matters into her own hands. After months of trial and error experimentation she invented her own pain relief remedy that has proved incredibly successful. It has helped her mother and countless others.

Michelle told her own story of recovery on my radio show that aired September 10, 2009. You can also read additional information about her remedy by visiting www.iwokeupwell.com. She concocted the remedy by combining together every known analgesic including the natural form of aspirin which is derived from willow bark.

Call Michelle and talk with her about her remedy. Her phone number is on the contact page of her website. Michelle invented Willow Balm. She makes it herself. She helps people get immediate relief from their pain so they can attend to the underlying cause of it. It you are experiencing pain, this remedy is worth investigating further.

Will Willow Balm really help you get relief? Who knows? Everyone is different. But with free samples to try, why not experiment and see for yourself. Michelle is so proud of her natural product that she gives me free samples to give all Jump Start to Wellness participants.

Restless Leg Syndrome

Nutritional Counselor and Pharmacist Randy Mentzer offers the following recommendation for Restless Leg Syndrome.

> *"I lean toward trying natural products first. We find that magnesium glycinate works really well for restless leg syndrome. It is natural. It is a muscle relaxer."*

Music Medicine expert Suzanne Jonas, PhD, has developed an acoustic CD to treat restless leg syndrome by ear rather than mouth. Is that cool or what?

Salivation

Excessive salivation can certainly become one of the most troubling and at times embarrassing symptoms. Foot Whisperer Randy Eady suggests that you can always press on the acupressure points on the face that are directly linked to the function of salivation glands. He reports you can get relief for about 15 minutes (until the same points are pressed again). Press the jaw joint on each side of your face at the same time for 5-10 seconds. There is also a pressure point just below the ear hole on each side of the head.

Acupuncturists are of course the perfect resource in this regard. They can help you find the precise location of the acupressure points you need to press when relief is needed. Acupressure is a sweet self help therapy, something you can do for yourself whenever salivation becomes problematic.

STRESS

What can you do to get relief from stress? You are probably thinking to yourself –

> *I know what I can do to get relief from stress – but it costs me money. If I spend money – I will be even more stressed.*

Why not consider ways you can get relief from stress without spending a cent? Of course, it will still take a little time and effort on your part – but the outcome is well worth the effort. Learn how you can reduce your stress level (and see an immediate reduction in your own symptoms) by listening to my radio program interview with Keith Zang from the Moonglow Enlightenment Center that aired on January 28, 2010. Oh – I suppose I should clarify – it does not cost you a cent to listen to Keith's suggestions. You can always download any of my radio shows for free from the radio program website by visiting the show page. Scroll back to the February 28th show to hear my interview with Keith:

http://www.blogtalkradio.com/parkinsons-recovery

Most people anticipate a happy retirement because the stressful demands of having a full time job can be terribly stressful. Some people count down the days until they will be free of the life style restrictions that are imposed by a 40 hour a week job.

Unfortunately, the expectation of a happy, stress free retirement is seldom realized. Most people are blindsided by the discovery that retirement itself is stressful. Here is the common sequence of events.

- *You just retired last month.*

- *You wake up in the morning.*

- *You confront the first decision of the day.*

- *You evaluate the possibilities: Walk the dog of take out the garbage.*

© 2013 Parkinsons Recovery

- *Then what?*

Such simple choices can be extremely stressed for a person who is used to making far more challenging and demanding decisions.

A passion is critical to managing stress successfully. If you have no goal for the day or week or month – if you have no reason to get out of bed in the morning - your hormones also have no reason to get out of their cozy beds either. It is hard to feel good when those hormones are always sleeping.

One successful approach for managing stress is to become more mindful each and every moment. Instead of anticipating the future (which creates stress) or regretting the past (which sustains past traumas), focusing on the present moment is a guaranteed way to reduce stress in your life. Becoming more mindful happens when you set your intention to live in the present. Becoming more mindful costs absolutely nothing!

Because I have such trust in mindfulness as a powerful, yet simple way to reduce stress, I created a Mindfulness Program which sends a challenge each week in the form of an email to become more mindful. Quite honestly, I developed this program because I was personally teaching myself to become more mindful. The Parkinsons Recovery Mindfulness Program costs a little money each week – the equivalent of one latte a week – so if paying out money for anything tends to create more stress in your life – the Mindfulness Program is clearly not the right solution for you.

Davis Phinney, the famous Tour de France cyclist who developed symptoms of Parkinsons, says that what has helped him is to take each moment as it comes. When you string the moments together, you wind up having a good day. If you spend your entire day thinking about what you cannot do, your chances of having a good day are slim. The mission of the Davis Phinney Foundation is to help people living with Parkinson's disease to live well today.

Most people believe that their minds activate stress hormones. Actually, the heart plays the leading role here. The mind is simply a "walk on" to the drama at hand. The opportunity to manage stress resides in the heart. When the heart relaxes, a signal is sent to the brain to relax. Open up your heart and watch stress in your life dissolve like a snowball in the sunshine. This therapy also costs nothing. Better yet, you pay nothing out and receive immense pleasure in return.

Sweating

Here is what I see is happening with sweating. Remember I am a researcher, not a medical doctor, so be sure and consult with your doctor before taking any action.

Your body is sending you a strong signal. What is the message? I have a strong hunch that the lymph system is clogged. The system is simply not functional at present.

Why is it clogged? You may have an overabundance of toxins. Please do not be offended if sweating is one of your symptoms. First, my guess may be wrong. Second, everyone has this problem because we all live in a very toxic world.

When the body is attempting to do its work of eliminating toxins (which remember is one of its many jobs) and there are too many toxins for the body to eliminate through the kidneys, liver, bowels, etc) the body will use whatever means available to release the toxins. If the lymph system is clogged, the sweat glands are the alternative outlet.

Looked at from this perspective, sweating may be critical for the organs in your body to continue functioning. In other words, it is actually a good thing to sweat even though it is making you miserable.

What do you do about this? First, you can evaluate everything you put on your body, everything you eat and everything you touch. It is possible you are contaminating yourself in a most innocent way. It may be the shaving lotion you use. It may be your laundry soap. It may be the furniture you sit on has toxins.

Consider all possibilities. Eliminate any and all possible sources of toxins. Make it a project for the month. The source of the problem may lie in a most strange or obvious place, one that you never thought about before.

Second, you can purchase a small trampoline and jump on it for 4 or 5 minutes a day (unless balance is an issue for you). Jumping on a trampoline every day helps to clear out the toxins and clear your lymph system. I jump regularly. It is fun. It jiggles out the junk. The only way for the waste in your lymph to move is if you move. There is no internal pump that moves it out for you.

Third, you can contact a naturopath or medical doctor who can help you to detox gently. Or you can visit your health food store where there are usually people available who can answer your questions. There are many other natural options that can help you detox (infrared saunas, steam rooms, homeopathic treatments, etc.)

You also probably need to be especially careful to hydrate your body. You may have the thought that you do not want to drink water because it will make the sweating worse. Without adequate hydration, you cannot detox your body and your lymph system will remain clogged. I personally use a homeopathic treatment that was designed to address the problem of dehydration which works beautifully for me.

© 2013 Parkinsons Recovery

Herbal treatments can be helpful. Magnesium in the form of lotions or oils will facilitate the elimination of toxins in your body. A number of herbs will help clear out your lymph system and help you detox your body. I interviewed an amazing herbalist in Pioneers of Recovery, Andrew Bentley. Kate Tossey (www.katesherbs.com) has also been a guest on my radio show who is an amazing resource. Both herbalists are resources I would approach to get the best advice on herbs to try for detoxing my body. Consider essential oils as an option too. Aroma therapists like Jean Oswald, also a Pioneer of Recovery, are also wonderful resources.

Once the toxins have been cleared to a manageable state, your lymph system will begin to function normally and the symptom of sweating will hopefully subside.

SWALLOWING PROBLEMS

Why are swallowing difficulties so serious? The primary cause of death among people who have been diagnosed with Parkinsons Disease is pneumonia, a serious infection of the lungs. When food slides down the trachea (which leads to the lungs) rather than the esophagus (which leads to the stomach) the lungs are the recipient of food that create the conditions conducive to infection. Once food enters the lungs – there is no exit pathway other than back up the trachea by coughing.

You may not recognize you have a swallowing problem. Do tears flow from your eyes when you eat? Does your nose run when you eat? Do pills get stuck in your throat? Does your voice sound funny after you eat? If the answer is yes to any of these questions you probably have a swallowing problem.

I have problems swallowing pills, so I have recently become aware I have a swallowing problem. Roya Sayadi, Ph.D. and Joel Herskowitz, MD, authors of Swallow Safely, offer a recommendation which has helped me enormously. When I swallow it helps to tuck my head to my chest and turn my head to one side.

If you have a swallowing problem, make it a high priority to heal it. Sayadi and Herskowitz's Swallow Safely book is an excellent resource. I also suggest that you take the time to hear my radio show with them as my guests which aired on July 22, 2010.

Swallowing problems may be caused by TMJ disorders (jaw bone misalignments). If you have a swallowing problem consider having a dentist qualified to diagnose and treat TMJ problems do an evaluation.

© 2013 Parkinsons Recovery

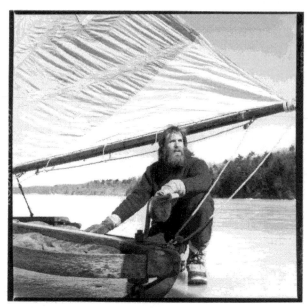

Iceboater, Hudson River by John Fasulo

WHAT PEOPLE DO TO FEEL BETTER

What helps people who have Parkinson's disease feel better? Everyone is different of course and the origins of one person's situation can be dramatically different from someone else. Still, it is nice to learn what has helped other people get relief from their symptoms.

FRANK

Frank (not his real name) was diagnosed in 2003. He currently takes small doses of Maripex and Propanonol.

Frank has had one dominant symptom over the past half decade – a tremor in one hand/arm. His symptoms have not "progressed" since he was diagnosed. Why not? Aren't symptoms supposed to "progress"? After all, that is what the textbooks say.

So, what does Frank do for himself to maintain his active life as a web designer and photographer? Here is his list: regular exercise, green tea, blueberries, meditation and QiGong once a week. He also listens to guided imagery meditations by Belleruth Naparstek which have been extremely helpful.

Everyone has their own way of feeling better. This list may not work for you, but it is clearly a winner for Frank.

ALAN

Alan is an ace photographer and web designer. Aside from his tremor, most of Alan's symptoms have gotten only a little worse since he was diagnosed in 2003 and seem to be very slow to progress.

"I'd like to think it's from the things I'm doing, but the truth is I don't really know. I may just have a slow progressing version (which tremor dominant PD often is). I'll take it - either way."

Here is Alan's story about what has helped him feel better and find relief from his symptoms.

"I was diagnosed in Oct 2003. Initial symptoms included right side hand tremors (I actually have 3 different types, lucky guy that I am), fine motor control klutziness, bradykinesia (slowness of motion), lack of arm swing, facial mask, beginning of stooped posture, micrographia and weak sense of smell."

"In early 2004, I began to sink into depression, a common Parkinson's disease symptom. I found Parkinsons depression different than the couple bouts with depression I'd been thru earlier in my life. It's not only that you have this lousy progressive disease (depressing by itself), but there's also a depletion of the important mood altering neurotransmitters - dopamine, serotonin and norepinephrin."

"Anyway, depression sinks all your boats, so in a rare moment of clarity I decided to make losing the depression job one. That decision was extremely important - a life-affirming, take control moment that began the arc of healing the depression so I could try to deal with everything else."

"I tried Prozac for a little while, but then the tremor got worse and I happened to see on the Prozac insert, one of the possible side effects was, you guessed it, tremor! (&^%#$). I did some talk therapy which helped a little, but what really turned things around for me was I resumed smoking cannabis which I had stopped for 6 months after my diagnosis. That largely took care of most of the depression. (I don't seem to get the negative effects that others experience - I feel more energized and creative and able to do everything I need to do)."

"Another thing that helped make me feel better was to take charge of my disease and treatment. I did enough research to feel comfortable making important decisions about what treatments to pursue. I saw the appropriate doctors and others as needed, and I value their expertise and advice, but the decisions are mine to make. I subscribe to a couple online email lists and visit a forum or two. I also get daily "Parkinsons" news alerts from Google. I don't read it all, just spend 10 or 15 minutes a day on it, but over the last few years, I've collected lots good info on subjects like potential tremor treatments and how to survive the process of getting SS Disability, etc. For me, this stuff is both useful and empowering (which makes me feel better)."

"In Jan, 2005, I started seeing Janice Walton-Hadlock, a Santa Cruz, CA Acupuncturist who has developed a Parkinson's treatment protocol using Chinese Acupressure and continued seeing her every 2 or 3 weeks or so for 2 yrs. Although I learned much, and have no regrets, for the most part, the treatment didn't help much. The disease progressed some, my symptoms got worse - especially the tremors. My sense of smell, however, got better."

"During this period I started other alternative work. Meditation, a guided imagery CD, QiGong - these helped with stress reduction and a bit with the depression. I'm still doing the QiGong, but not the other two (for now)."

"Then in Jan 2007, I decided it was time to try meds. I started with Mirapex and settled on a medium dose. It's worked very well for me, knocking back most of my symptoms to where I hardly notice them (except the tremors, which it doesn't help). It has also boosted my mood and energy. The only side effect has been some stomach stuff - light nausea and excess acid/reflux - nothing too serious. Also Mirapex may slow progression."

"For the tremor I tried a couple meds that did nothing for it - then I decided to focus on the worst of the 3 tremors - called a postural tremor. I requested Propranolol and it has helped some - kind of knocking the wind out of it. I have a little room to up the dose. Sometimes - and I don't know why - all the tremors disappear for a half day or even a day. It's really amazing to put my hand out and watch it remain steady as a rock!" As a side effect, the propranolol seems to have stopped my migraine headaches which I used to get a couple times a month."

"So here's the list of things I do or take to feel better - most of which are thought to be neuro-protective and may slow down the disease progression."

- Mirapex

- Propranolol

- CoQ10 @1200mg/day

- Vit E @ 1000

- Omega 3

- Green tea

- Blueberries

- Exercise -- stretches, walks, resistance

- QiGong

- Medical Cannabis

"The other thing that has really energized me and made me feel better has been the realization that I could use my tremors as a photographic technique. It's been extremely empowering. I feel I've taken back a bit of control in a situation where losing control a little at a time is normal. And it's very gratifying to hear people tell me that what I'm doing is inspiring to them. That's the best!"

"It also doesn't hurt that I'm blessed with a loving and very supportive wife (and good friends)...which reminds me that I found meditating on gratitude a very powerful technique."

Alan Babbitt PD History - March, 2008

The cover of this book is a superb example of Alan's "tremor enhanced" photography. You can see more images at: http://abproductions.com

SALLY

The following is an excerpt taken from an interview I had with Sally (not her real name) who has Parkinsons and who talks about using a technology for meditation and stress reduction called holosync.

I have personally used holosync for several years and found it helped me to reduce stress and maintain a deep meditative state. Read what Sally says below:

"A friend of mine told me about Holosync. It is supposed to help you get into a deeper meditation. It's expensive but I decided that I needed to try whatever means I could to help myself. So I bought this tape or CD and I've been listening to it about three weeks. I will not go to bed - I don't care if I'm home at 11:30 at night - without listening to it. I do fall asleep during many times but they say that's ok."

"They say it helps you in a lot of ways. Certainly they don't talk about any illness that they're going to help you with, but it just really helps you get into a deep meditative state."

"I would say that when I am meditating I do not shake. When I lie down I don't shake. When I sleep I don't shake. I guess it is pretty symptomatic that you're not supposed to shake. I don't have a problem sleeping. They say that Parkinson's patients have a

problem sleeping. I never had a problem. I don't know if it's the meditation tapes that I was listening to or the relaxation tapes but I just don't have a problem."

"The CD tape is like $179.00. What I've come to understand is that you listen to different levels. Now I realize they're going to try and sell you more levels. I just started with this and even if I keep the same one over and over, it seems to be helping."

"They don't claim and I don't claim that it's going to do anything, although I did have a great business idea, so it helps you on all kinds of levels. You know I thought, oh my God, this is terrific. I came up with a great business idea."

WORDS OF WISDOM FOR THE NEWLY DIAGNOSED

Imagine you had the opportunity to gather people together who have had Parkinsons for many years. Hear the advice now they would offer to anyone who has just been diagnosed with Parkinson's disease.

John Coleman , ND:

"I want to say to everyone diagnosed with Parkinsons it's your life, your body and your symptoms. Take control and change things. You can choose to live a healthier life. When you do, your body will become healthier.

Don't listen to anyone who says you can't. In fact, delete "can't" from your vocabulary. You can change if you choose to, and healthy changes will make you healthier".

Carol Meenan, Senior Advisor for Newly Diagnosed, Parkinsons Action Network.

"Don't give up. Don't give in to this disease. Fight it with all your might. Have a positive attitude and go on. Don't let it take your life over."

Mary Pauer:

"Love yourself. We are really hard on ourselves. I think I blamed myself for having the disease, that it was my fault, I did something wrong. Have hope. Pray."

Sandy:

"I think it is most important not to act as if you have a disease. In other words, continue to do all the activities that you enjoy or want to do or have to do even if you are a little slower or not as good at it.

I used to play a little golf – I never was good and I am worse now – but I just keep doing it. Just keep living a normal life. That will help you both physically and emotionally. I

© 2013 Parkinsons Recovery

think the emotional part is real important. Attitudes come from that. It reinforces the idea that you are normal. Just keep being normal."

Stan:

"Well, I'd want to tell them that first of all, Parkinsons is not in itself fatal. They do not have a fatal disease. They have a disease that might dis-accommodate them. Might make them feel uncomfortable. Might make them feel some pain.

There is hope to cope with all of this by getting your mindset and learning to just numb yourself out to the interference of Parkinsons and see what you can do to cope with it yourself."

Mary:

"Start your alternative therapies early. Everyone says

> *'I wish you had come to me five years ago.'*

And I was like – well, I was in another office. I would definitely try this Glutathione right away."

Nathan:

"First and most significant thing I would say to someone with Parkinsons is - get the Ayurvedic from <u>Dr. Paneri</u> *who has a thousand people under treatment and has cured close to a hundred of them I believe. Cured, meaning cured, final cured. How many people? In various degrees of improvement everyone is improving."*

<u>Marie Judd</u> *(Husband has Parkinsons):*

"The sooner they make these changes, open their minds and open their hearts to the idea of healing, the more likely they are to come to total recovery.

There is a new age of Parkinsons discovery coming about...Our understanding is expanding. Our capacity to back this up on our own with a lot of good health support is something I would dearly love for all of the people who are facing this situation to know.

The earlier they get at it, the better they will be. We know that we are on a correction direction. That is where we plan to stay. It took us 17 years to reach that brick wall and realize:

> *'Oh My goodness. We have to do something different'.*

John Carlin:

"When you first get diagnosed, the best thing you can do is get off the window sill and get back into the room. Keep trying. Deal with this as sanely as you can.

Depression is a big function early on. At least it was for me. I was able to get rid of the depression successfully. It wasn't one acupuncture needle that solved the whole thing. I went back every week for a month. Then every two weeks every month. After that I was shall we say cured.

I look forward to every year being better than the one before. You treat it like an elephant in the room. Your job is to shrink that elephant to smaller sizes so you can deal with it better. The elephant is always going to be there. It is your job to shrink it down. When you are having a bad day because the elephant farted it is your job to fan it.

Try and do as much research and educate yourself as much as you can. Do searches on the internet. You will come up with tons of information. The Michael J Fox Foundation is good for information. That is big money going after possible cures.

You've got to find a good set of health practitioners like I have put together. I know you cannot put those together immediately. Try and keep your head about yourself and not go off the deep end because you don't have to.

When you do go to your health care practitioner - your internist or neurologist or naturopath - bring another set of ears along. My wife comes to all of my appointments with me. You will be sitting there and your practitioner will say something and you will get fixated on that. The practitioner continues on with the conversation. You have totally fixated on the first part of the conversation and missed all the rest. Having another set of ears is very important when you go see your practitioners."

Lee Bender:

"Number one: You must develop hope in your mind. Whatever it takes to do it - however you talk to yourself - develop that hope and a good attitude that you are going to whip it. Don't be afraid to try some things.

Keep up the hope. Keep smiling. There is always a better day out there."

© 2013 Parkinsons Recovery

Cynthia Gilbertson:

> _"Keep trying different things. You don't know what is going to help you if you don't try. People sit in their rooms waiting for something to happen to them. You have to go out there and find it._
>
> _Don't wait until your symptoms are not responding to the drugs. The drugs will respond beautifully for a certain amount of time. Then they stop being effective. If you wait until then to deal with your situation with supplements or detoxing your body from the pesticides or whatever may be causing the problem it is a little bit too late. You have to start right away."_

Poet Kenneth Allen Patrick has a sister who has been diagnosed with Parkinsons. Kenneth wrote a book of poems titled _Parkinsons Won't Win_ which you can order from his website. It is a divinely inspired book of poems that offer hope to any and all persons who confront the symptoms of Parkinsons. You can also catch my radio interview with Kenneth who was a guest on my radio show October 1, 2009.

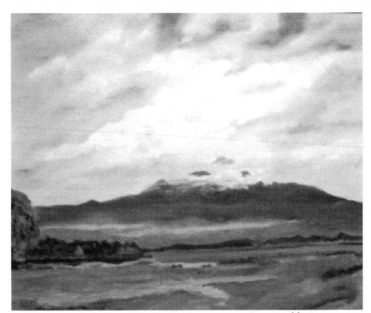

Cloudy Mountain by Edwin Ferran[14]

PARKINSONS AND CREATIVITY

If you happen to have the symptoms of Parkinsons, there is a near perfect chance that you have already been very successful with whatever you chose to do with your life. I validate this truth over and over, week after week in my conversations with people who have Parkinsons.

I now have a very strong suspicion that when the symptoms of Parkinsons creep into your daily life, many people become significantly more creative. They begin doing things they have never done before in new and innovative ways. Their creativity skyrockets (and it was already off the scales to begin with).

Something happens - perhaps to the soul of the brain - that is magical. Here is a snippet from one of my interviews with a man who has the symptoms of Parkinsons.

> *"Although I have always been creative when it comes to ideas, I had never written poetry before nor children's books and after I was diagnosed, I started doing both. It also seemed very easy for me to do so. When I sat down and started writing, the words flowed very quickly."*

For reasons unknown to me, I have observed that people with Parkinsons expand their horizons, make choices they never imagined taking and do things they had never planned on doing. The world is a better place because of it.

---

[14] **"Cloudy Mountain reminds me a little of a recent trip to Alaska I took with my wife Susan."** Edwin Ferran

Parkinsons is a gift in disguise. It is not a question of recovering the life that you had before the symptoms of Parkinsons. It is a question of honoring a new life that is gifted with unbounded creativity, wisdom and power.

> "I have experienced the same enhanced creativity as others. After being diagnosed 10 years ago I was laid off from my job after 9/11. It was during this time I began to use my father's tools he left me and started building things out of wood.
>
> So far I've built two blanket chests, one for my daughter, another for my wife, a toy chest for my niece, an outdoor barbecue table and a kitchen center island. In addition, I completely tore down our old deck and rebuilt it with composite boards, added all new vinyl railings and topped it off with deck lights. These things never entered my mind before being diagnosed."

I believe everyone has an inherent passion to create whether it is a new idea, furniture, art, comedy - the list is endless.

If I have been unable to create something new for even a day, I begin to have an empty feeling deep inside. It is a familiar feeling, a sense of sorts that I am wasting my life. When I can write as I am now, my juices flow. My energy expands. My steam for living bursts at the seams.

For many of us, there is too little opportunity for creativity to have a place in our lives. Jobs, family or other commitments have a way of commanding our attention and energy.

The body eventually insists that we devote the time and energy to create. If we do not allow an expression of our creativity our body inevitably gives us a reason to change our priorities, habits and passions.

Symptoms of Parkinsons cut away at the ego's insistence on being in total control. Neurological difficulties soften us. They tame a life time pattern of self-control. The endless reservoir of creativity which has remained dormant and silent is nudged to blossom. A renewal of impulsivity nurtures creations we never realized we were capable of manifesting.

What does our body do when confronted with neurological challenges? It sends us a clear signal to slow down, change our habits and do things differently - out of necessity. If the choice were up to us we would probably not initiate any changes.

The symptoms of Parkinsons slow down the time spent on addictions that do not feed our creativity. When the furious pace of activity is sufficiently slowed the creative juices that simmer from deep within our souls have time to ferment.

© 2013 Parkinsons Recovery

This in no way implies that we were uncreative previously. The focus and intent of the creative impulses shift. Let me explain.

INNOVATION VERSUS CREATIVITY

One form of creativity is to be innovative which involves generating creative ideas and applying them to a specific context. With innovation the problem is clearly defined and the solution set is clearly bounded.

This form of creativity takes a given problem or challenge and solves it. For example, how do I invent a car that runs on water? Or, how do I motivate my secretary to come to work on time? Or, how do I fix my clothes washing machine that is so old the part I need is out of stock?

When lives are busy and demanding, a second form of creativity lies dormant just below the surface of our consciousness. It waits for a chance - any chance - to pop out and claim its birth right to be heard.

This is the form of raw creativity where something entirely new pops out of our brains for no reason whatsoever. There is no pre-defined problem to solve. There is no deadline to meet. Instead there resides a massive body of creative urges and ideas deep inside each of us that are patiently waiting their time to be acknowledged.

THE PROCESS OF CREATIVITY

What is the process that makes this happen? Control does not work. If you try to order the creative ideas to be revealed they will drill a hole even deeper into your subconscious and cuddle up for the long haul.

Using brute force to dislodge creative thoughts does not work. You will have just as much luck trying to break through the walls of Fort Knox with a jack hammer. Setting a schedule for creative ideas to be revealed does not work. Creativity does not obey a time schedule.

Enough. How do thoughts that seemingly have no origin or history find their way out of our own consciousness? How will we know them when we see them? They are revealed in their own time and place as we quiet down the mind babble that controls our lives. They pop out in the most unexpected ways during the moments of living when we are at peace with ourselves.

We become creative when we quiet the chatter of our minds and allow the part of us we have stuffed for too many years to emerge. It is the ultimate calling to become whole again.

For many people this opportunity comes because our bodies make us slow down the quick pace of activity and force us to take in the mysteries of the world. We appreciate our friends and spouses in new ways. We see life differently.

Once the feverish activity of our minds slows to a snail's pace the creative juices begin to percolate. At long last we recognize a good idea when it pops out of our minds because we can feel the surge of energy that bubbles up from inside.

The same creative ideas may have peaked around the corner to be noticed by us before, but we were too busy to notice. The faucet of adrenaline was wide open and all of the associated hormones were being manufactured by our body 24-7. No rest for the restless.

To summarize, the symptoms of Parkinsons slow down the pace of life. An opening is created for the creative juices to flow and the fresh ideas to emerge. We begin to do things we have always wanted to do in our lives, but did not know it until now. We stuffed the creative urges before because there was no time. Now, with a little more space for new things to happen, we become whole again.

RECEIVING THE CREATIVE ENERGIES OF OUR MOTHERS AND FATHERS
Men need to feel the support of their fathers for true creativity to blossom. Women need to feel the support of their mothers. When we genuinely receive and accept that support, we come into our full creative power. We manifest creations we never before thought were possible.

When we take in the support of our father, we are also receiving the creative energies of all fathers who came before him - all our grandfathers, great grandfathers, great great grandfathers (and so forth and so on) that go back in time generation after generation.

When we fully receive the support of our mother, we are also receiving the creative energies of all mothers who came before her – all our grandmothers, great grandmothers. great great grandmothers (and so forth and so on) that go back in time generation after generation.

I have personally noticed a profound shift in my own energy and attitude toward life after I fully took in the support from my own father. I had resisted his support for years, having convinced myself I could do everything on my own. I distanced myself from him. It is much easier and more truthful to acknowledge and honor the truth that I am just like him. I acknowledge his creativity and thus become more creative myself.

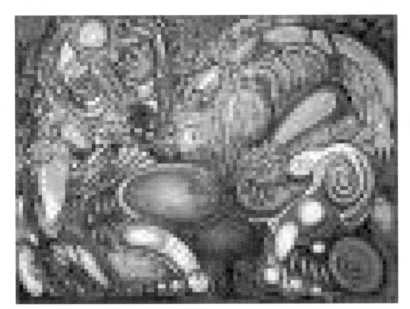

COMMITMENT IS THE KEY

Creation by

Carol McLeod

One of the Pioneers of Recovery is the well known comedian and juggler Chris Bliss who has appeared on the Tonight Show countless times. While Chris does not have the symptoms of Parkinsons himself, I have reflected often about his answer to being asked the following question I asked him:

> *"What practical suggestions do you have for people who are trying to live their lives in that very same space you are in when you are juggling?"*

I found his answer inspirational.

> *"I was doing a conference with Sir Bob Geldof in Scotland. His story is pretty remarkable. He was sort of a washed up rock star. Now he has became the first Bono with the first Live Aid concerts.*
>
> *He was telling the story of how he got to be this person of tremendous impact in the world. Basically it was just by putting one foot in front of the other and making the commitment.*
>
> *He read a great quote about commitment from a Scottish Mountaineer named W.H. Murray*
>
> > *'...Until one is committed, there is hesitancy, the chance to draw back, always ineffectiveness concerning all acts of initiative and creation. There is one elementary truth, the ignorance of which kills countless ideas and splendid plans: that the moment one definitely commits oneself, then providence moves too. A*

whole stream of events issues from the decision raising in one's favor all manner of unforeseen events, meetings and material assistance which no man could have dreamed would have come their way. I learned a deep respect for one of Goethe's couplets:

> *'Whatever you can do or dream you can, begin it. Boldness has genius, power and magic in it. Begin it now!'*

It is just something I have seen take place. Once you lose the fear and make the commitment, providence moves with you. All manner of resources and opportunities appear that didn't exist before. Just making the commitment unleashes all sorts of things whichever among those commitments it is, whether it is (like you said) to exercise, to diet, to just being as proactive as possible in the face of Parkinsons and what people are facing. I think commitment is just the most enormously empowering thing. It has always been my issue in life. It is a real key."

Take action today. And tomorrow. And the next day. There are many ways to get relief from your symptoms. I have documented them in this book. You have taken the first step by reading **_Road to Recovery_**. Now take action on one therapy or approach that calls out to you. If that one does not help, choose another.

The world needs you to hang around for a little longer. The world needs to benefit from your gifts and your talents. The world needs you to recover so you can fulfill your passions and your dreams.

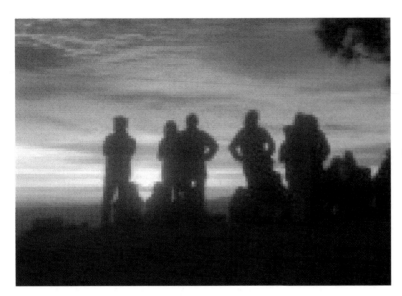

People gathering by Peter Thompson

WHAT ARE SOME TREATMENTS WHICH RELIEVE TREMORS?

I am very hesitant to answer this question directly. You can obviously review my general suggestions on treatments for tremors in this book, but I have a problem with offering specific suggestions. I know nothing about your actual situation. More to the point, your question smacks up against the unrewarding strategy of masking symptoms rather than identifying the root cause.

When there are tremors - as in your case - your body is sending you a strong message that something is seriously out of balance.

- *Perhaps the imbalance involves exposure to toxins.*
- *Perhaps it involves a past trauma that is unresolved.*
- *Perhaps it involves living a stressful life that offers your body little relief from a continuous adrenaline rush.*
- *Perhaps it is due to an insufficiency of certain substances the body needs to create energy.*
- *Perhaps it is due to an overabundance of dopamine which is not being properly assimilated by the body.*
- *Perhaps it is due to a deficiency of dopamine.*

And to make matters even more complicated, this is a short list of possibilities! I think the better questions to ask first are:

© 2013 Parkinsons Recovery

- *Why is my body sending me this strong signal?*
- *What is causing my body to react as it is reacting now?*

There is indeed a long list of possible answers to these questions. How do you find the answers?

A variety of assessments are available to you that can provide rich information about any and all imbalances in your body. These include (among others) bioenergetic testing, saliva tests, voice analysis, hair analysis to ascertain the presence of toxins and a wide variety of standard medical tests.

Health care practitioners have creative ways of ascertaining the root cause using muscle testing. We teach people how to use muscle testing at our Jump Start to Wellness programs because it is an approach that is free, easy to do and reliable.

In summary, I would say in response to your question that yes - it is certainly possible to mask a tremor with a wide variety of approaches including prescription medications, natural herbs and exercise. With most such treatments (other than exercise) more of the medicine or herb or supplement is needed over time to get the same effect. You ultimately wind up creating more problems for yourself as the imbalances become more pronounced.

Why not ask a different question here which is:

What is the underlying cause here?

Once you figure out the answer to this question you can search for a treatment or therapy that will address the cause. With this approach masking the tremor becomes irrelevant. It may take longer to find relief from the tremor but in the long run the outcome will be far more rewarding.

I WOULD LIKE TO TRY FAVA BEANS TO BOAST MY DOPAMINE LEVELS. I FOUND BLANCHED AND SHELLED BEANS BUT I DON'T KNOW IF THEY HAVE ENOUGH DOPAMINE TO MAKE THEM WORTHWHILE OR HOW TO PREPARE THEM.

Eating fava beans are a delicious, natural food in themselves that also happen to enhance dopamine in the body. For regular updates on fava beans be sure to become a regular visitor of the Parkinsons Recovery Fava Bean blog sponsored by Aunt Bean who has a four acre farm in Tennessee where she grows fava beans and mucuna.

http://www.favabeans.parkinsonsrecovery.com

You will get the most mileage out of the value of fava beans if you sprout them first. Aunt Bean formulates a homemade tincture using the tips of the fava bean plants. Why not consider growing your own - as does Aunt Bean?

Keep in mind that ingesting fava beans in whatever form may have an effect on your medication, so be sure and consult with your doctor about any adjustments that may be required if you decide to add fava beans to your diet.

DO YOU HAVE ANY INFORMATION ON LYME DISEASE AND PARKINSONS? I WAS BITTEN BY A TICK IN 1998 AND DIAGNOSED WITH PARKINSONS 30 MONTHS LATER.

Oh my goodness. This sounds like a huge clue regarding a probable cause of your symptoms. The symptoms of Lyme disease are very similar to those of Parkinson's. Many people get misdiagnosed with Parkinson's when the true culprit is a Lyme infection.

The treatment for Lyme is a long term use of antibiotics. The challenge of the treatment is that antibiotics destroy the immune system and the digestive system which also create other disruptive imbalances in the body. Naturopath doctors treat infections using homeopathic treatments and natural herbs which are typically not as disruptive to the digestive system.

We know that the factors which cause neurological complications are multi-faceted and one of the root causes turns out to be bacterial infections of one form or another. There is a particular bacterial infection which is horrendously difficult to detect called mycoplasma. These are tiny bacteria that create a neurological disaster in the body. From my recent research, it appears many people have these bacteria and do not even know it.

The best resource I have found on treating the Lyme infection which is far more common than most people realize is Dietrich Kinghardt, MD:www.klinghardtacademy.com

DO OTHER PD PEOPLE NOTICE A CHANGE/WORSENING OF SYMPTOMS SEASONALLY? I JUST REALIZED THAT FOR SEVERAL YEARS NOW MY SYMPTOMS SEEM TO INCREASE ABOUT DECEMBER OR JANUARY. THIS TIME PERIOD IS WHEN I HAVE BEEN STARTING OR CHANGING OR INCREASING MEDICATIONS.

Yes - my experience is that many people experience a flare up of symptoms during the winter. I suspect there are several reasons:

- *Diet - the holidays trigger unhealthy eating.*
- *Lack of exercise - the winter months can mean colder weather with more rain and snow.*
- *Lack of sunshine - Although you live in a rather hot climate, vitamin D3 may not be an issue - but Naturopath Doctor Laurie Mischley finds most people with Parkinson's*

symptoms have severe vitamin D3 deficiencies. If there is less sunshine - your body will be getting less D3 the natural way.

- *Change or addition of medications - If you have been adding new medications or increasing the dosage, that could also be a possible cause of a symptom flare up due to interactions and side effects.*

All in all - there are a multitude of factors that can potentially contribute to shifts in symptoms seasonally. Since there are typically fluctuations - you can always celebrate improvement down the road.

CAN YOU RECOMMEND ANY TECHNIQUES TO IMPROVE MY WALKING? AT PRESENT I TEND TO DRAG MY RIGHT LEG. IF I GO FOR A WALK I AM OK AFTER ABOUT HALF A MILE. I TEND TO DRAG MY LEG ON SHORT RUNS AND AROUND THE HOUSE

First, consider doing Tai Chi on a regular basis. It is a good idea to connect with a teacher who is proficient. There are excellent DVDs on Tai Chi that are also extremely helpful if accessed on a regular basis.

Arieh Breslow in particular has produced an outstanding DVD - When Less is More - that is mindful of the mobility challenges that confront individuals who currently experience the symptoms of Parkinson's.

Second, I have a suggestion offered by professional dancer Pamela Quinn during my radio show interview with her on September 30, 2010. The entire show is worth hearing from start to end. Pamela offers a number of suggestions to persons with mobility challenges. She suggested that you practice kicking a soccer ball using the leg that drags. It helps to wake up that lazy leg.

You obviously do not want to kick a soccer ball while going to work or doing errands. Instead - you simply pretend that you are kicking the soccer ball as you walk from one place to the next. It works just as well as if you were actually kicking it.

Third, try bouncing a ball as you walk - just as you did when you were a boy. Your foot is dragging because your body is navigating through neural pathways that are dysfunctional. When you bounce a ball while you walk - you create new neural networks. This short circuits the old pathways that are presently hindering that lazy leg's functionality.

I AM WONDERING ABOUT HOW TO DEAL WITH SLOW MOVEMENT. ARE THERE ANY WAYS TO OVERCOME THIS? IT IS MY WORST SYMPTOM.

The big picture is to reprogram your neural networks. It appears that your movements are being controlled by neural pathways that are a bit rusty. There is no reason for panic!

© 2013 Parkinsons Recovery

The brain has an incredible capacity to reconfigure pathways. You just have to begin moving a bit differently to configure the new pathways which will make walking easier and require less effort on your part.

First, I suggest that you listen to my interview with Professional Dancer Pamela Quinn from New York City. Pamela offers a number of suggestions you will find helpful during my radio show which aired September 30, 2010.

Second, I suggest that you add a little music (with a hefty beat) when you walk. Use an MP3 player or IPOD or any portable device. Find some music you like to listen to which has a marching type of beat. Music with a strong beat does wonders for movements that are slow and cumbersome. Michael Jackson recorded some great songs with incredible beats.

Third, there are a number of brain challenge exercises and programs which provide great ways to forge new neural pathways. You might try out a few. They always have free ones to try out on the websites. I post information on the Parkinsons Recovery blog about such programs from time to time and a number of posts are archived there.

Fourth, inside of thinking of walking from point A to point B, think to yourself that you will dance from Point A to Point B. You may be surprised by your body's response to a shift in your thinking.

THE MEDICATIONS ARE NOT WORKING FOR ME NOW. CAN I GET A BLOOD TEST OR A SCAN OR ANYTHING ELSE IN THE WAY OF A TEST TO TELL ME HOW GOOD OR BAD I AM AND WHAT CAN I DO FOR MYSELF. I FEEL SO USELESS, NOT KNOWING WHAT TO DO NEXT.

First, person after person with Parkinsons on the road to recovery tell me it is extremely important to find health care practitioners who are trustworthy, professional and helpful. They need to be there for you. They need to be available to answer all of your questions. If they are not, find someone else to be a member of your medical team.

Second, it appears you have focused all of your recovery efforts on prescription medications. This program of recovery is not helping you now, though it may have been helpful in the beginning. When a person begins to take more than one prescription medication, side effects and interactions can be very problematic. Where do you go from here?

I recommend that you launch a search outside the domain of prescription medications. The option of prescription medications works well for some people and poorly for others. Everyone is different.

There are a multitude of therapies - some thousands of years old - that people with Parkinsons say give them relief from their symptoms. Most therapies are natural, safe and offer the potential for improvement in your health on some level. Take time to review the therapies that

© 2013 Parkinsons Recovery

are discussed here in Road to Recovery that have helped people get well. There is a wide range of choices to consider from sound therapy to vibration therapy to herbal remedies to quantum healing to energy healing to biofeedback to Emotional Freedom Technique to ... The list goes on and on.

I would recommend that you find another health care provider - perhaps a naturopath or osteopath or an MD or a neurologist - who you can connect with. I also recommend that you listen to some of the Parkinsons Recovery radio shows that are archived. All downloads are free. You will find useful suggestions in virtually every show I have aired over the past two years. You can always listen to the radio shows live and call in with your questions.

There is no definitive test for Parkinson's. Scans simply rule out other possible causes. There is no blood test. Instead of focusing on what is out of balance in your body – focus your thoughts on what is in balance. Be delightfully surprised to realize how many functions of your body are actually functioning quite well indeed.

Set your intention to transform your thoughts. When we focus on what is wrong - we feed the illness with more energy. We give it food to digest. This makes the symptoms get worse. When we focus on what is right and strong - we get stronger inside and out.

The people who are recovering realize that they have to take responsibility for their own health. When our bodies get out of balance we have to take responsibility for our own health and wellness. In the end, we are really the only one who can figure out what is happening to us and how to heal it.

DO YOU KNOW WHETHER THERE IS A CURE FOR THE DISEASE WITH THE INVENTION OF A NEW PILL AT THE FOREFRONT?

Will there be a cure for the symptoms? No. There is not now nor will there be a single factor that causes the symptoms associated with a diagnosis of Parkinson's disease. If there were a single cause, then it might be possible to see a "cure" down the road.

There will never be a cure because the conditions that create the symptoms are multi-faceted. There are a minimum of five unique cycles in the body involving dozens of pathways that are critical to a healthy neurological system. When any link in any one of the causal pathways is compromised, symptoms will emerge.

Each person's situation is entirely unique to them. That is why the symptoms vary so widely across individuals and why the "solution" will be unique to each person.

Please take note of my writing here. I am not qualifying my answer. I am not even saying this is my belief or my idea regarding a cure. I am so certain that I am right that I am flat out saying - no. There will never be a cure.

Trauma creates havoc with the neurological system. Stress damages neural connections. Toxins blow the neurological system up. When you realize the complexity of the factors that cause the symptoms, it is easy to see why no single solution will ever be found.

From my contact with hundreds and hundreds of people who currently experience the symptoms of Parkinsons I have observed the following. The people who are hoping for a cure or are looking for someone to fix them feel worse and worse with each passing week. The people who are taking responsibility for their health and take it upon themselves to figure out what their body is telling them feel better with each passing week.

Davis Phinney, founder of the Davis Phinney Foundation, believes that it is a huge mistake to wait for a cure. Waiting means that you are not living. Embrace what you can do for yourself each and every day – whatever that might be. In a small way, you discover your own cure.

The bottom line: Take responsibility for your life and you get better. Expect someone or something to fix you and you get worse. When we stop holding on to the hope of a cure, we suddenly realize it is up to us to heal ourselves. It is very empowering to realize all healing comes from within, not from without.

WHAT IS THE BEST WAY TO TRIGGER A PLACEBO EFFECT AND MAINTAIN IT TO REACH THE RECOVERY?

The placebo effect is simply a way of installing the belief that you are going to get better. But how do you maintain the belief that recovery is possible, especially when symptoms can flare at any moment? It is easy to switch a positive outlook into a negative one in a matter of seconds.

The key is to acknowledge that maintaining the belief that recovery is happening is a moment to moment process. In any given moment we can choose to criticize, judge and be negative about our situation or instill thoughts that embrace hope, new possibilities, new visions and new life for ourselves and our family.

We have over 60,000 thoughts a day. An interesting twist for most of us is that 90% of those thoughts are the same thoughts we had yesterday, the day before and a year ago. We trash ourselves with negative thoughts day in and day out.

Simply put, we humans are really not very creative when it comes to the thoughts that we express silently to ourselves. Perhaps we have an affinity for being redundant. Perhaps we get negative pleasure in beating up on ourselves.

Make it a practice to recognize the hamster wheel of negative thinking when it starts to churn. Acknowledge the power of negative thought forms when they rear their ugly head. Release, remove, detach, eject and shield those thoughts from pestering us again. Hop off of the hamster wheel. Hop onto a vehicle that takes you on the road you do want to travel down - the Road to Recovery.

© 2013 Parkinsons Recovery

Maintaining the beliefs that will make us well depends on a steady focus and unwavering intention. Day by day negativity is released, allowing new possibilities to become manifest. This is not an easy process. It takes time and focus, but it is doable when a clear intention is set.

At Parkinsons Recovery we devote time and attention to helping people who attend our Jump Start to Wellness programs with just this type of transformation. It makes the difference between coming back into balance and nurturing the spirit of our souls or sustaining a state of disharmony that nurtures the symptoms of discomfort and disease.

CAN YOU GIVE ME A SUGGESTION FOR HOW TO REVITALIZE MY SUPPORT GROUP? PEOPLE ARE LOSING INTEREST AND DROPPING OUT LIKE FLIES.

Here is an activity Pamela Quinn uses in her own classes that is the perfect kick off to a support group meeting. To prepare, you will need to purchase three gamma tennis balls from a sport supply store. The soft gamma balls are used by novice tennis players. Here is how Pamela describes the game:

> *"You get in a circle and you establish a pattern. Pam throws to Joe. Joe throws to Leo. Leo throws to Martha. Martha throws to Dorothy. Dorothy throws back to Pam. You then keep that pattern going.*
>
> *Once you accomplish that with one ball you add in another ball. Once you accomplish that with two balls you add in a third ball. You just have to know who you are throwing to and who is throwing to you. As you toss the ball the excitement increases. It is a fun game to play - all the while having the idea of helping your reflexes stay in tune and helping your body control as you have these little shifts of weight."*

Ball tossing offers support group members an opportunity to develop better hand - eye coordination. It also entails the challenge to shift weight quickly. You have to reach to get a ball that is being thrown to you or you have to lean forward or backward. It deals both with quick reactions and hand eye coordination. It is also total fun for everyone.

WHAT HAPPENS IF YOU TAKE SINEMET AND MUCUNA AT THE SAME TIME?

The following account was written by Max. Max has Parkinsons and lives in Canada.

> *"I'm 53 years old (or young). I was diagnosed with PD back in March 2001. I had a minimal exposure to PD meds back then, just long enough (one month on Sinemet) to see an improvement. That convinced me that I have PD. Whatever PD is."*
>
> *"I started taking lots of vitamins, antioxidants, eating better, exercising the best I can, meditating, acupuncture, Ti-Chi, tried PDrecovery, QiGong, visualizing techniques, energy work, etc. etc. I'm sure it all helped, but eventually I needed a walker and could barely take care of myself."*

"By February of 2006, 5 years later, I was having a hard time using a walker and was looking into getting a wheelchair. I couldn't take it any longer, so I regrettably broke down and decided to take Sinemet. "

"In about a week, Sinemet started to work. And in about a month, I was a completely different person. I could walk, got my balance back, started to gain back my normal weight and I could even ride my mountain bike again.""

"But in only 6 months of taking Sinemet, I found it was taking longer and longer to kick in, not lasting as long and sometimes it wouldn't kick in at all. Sometimes I would take 1 1/2 tablets of Sinemet CR 200/50, at time, with no effect at all."

"Talk about being scared all over again. I knew getting on Sinemet would be a limited ride, but I never thought it could be this short for me."

"When I heard about "Mucuna Pruriens" (Zandopa also called HP-200), a natural herb from India, in the fall of 2006, I got very interested. The first time I tried it, I felt some improvement. In about two months, I gradually reduced my Sinemet CR 200/50 from 5 tablets a day to only 1 tablet a day (break it into 1/3's) and I take it with Mucuna. "

"I feel like this "Mucuna" (Zandopa) is REALLY HELPING me a lot. I take it 3 or 4 times a day and can pretty well function normally when the herbs kick in - not bad considering that I was ready for a wheelchair. When the herbs wear off, my PD symptoms still come back, but not nearly as bad as before. "

"I've been taking Mucuna and Sinemet for the past 1 1/2 years. I'm currently taking 1/2 a tablet of Sinemet (200/50) with 1 tsp of powdered Mucuna (Zandopa) 3 or 4 times a day. In 3 hour intervals."

I also take Ashwaganda & Brahmi. I try not to take anything in the evening or before I go to bed. I like to give my body a break and give it a chance to build up its own dopamine over night. It seems to work because I can go for an hour walk in the morning before I take my herbs."

"I purchase Zandopa directly from India:

http://mall.coimbatore.com/bnh/zandu/zandopa.htm

"From my own personal experience, if anyone with pd wants to try Mucuna, I recommend that you take it slowly. You might want to get some small measuring spoons, the kind used for cooking. I've started taking a level 1/4 tsp of powered Mucuna (Zandopa) 3 times a day for the first week. A 1/2 tsp 3 times a day for the second week. And I worked my way to 3/4 tbsp 4 times a day by the 4th week."

"I also gradually reduced my Sinemet from 4 (200/50) tablets per day to only one pill a day in a couple of months. I break the Sinemet pill into quarters. I take the Sinemet at the same time as the Mucuna."

"It works best if you take it at least 1/2 hour before meals or at least 1 1/2 hours after a meal. I mix the Zandopa in half a glass of water. I use a small hand held blender to mix it, it gets rid of the sludge at the bottom. Personally I don't mind the taste, but I do add some juice to it cranberry, etc."

"I'm doing all this on my own right now, but you should let your doctor know what you're doing. I keep a record (date, time of day, amount, when it kicked in, faded out, and effects (good or bad) meals time, etc."

"Just take it slowly. If you feel anxious, hyper, antsy, or have a lot more energy than normal, you know you're taking too much."

"I space the doses by three hours 'till the next one. I take just enough to be normal without feeling anxious. It works extremely well for me; I'm really surprised more people with pd don't take it."

"My pd hasn't gotten any worse in the past 1 1/2 years of taking Mucuna. If anything I've gotten better in some areas.

I no longer have any balance problems, haven't been constipated for over a year now. No longer have any tremors unless I'm stressed. Can ride a bike, jog, walk normal etc. when the herbs are in my system. But I did have to increase my intake of Mucuna. I'm now taking 1 level tsp. And 1/2 a tablet of Sinemet (200/500) 3 or 4 times a day."

"I'm not having any negative side effects at all from taking Mucuna. My body has adapted to it. I believe the body can repair itself; taking Mucuna is a natural plant product. It helps me regain my strength so I can take care of myself.

I AM CURRENTLY ON A REGIMEN OF STALEVO, AZILECT AND CoQ10. MY MAJOR PROBLEMS ARE BALANCE, MUSCLE WEAKNESS (MOSTLY LEFT SIDED), WORSENING MANUAL DEXTERITY AND SOME COGNITIVE DETERIORATION (INCLUDING SHORT-TERM MEMORY PROBLEMS). ARE THERE ANY SUPPLEMENTS TO ADD OR ANYTHING I SHOULD BE DOING TO HELP SLOW PROGRESSION OR REVERSE SYMPTOMS?

There are four parts to my response.

1. When you take more than one prescription medication and/or supplement there is always the chance of a drug/supplement interaction.

2. Supplements may not help people with Parkinsons because their digestive systems do not work properly.

3. An alternative to taking supplements is to have a nutritional IV. This therapy involves infusing vitamins and minerals directly into the blood stream, by passing the digestive system altogether.

© **2013 Parkinsons Recovery**

4. Pay very close attention to what you eat. What we put into our bodies has a much more significant impact on how we feel than anything else we can do.

Every one's situation is unique. I may have a deficiency in magnesium. You may have a deficiency in calcium. The critical issue turns on how you can determine what your body needs, not what my body needs.

One alternative that works for some people is to ask your doctor to run a set of lab tests to determine if any deficiencies exist. You will then have an idea of what foods to eat and what supplements you should be taking.

The downside of this alternative is that it is very expensive and the results are only applicable for the present. Needs of your body are always changing, so what your body needs today may shift by tomorrow. Our bodies are in a constant flux of change.

A second alternative is to give your body the basic vitamins and minerals that it needs to maintain balance and vitality. It is a good idea to take a multi-vitamin supplement as we age. There are also super antioxidant foods and vitamins that help the body maintain hormonal balance (e.g.: vitamin B6, B12, folic acid, amino acids, fish oil, etc.).

The downside of a decision to take supplements that one expert or another suggests is this: There may be adverse reactions with the supplements and the prescription medications that you are taking. It is not necessarily a good idea to pour one supplement after another into your body without taking into consideration the consequences.

When you take more than one prescription medication and/or supplement the possibility of an adverse interaction always exists.

I believe that one of the best choices a person can make who takes more than one prescription medication is to have a comprehensive nutritional consultation. Our nutritional consultations are done over the phone by Randy Mentzer, a licensed pharmacist in Washington and a certified clinical nutritionist.

My experience is that people with Parkinsons often feel lousy because their medications are working against one another. Randy does a comprehensive review of your medical history and offers a set of individualized recommendations that you can take to your doctor for further review and discussion.

I personally do not have any idea if there are any contraindications from the medications and supplements you listed in your question. Randy helps out our clients with all such questions.

© 2013 Parkinsons Recovery

Randy tells me that there is a good chance of problems if a person takes two prescription medications. He also tells me that there is a 100% chance of adverse interactions if you take five or more medications.

I believe that a good step to take on the road to recovery is to request a thorough investigation of any potential interactions that may be coexistent with the medications and supplements you currently take. Ask a certified clinical nutritionist for a full evaluation. They are the health care providers who know about drug interactions and are in a position to recommend good alternatives if problems with interactions are identified.

Any prescription drug may be perfectly safe and useful when used alone. But when combined with a second drug, the same drug can create horrible problems for a person. Randy often has to do additional research to understand the implications of combining certain medications together.

So, let's say that you have checked out the medications that you are currently taking and have resolved any issues and problems that have been identified. Perhaps you reduced doses or switched medications at the recommendation of your doctor. Or, perhaps what you are taking now is not creating any problems.

You now decide to bite the bullet and take vitamins and supplements that one expert or another says should offer you relief from the symptoms of Parkinsons. You spend $300. You take the supplements for a month.

To your grave disappointment, there is no improvement. You don't feel worse but you certainly do not feel any better. What is happening here? Might you just as well have poured the $300 down your kitchen sink? The answer to this question may be yes!

Supplements often do not help people with Parkinsons because their digestive systems have shut down. I of course have no idea if digestion is a problem for you. You do not mention digestion as a problem in your list of symptoms. I do know that digestion is a problem for many people as they age and for many people with Parkinsons.

For example, when we eat wheat, the walls of our intestines gradually become crusty with a cement like paste. Nutrients pass through the entire digestive track without being absorbed. They are discharged from the body in tack - literally. Many people have colons that are plugged up with undigested food.

A second step on the road to recovery is thus to take an assessment of any digestive blockages you might have. Excellent alternatives exist on ways to detox and clean out your digestive system.

© 2013 Parkinsons Recovery

Naturopaths are skilled at being able to help you detox your digestive system. Colon Therapists are trained to clear out the debris and pathogens that may have been residing in your colon since you were 12 (or 20 or 30 or...). There are nationally certified programs that train people to do a colon cleansing safely and effectively.

Depending on the therapy you choose, it can potentially take months to get your digestive system back on track. What do you do in the meantime? How do you help yourself feel better now?

An alternative is to bypass the digestive system altogether by having a doctor or naturopath administer nutritional IV's. This therapy involves the infusion of vitamins and minerals directly into the blood stream through an IV.

With nutritional IV's you are mainlining the nutrients directly into the blood stream. The digestive system is bypassed, so it does not matter if it is not working properly. Nutritional IV's should be done only to jump start the systems in your body so that you can begin to feel better quickly. The idea is to get your body back on track so it can do the work it knows how to do so well: Keep your hormones in balance and your spirits high.

Do not plan to receive nutritional IV's for long. They are simply a way to help you feel better quickly so that you have the energy needed to heal.

There are many experienced and highly qualified doctors (MD's and naturopaths) who administer nutritional IV's to patients. If you choose this path it is important to find someone who is certified, experienced and equipped to administer nutritional IV's in a sterilized environment.

What we put into our bodies has a more significant impact on how we feel than anything else we can do for ourselves. The one single thing you can do to feel better is to maintain vigilance on what you eat and drink. What we eat has everything to do with how we feel.

Imagine a large circle in your mind's eye. The circle represents the sum total of everything you can do for yourself to feel better (exercise, laughter, mind challenges, stress and trauma release, etc.). Now place a single dot somewhere inside your imagined circle. This dot represents the contribution supplements typically make to helping people get relief from their symptoms.

The far more significant factor is the food we put into our bodies. Good nutrition consumes a huge chunk of this circle. All things considered, the best thing you can do for yourself to get relief from the symptoms of Parkinsons is to be mindful of what you put into your body.

Eat well and I promise that you will feel better soon.

© 2013 Parkinsons Recovery

DO YOU THINK THAT USING THE MEDICATIONS CAN MAKE YOUR SYMPTOMS WORSE? I HAVE BEEN TAKING L/DOPA FOR 6 MONTHS NOW AND JUST INCREASED MY DOSE IN THE LAST COUPLE WEEKS AND I HAVE NOTICED MORE TREMORS IN MY LEGS.

Unfortunately, taking medications is a two edged sword. Yes, they can provide relief from some of the symptoms - especially in the short run. And yes, all prescription medications have side effects. If you list all of the side effects associated with the prescription medications that are available to treat Parkinson's disease you will actually see a list of the symptoms that are associated with Parkinson's.

Some people experience few side effects. They find the medications provide them with welcome relief. Other people report that the side effects are worse than the symptoms they experienced before taking the medications.

As you know, I am not a medical doctor. I am not qualified to diagnose what is happening to you. I can offer a simple observation. If you increase the dose of a medication and the symptoms are worse than before, your body is giving you a strong message. For whatever reason, the medication(s) you are presently taking do not appear to be helping.

It could be a single medication. Or, it could be the side effects created from taking more than one medication. It is time to have a follow-up consultation with your doctor.

WHAT IS THE BEST EXERCISE FOR PEOPLE WITH PARKINSONS DISEASE?

The following answer to this question was offered by professional dancer Pamela Quinn during my radio show on September 30, 2010.

> 1 "*Do an exercise or a sport that you used to do as a child. There is a neurological memory, a neurological map built into you that is already there - the old saying that once you have ridden a bike you always know how to ride a bike routine. If you used to play tennis you will still know how to do that forehand and backhand. You won't necessarily be as good as you used to be but the elements will be there. If you can do something and take pleasure in it, you are more likely to do it more frequently.*"

> 2. "*Do a kind of exercise you have never done before as a way of having to learn something - to create new neural activity in the brain.*"

> 3. "*Whatever you do, try to do it with someone else - whether it is a friend, a personal trainer, a family member, your pet. You can make a commitment to yourself to do something but you won't keep it. If you make a commitment to someone else, the likelihood of your keeping it is much improved. It is much more likely you will get out and do what you planned to do*

There is no one exercise program that is going to be the best for everyone that has Parkinsons. Don't think of it that way. Think of it as:

"What is best suited to me?

It depends on what you like. It depends on what your history is. It depends on your climate, on where you live. It depends on how close you are to something. It depends on who will do "X" with you. There are a whole bunch of factors that go into helping you get going. Just do it. That is what is important here."

WHAT ARE EXERCISE AND DIET REMEDIES THAT WOULD HELP MY HUSBAND WHO HAS PARKINSONS?

From my extensive review of the research literature on Parkinsons you have asked the right question. Diet and exercise have a compelling influence on how your husband feels every day.

- Eat healthy food. Exercise. He will feel better.

- Eat junk food. Be a couch potato. He will feel lousy.

It is as simple as that. This is not rocket science.

The research on exercise and Parkinsons is unequivocal. Exercise helps people feel better and get relief from their symptoms.

WHAT NATURAL METHODS CAN HELP ME WALK BETTER?

Bounce a Ball

Do you have a tennis ball or a rubber ball of any type? When you walk, bounce the ball just like you did when you were small. Bounce the ball on the ground as you walk. If that doesn't help – throw it into the air as you walk.

There is a plastic ball (filled with water) which you find at fairs which has a rubbery string or chain that is attached to the ball itself. You put the rubbery string around your hand and throw the ball toward the ground as you walk (though the ball does not touch the ground). It is great fun – and it helps mobility greatly.

This suggestion was inspired by Hans from Holland. He explains that instead of walking with a cane or walker (where people perceive there is an old person attempting to walk) you bounce a ball like a child. People perceive your youthful energy – and so do you!

Listen to Music

Listen to music with a strong beat while you walk. Your mobility will improve. Listen with an ipod to make it easiest.

© 2013 Parkinsons Recovery

Nitendo Wii

Ever heard of it? Young people know about it. You play games like tennis, football, bowling and soccer which require you to use your body as you play. The games require eye-hand coordination and movements that must be sequenced. As such they afford the opportunity to have ongoing physical therapy treatments that are self administered. Associate Professor Ben Herz announced remarkable results he found in a recent study that evaluated the use of Wii games for persons with Parkinsons. For a discussion of his excellent study and his findings, listen to my radio show November 21, 2012.

I understand you can always purchase a WII on a 30 day warranty so if it doesn't work for you, just return it. Play a game – whichever one you are called to play - every day. Have fun. The Herz study results suggest that you will celebrate an improvement in your mobility in addition to seeing a reversal of other symptoms. I like this approach because you reverse symptoms and have fun at the same time.

Herbs

Natural herbs can be a huge benefit for the problem you describe. One of the Pioneers of Recovery, Herbalist Andrew Bentley, suggests promising results with one herb in particular:

> *"With certain herbs like the Barley Malt Extract – I have definitely had times when people came to see me in a wheel chair and were able to walk out because it makes a big difference pretty quickly in how their nervous system is functioning. It can be the difference between having a good day and having a bad day or having a lot of good days and a lot of bad days".*

Tai Chi

Tai Chi helps strengthen your inner core which enables you to stabilize your balance. Some people who make Tai Chi a habit tell me that they are virtually symptom free.

Strengthen Your Hara

The Hara is a stream of energy through the body from top to bottom that connects a person's tan tien (the source of martial arts power) to the earth and to the Divine. The ability to walk with ease is challenged when the hara line is weak, broken or dissipated. We teach self help methods at Jump Start to Wellness which help people learn how to strengthen their own hara lines. When a person's hara is strong and vibrant, walking becomes much easier and effortless.

© 2013 Parkinsons Recovery

MY CREATIVE WRITING HAS COME TO A STANDSTILL BECAUSE MY HANDS AND FINGERS ARE CURRENTLY NOT FLEXIBLE ENOUGH TO TYPE. I AM TRYING TO FIND OTHER CREATIVE OUTLETS, BUT I REALLY LOVE TO WRITE. ANY SUGGESTIONS?

The symptoms of Parkinsons can include cramping. Tightness and weakness in the hands and fingers make typing much more challenging. It certainly sounds like you are worried your creative writing career is dead because you are having such a tough time typing on a keyboard.

I have a great suggestion for you. Actually, it is an awesome suggestion. There is another way to write without having to punch the keys on a typewriter or computer keyboard. You can talk into a microphone and your e-mails, letters, articles and books will be produced automatically using speech recognition software.

It is simple. You talk into a microphone that is connected to your computer. The words you speak are automatically translated into written words and sentences that magically appear on your computer screen. Really! If you can talk, you can write anything to anyone. And I do mean anything.

I should be using speech recognition software right now to write my book, but I am not. Why? I am stuck in my old habits of using my fingers to think. My writing would probably improve if I started using my mouth to write. I have always had a big mouth.

There is a big advantage if I start talking out my blog entries and newsletters rather than typing them. Why? I can talk much faster than I can type. My Parkinsons Recovery book would have been written in a month if I talked it rather than typed it. Instead, my book has taken several years to write.

I need to disclose a little truth and advertising here. I have not personally used this software but a friend of mine has. He tells me it works beautifully. My friend does give me one warning: Do not look at the computer screen as you talk. It is totally weird to read what you have just said as you are thinking about what to say next.

A little work on your part is required before the software will work. You have to train the software program to recognize the connection between your voice and the words. The creators of this software accomplish this by having you read several pages of a story so the software can identify how you say words. The program can then correctly connect the dots between what you say and the written words you are speaking. Once you are set up, you are good to go.

The software is called Dragon Naturally Speaking at www.nuance.com/talk. I just watched a video that demos the software which is very informative.

The other good news is that the more you exercise your voice the better your ability to speak forcefully and clearly will become.

Sorry. No more excuses for not writing to your friends and family. The world needs to hear from you so start talking, or should I say writing?

SOMEWHERE I REMEMBER READING THAT PD PEOPLE SOMETIMES BECOME MORE ARTISTIC. IS THIS REALLY TRUE?

Yes indeed - the gift of symptoms associated with a diagnosis of Parkinson's disease is that many people shift gears in their life as they become incredibly creative. In some cases this translates into artistic endeavors. All pictures and images you see in this book were created by persons who have been diagnosed with Parkinson's disease.

Why does this happen? I suspect the body demands that mental (as well as physical) activity slow down several notches. The body demands that standard routines of the past be interrupted. We often get so busy with the demands of work that does not challenge our creative juices. With Parkinsons our soul begs us to change how we live our lives.

When symptoms smack us in the face, the questions change: *What now? What do I do with my life now?* With a little reflection, many people realize that they have not been pursuing their life's passion. A creativity switch gets activated. Off they go into the world of art or some creative endeavor that puts them on a path where they are finally willing to acknowledge what gives them inner joy because it emerges from the seat of their soul.

What helps people with Parkinsons?

> *"After reading a number of your helpful articles, I am writing to ask your opinion regarding a difficult case of Parkinsons disease or similar disorder (as described below, the symptoms are somewhat atypical for classical PD).*
>
> *The person in question, now 63 years old, was diagnosed in mid-2005. The symptoms include right arm/shoulder pain, which has worsened over time, along with a mild tremor in the right hand. This is accompanied by a feeling of internal tremor or other unpleasant sensations which are difficult to describe but are all the same extremely and increasingly difficult to experience, sometimes like a feeling that his entire body is disintegrating (but he is otherwise healthy).*
>
> *On observation, he has a slow or shuffling gait and decreased facial expression at rest and mild tremor of the right hand, but otherwise few other noticeable signs to indicate PD. This person has been on Dopicar (L-dopa/carbidopa combination) for over a year,*

© 2013 Parkinsons Recovery

which helped for the first 3-4 months. However, over a short time the beneficial effects of L-dopa have diminished greatly, so that now it sometimes doesn't help at all, and when it does, only for a very short period of time (an hour or less). The present dose of L-dopa varies between 300 and 600 mg 2-3 times daily, depending on the particular symptoms and feelings on a given day. When the effect of the L-dopa wears off, the right arm becomes stiff like a log and very painful (worse than before taking it). This means that most of the day he is feeling bad, with little relief from L-dopa.

He has also been taking Azilect with little noticeable benefit. This was stopped recently after hearing John Coleman's teleconference, but pain and other symptoms have worsened since that time.

My question is: Have you ever seen anyone like this who responds very poorly to medications after such a short period of time, and whose primary symptoms are pain and a very unpleasant internal tremor or other sensation? "

At the top of my response to your fascinating question is a brief explanation of my qualifications. It is true that I am a doctor, but I am not a medical doctor. I have a Ph.D. and am a researcher. I need to be clear that I am not a medical doctor and so I am not qualified to diagnose or treat any disease. I regularly interview people with Parkinsons (like John Coleman) and conduct interviews with experts in various modalities regularly that are aired on my radio program. I am in a position to provide insights based on the interviews I do.

Please do not interpret anything I might say as medical advice but rather as simply information. It is always important to check with your doctor or health care provider before making any changes to a health care program.

From my research, your experience with medications after 3-4 months is typical but it is probably at the low end of the range. Qualitatively speaking, the average time appears to me to be around 7-8 months. Some people get no relief. Some get good relief for 2 years or more. I hear many reports of good relief for 6 months. Everyone is different. It does not help to compare yourself to anyone else.

Regardless of the length of the honeymoon, I have not interviewed anyone yet who has been on medication and not had to increase the dose after a period of time. The brief honeymoon suggests to me that the primary cause of symptoms may be rooted in factors that are not directly connected to the level of dopamine in the body.

YOU DO NOT BELIEVE THAT PARKINSONS IS A DISEASE? DO YOU NOT BELIEVE THAT THERE IS PHYSICAL DAMAGE TO THE PART OF THE BRAIN THAT PRODUCES DOPAMINE? DO YOU NOT

BELIEVE THAT THE DAMAGE HAS BEEN VERIFIED BY EXAMINING BRAIN TISSUE FROM DECEASED PARKINSONS PATIENTS? IS THE BRAIN NOT PART OF THE BODY? IS THE BRAIN JUST "OUT OF BALANCE"?

The Road to Recovery involves examining our thinking about "disease" - any disease. In this case of course it is Parkinsons "disease". If we focus on the "disease," we are holding very negative thoughts about what is happening by thinking:

"My body is broken."

Since thoughts can manifest anything our heart desires, holding this thought will ensure that our body will forever remain broken.

What percent of the body is "broken" in the case of Parkinsons? I assure you that answer varies widely across persons. My hunch is that a tiny proportion of cells are problematic: perhaps 1%; maybe 3% for some people. At least 97% of the cells are working perfectly. I would say that is close enough for me to say that the body is working perfectly. Speaking for myself, I get much more energy by focusing on what is working than what is not working.

You say that damage has been verified by autopsies. This is certainly true, but only in a minority of autopsies. For a majority of autopsies, they find no substantia nigra damage. Don't take my word for it. Do your own research on the matter. I have been surprised myself to see how low the percent actually is.

My point is that you are holding the belief that cells in your brain are dead. It may be the case that a tiny fraction of cells in your brain are dead, but cells are dying throughout the body all the time. It is the natural process of life and death.

It is also possible you are one of the majority where there is no damage to your substantia nigra. There is no way to tell without an autopsy.

A third of the people who have a diagnosis of Parkinsons are misdiagnosed. It happens. There is no definitive test for it. Perhaps you are one of the one third who have been misdiagnosed? There are certainly many possible causes for the symptoms. For example - perhaps toxins are the culprit and not cell damage in the substantia nigra.

Let's say all of these speculations are wrong and that yes, you do have neural damage in the substantia nigra and that yes, you do have Parkinsons Disease.

© 2013 Parkinsons Recovery

New cells can be created anywhere in the body anytime. If you happen to have an overabundance of dead cells in the substantia nigra for the moment, you can set your intention to grow new ones. If the body can make new cells, I would say it is working perfectly.

Here is the rub: If you focus on the dead cells (assuming they even exist) you are assuring that new cells will not be created. Your thoughts are centered in a negative sphere. If you focus on the reality that your body can heal itself, it will heal itself.

This is what I have learned from my research. At the core of all healing are our thought forms. If you think your body is broken I can assure you it will remain "broken" and become more "broken." If you believe your body can heal itself, new cells will be born, hormones will be balanced, and your body will return to health and wellness.

The most powerful force in the universe are thoughts. When we change how we think, we change the course of our lives. This is what motivated me to write The Five Steps to Recovery which is all about how to transform our thoughts.

HAVE YOU EVER SEEN ANYONE WHOSE PRIMARY SYMPTOMS ARE PAIN AND A VERY UNPLEASANT INTERNAL TREMOR OR OTHER SENSATION? I HAVE GONE COLD TURKEY ON MY MEDICATIONS AND MY SYMPTOMS ARE MUCH WORSE. WHAT CAN I DO NOW?

If I have learned anything from my research, it is that each person's symptoms are entirely unique to them. I interviewed a man recently whose primary symptom was pain. Internal tremors are also common among the many people I have interviewed. It is a clue that the neurological system is not functioning at full capacity.

Your symptoms are worse after going cold turkey off the medication. This too is very typical from the people I interview. Some people who go cold turkey without gradually reducing the dosage often wind up deciding to start taking the medication again, but at an even higher dose. You can probably expect a period of time for the body to adjust. From my research, what has happened to you is typical and very difficult to deal with.

Most people begin feeling better slowly and gradually when they make certain changes in how they eat and live. Finding ways to reduce stress and release trauma have also helped many people. Finding ways to help the body release toxins has certainly helped many people with Parkinsons. Another place to look is your digestive system. My guess is your digestive system may be compromised. Ayurveda has offered some people with Parkinson's wonderful relief. Please note that I say some.

© 2013 Parkinsons Recovery

My suggestion is that you begin to experiment. Check out what is working for other people. Try out something that calls to you (a herb, a form of body work, a detox method, etc.). If it begins help, stick with it. If not, turn to something else. The people who are having the greatest success with recovery do just this. They are always experimenting.

I might mention that this is precisely what John Coleman did. He experimented with a number of therapies. Some helped and some did not.

Give whatever is tried time to take effect. Most people are not aware they are getting better, so they abandon therapies too early because they falsely convince themselves the therapy is not helping. The process of healing involves a period of feeling worse before you begin to feel better. Most people abandon a therapy because they do not instantly feel better. This is a huge mistake.

The one thing that will help the most is to acknowledge no single medicine or pill exists that can fix the problem. The causes of the symptoms are far too complicated and delicate for this to be true. It takes a dedicated commitment to give the body all that it needs to heal itself.

DO EMOTIONALLY HEALTHY, WELL LOVED PEOPLE, WHO HAVE HAD THE ADVANTAGE OF DIET, GET PARKINSONS DISEASE?

What an interesting question. I asked John Coleman what factor was most important to his own recovery from Parkinsons. His answer was learning how to love himself. Perhaps it is more a question of the love we send to ourselves than the love we receive from others.

How about people whose diets and nutrition have been excellent? Since stress and trauma contribute to the symptoms, my guess is that people whose diets are excellent and who love themselves may still have symptoms if they find themselves in a sustained state of stress and fear.

CAN YOU COMPARE ALZHEIMER'S AS A CONDITION WITH PARKINSONS? IS ONE OR THE OTHER EASIER OR HARDER TO ADDRESS WITH REGARD TO ALLEVIATING SYMPTOMS?

The following response is provided by Steven Fowkes, Executive Director of the Cognitive Enhancement Research Institute in Menlo Park, California.

> "I would say there is a mechanism they have in common right down the line. That has to do with the mitochondrial energy systems. There is a "brown out" that happens with Alzheimer's disease and there is a brown out that happens with Parkinsons. By this analogy, the voltage of the body is failing.

On this level, there is no difference, so the treatments would be the same: Energy related nutrients, mitochondrial nutrients, exercise, aerobic capacity, coconut oil, thyroid hormones, hormone replacement therapy with testosterone in men or progesterone in women. These are kinds of things that would be universal to both diseases.

Steven Fowkes, 2008

I WONDER WHY SOME PEOPLE CAN INGEST SO CALLED TOXINS AND NEVER GET PARKINSONS DISEASE, AND OTHER PEOPLE LIKE MYSELF DO. IT CAN'T BE THAT SIMPLISTIC. IT HAS TO BE A COMBINATION MANY OTHER FACTORS.

I totally agree with you. There are a complicated set of factors at play which determine which people will experience more troubling symptoms.

We all ingest toxins every day – from the breaths we take to the food we eat to the toxic substances we put on our bodies as cleanses and washes. The body has a limited capacity to eliminate toxins. Only so many toxins can be discharged from our bodies in any given day. When the body gets too clogged with toxins, symptoms will present themselves.

I believe the symptoms of Parkinsons will present themselves for everyone whose system becomes "clogged up." Everyone has experienced tremors at one time or another. Most people have felt a deep sense of depression. Everyone has experienced pain. Most people I know have been "frozen" in the sense that they are unable to take positive action. Most people have experienced balance problems at one time or another. Symptoms at any particular time may not be so problematic that a formal diagnosis of "Parkinsons" is offered, but symptoms nonetheless can present themselves for everyone from time to time.

When the body's immune system, lymph system and elimination organs are healthy, the body releases toxins efficiently and expeditiously. When any of these systems are compromised, symptoms are likely to emerge.

I WONDER WHEN PARKINSONS DISEASE STARTED. I WONDER IF IT STARTED WHEN THE INDUSTRIAL REVOLUTION BEGAN, IN THE LATE 18TH CENTURY, OR BEFORE THAT?

The individual who is credited with isolating the symptoms of Parkinsons disease is James Parkinson who wrote a seminal article entitled "An Essay on the Shaking Palsy" in 1817. Forty years later the symptoms of Parkinsons were identified as "Parkinsons disease" by Jean Martin Charcot. Parkinsons is now widely accepted as the diagnostic term for the neurological disorders associated with what is known as Parkinson's disease.

© 2013 Parkinsons Recovery

Did the symptoms exist before then? Obviously we do not know for sure, but there is evidence in early writings of neurological problems that existed hundreds and hundreds of years previously.

Leonardo da Vinci from the 15th century appears to have observed the symptoms of Parkinsons and recorded these observations in his journals which contain descriptions of people who tremble "without permission of the soul." There is speculation that Leonardo himself had the symptoms of Parkinsons which explains why he was unable to paint during the later years of his life.

Since Parkinsons is affected by stress, I suspect that the prevalence of Parkinsons has been more pronounced during those periods of history which were tumultuous.

The neurological system is very delicate. It does not take much to challenge it. It would seem logical to me to conclude that the symptoms were present in one form or another throughout history.

Keep in mind also that there is a very long list of symptoms which overlap with many other "diseases." It is obvious that many of these symptoms have been present throughout history (e.g.: speech impairments, masked face, depression, constipation, etc.)

WHAT IS THE BEST WAY TO DETERMINE AN INDIVIDUAL'S NEED FOR SPECIFIC SUPPLEMENTS - VITAMINS, HERBS, MINERALS, ETC.?

What follows is Nutritional Counselor and pharmacist Randy Mentzer's answer to this question:

> "I look at a question like that and think - ok. The first thing we look at is: What are you eating? Are you eating organic foods? Are you eating things in a can? Are you eating things in a box? Is your food the problem?
>
> The other thing I look at is: Are you exercising? If you are not exercising, that may be the problem. The first thing we look at is your diet. The second thing is exercise.
>
> The third thing is: what medications are you taking? If you are taking aspirin, it is sucking about five or six different things out of your system such as vitamin C. In that particular case you might need more vitamin C.
>
> If you are really concerned about what to take and how much to take, there are tests that you can take to find out what your levels are. There again, you can talk with your compounding pharmacists or a health care provider who practices alternative medicine."

WITH RESPECT TO YOUR NUTRITION SUPPLEMENTS OF FOLIC ACID, VITAMINS B6 AND B12, HOW DO THEY HELP ANY FURTHER DETERIORATION SINCE THE BRAIN CELLS IN THE SUBSTANTIA NIGRA ARE ALREADY DESTROYED WHICH HAS CAUSED THE PARKINSONS DISEASE?

Many people believe that the symptoms of Parkinsons are caused by the death of brain cells that do not produce dopamine. As I feel into this thought form, it carries me into the pit of depression. If there are no more cells to produce dopamine, then no more dopamine will be produced. I personally cannot access any hope here!

This belief is clearly not the foundation of recovery. This belief is also blatantly false. First, the body has the capacity to make all the new cells we need. If there is a deficiency in the cells that produce dopamine, it is because there is no demand to produce dopamine for one reason or another. The body may be currently suspended in a perpetual state of fear. In this case, the body will be producing adrenaline and all the other stress related hormones. There may be little demand to manufacture dopamine.

Second, there are over 40 hormones in the body that must be delicately balanced in any given moment. Dopamine is one of these hormones. Focus attention on creating hormonal balance throughout the body and all systems in the body will return to health and wellness.

It is more healing to acknowledge that the body is working perfectly. It may be presently out of balance as indicated by the presentation of specific symptoms.

My thinking is that it gets us nowhere to hold the thought that something is wrong with our bodies which must be fixed. In this case, the belief is that all the cells needed to produce dopamine are dead.

If there is the demand to produce dopamine, the body will make the cells necessary to produce it. The body is working perfectly. It just sends us signals from time to time (as in the case of neurological challenges) which indicate an imbalance that needs to be corrected. It is possible a source of the imbalance comes from specific vitamin or mineral deficiencies like B6 and B12 which help the body cope with stress and trauma. Many deficiencies can be the cause of imbalances. These are only two possibilities.

I HAVE BEEN DIAGNOSED RECENTLY AND AM SHOOTING FOR FULL RECOVERY. PROGRESSION SEEMS TO BE SLOW. I CAN'T FIND ANYWHERE TO COMPARE PROGRESSION TO.

My suggestion is to compare your own progress against yourself. Forget about the progress of everyone else. This approach is called a "pre-post within subject design." This is a fancy, scientific way of saying that you create a baseline of your symptoms and then track your own symptoms over time.

© 2013 Parkinsons Recovery

The sample size is one – yourself. It is the most meaningful result you can ever get since your body is unique to itself.

Track your symptoms using the Parkinsons Recovery Symptom Tracker which will always be free to use and always accessible. It is easy to use. You will need to register by entering an email address and password. It is anonymous. No other information is required.

You then log on to the Parkinsons Recovery Symptom Tracker and answer 39 questions about your symptoms. Once your personal baseline is established, you can answer the same questions over and over, giving you a plot of your progression over time. Using Parkinsons Recovery Symptom tracker regularly is a great way to celebrate your progress toward feeling better.

Angela, my radio show guest on October 28, 2010, explains how she tracks her own symptoms on a regular basis using two self administered assessments. In the first assessment she records the time it takes her to stand up from sitting, take three steps, return to her chair and sit down. Shorter times indicate an improvement.

In the second assessment she challenges herself with taking five long strides. She measures the length of the middle three strides. The longer the distance of the middle three strides, the greater is the evidence of her recovery. It takes her five to ten minutes to complete these two assessments. Results often offer her the opportunity to celebrate her progress.

I AM WONDERING, HOW I WILL KNOW WHICH EXERCISES ARE THE MOST HELPFUL TO ME? WOULDN'T THIS BE THE SORT OF THING A PT (PHYSICAL THERAPIST) WOULD BE NEEDED FOR? OR NOT?

I have heard reports back from people who tell me David Zid's book, Delay the Disease: Exercise and Parkinson's Disease has been helpful, as is the work of Kevin Lockette who is a physical therapist, Arieh Breslow who has developed a DVD on Tai Chi and Qi Gong and Kristina Mauak who has created a DVD on Qi Gong.

In my opinion, it is a smart idea to involve a person like David, Kevin, Arieh or Kristina in tailoring an exercise program that suits your current needs. Coaches can help you sort out which exercises will be most helpful and provide the personal support that can be so helpful. Each of the incredible professionals I listed above develop personalized exercise programs for people with the symptoms of Parkinsons.

It is also about asking for help, which in itself is healing. You do not want to start with exercises that are too strenuous because you will likely get discouraged and quit. I believe the key is to find a form of exercise that you love to do. If it is a joyous activity, it will become a habit. Your body will love you for taking care of it every day.

WHAT DO YOU KNOW ABOUT THE EFFECTS OF CoQ10 AND VITAMIN E IN PD? IS IT CONSIDERED A DRUG OR A VITAMIN? CAN YOU SEND ME SOMEWHERE TO GET INFO?

I think of COq10 and vitamin E as food. Sometimes our body is deficient. Taking supplements can be very wise indeed.

Many doctors recommend that their patients take CoQ10. Quite a few studies now show that it can help provide relief for symptoms of Parkinsons. Low quality CoQ10 will provide little relief however. Laurie Mischley, ND, says you are better off paying for high quality CoQ10 than purchasing the budget brands.

The evidence on vitamin E is somewhat contradictory. Some studies show a large effect. Others don't.

I find information on the internet by typing in very specific search terms like:

"What is the research evidence on CoQ10 and Parkinson's disease"

Usually, the most helpful websites float to the top.

If your body needs either, you will know. Take it and you will feel better. Everyone will not feel better because everyone is not deficient in these two supplements. I have concluded that our bodies know the answer. Just ask your body. You can always get the answer you need to hear.

HOW DO YOU REDUCE STRESS?

Stress is directly connected to the symptoms of Parkinsons. When relaxed and care free, symptoms are minimal or nonexistent.

There are a variety of possibilities for reducing stress. They best way to approach the goal is on a moment to moment basis.

1. **Exercise.** Many people tell me that when they feel anxious or are worried, exercise does the trick of reducing anxiety beautifully.

2. **Meditate.** Be quiet and still for a minute. Focus on your breath. I am not talking here about a big deal. One minute will do during the moment when you need it. I have just finished a series of interviews with people who are experts on meditation for a book with Nancy Welch, Medicine Meditation.

There are many different approaches to meditation. The trick is to find an approach that works for you. Regardless of the method you are drawn to, the idea behind meditation is to still the mind babble which aggravates and inflames the stress.

© 2013 Parkinsons Recovery

3. *Laugh.* This is a simple suggestion, but it works. I post a joke a day on the Parkinsons Recovery member website. Laughing out loud gives an immediate dopamine rush. That is pretty cool if you ask me.

The irony is that you do not even have to think the joke is funny. Laugh out loud and you will get an immediate dopamine rush. The only side effect to laughter is improved health on some level.

4. *Holoysnc.* This method was created about 80 years ago by Robert Monroe. It consists of sounds that have slightly different frequencies which are sent to the two sides of the brain through headphones. I personally used this technology for about two years. I listened to tapes for about 30 minutes a day. Very gradually, the little things that stressed me out no longer had any impact whatsoever. I would listen for about a minute and instantly fall asleep.

5. *Body Work*. Craniosacral body work or energy work can be extremely helpful. There are physical blockages which twist and contort the body's tissues that are released and removed through gentle body work. Everyone has blockages to one degree or another and, in my opinion, everyone in a body should consider getting body work of one form or another.

I have used many different forms of body work for myself – energy healing, cranial sacral therapy, Reiki, healing touch, Zen Massage, Bowen therapy. I recommend you try some of these wonderful techniques out and see which one your body likes the best.

My concluding suggestion is to acknowledge that many stresses are external to us. We are impacted by our parents or children or spouses or partners or money or jobs or the world condition or the economy – you name it. When I feel the external world invading my internal space, I have a mantra which helps me.

"I honor the fate of [my child, my parents, etc.] What do I need now?"

The mantra instantly connects me to myself rather than responding to other external issues. Worrying about other people's issues is a clever way for me to avoid a connection with myself. When I ask myself the question,

"Why am I here on the earth?

Much of the stress I carry is instantly released. Combine the strategies and you get an even bigger result.

WHAT IS THE DIFFERENCE BETWEEN CRANIOSACRAL THERAPY AND BOWEN THERAPY?

© 2013 Parkinsons Recovery

Bowen Therapy:

- *Moves, positions and holds hands, feet, arms or legs into various positions for releases*
- *Gently rolls the body or positions the body for releases*
- *Focus is on the release of trauma and tension throughout the entire body*

Craniosacral

- *Touch is very gentle - more so than Bowen Therapy.*
- *The therapist may work on or off the body*
- *Focus is on cranial sacral system - the system that comprises the brain, spine and sacrum.*

The difference between craniosacral therapy and Bowen therapy depends in large part on the practitioner. Some craniosacral therapists are more technique oriented. They are trained to move through a standard series of adjustments.

Other craniosacral therapists are trained to listen to the person's body and allow the body to communicate how it needs to release the trapped trauma. There is no standard protocol that is used with any particular patient.

My personal experience with Bowen therapy involved a treatment I received from Naturopath doctor John Coleman and his associate at a workshop in Tacoma, Washington. Bowen therapy originated in Australia in the 1980's. I loved receiving the Bowen treatment from John. It clearly allows for gentle releases of stress, trauma and tension.

Bowen therapy is a wonderful therapy, as is craniosacral. Either one will work for some people and not others. It is more physical than craniosacral therapy, but both can generate similar outcomes. If one therapy does not help you, try the other!

John Coleman recommends Bowen therapy to persons with Parkinsons Disease because it was so helpful to him personally. Some people report back to me who have had Bowen therapy that is indeed the case for them. Others report they did not receive the releases that they had hoped for. Still others report relief is maintained for several days after the treatment, but symptoms tended to reappear.

Most therapists - whether they are Bowen or Craniosacral therapists - have extensive training with other modalities. When they begin working - they will employ other modalities as needed in addition to using the techniques associated with craniosacral therapy or Bowen therapy.

© **2013 Parkinsons Recovery**

I suggest that anyone who currently has the symptoms Parkinson shop around for a practitioner who provides the support that works well for you. It is a very personal choice. You might want to try several therapists so you can experience the wide range of treatments that are possible.

IS THERE ANY EVIDENCE OR INFORMATION ABOUT THE BENEFITS OF MASSAGE FOR PEOPLE WITH PARKINSONS?

What a large question which consumes one tiny sentence! I talk with people with Parkinsons who get massages regularly to help them release stress. To the extent that any therapy helps you release trauma and stress, you can rest assured your symptoms will become less bothersome.

Keep in mind that massage is a general term for many different therapies. People have told me that deep tissue massage is not helpful. The reason? I suspect that it is much too invasive. The body clamps down muscles in response to the intrusion.

If massage is coupled with energy healing (Reiki, healing touch, energy healing), the therapist is much more likely to be gentle with the body's response to the treatment as they invite the trauma and stress to be released. In my own experience everything depends on the therapist.

I would say this very simply: There is a massage therapist out there in the universe that can be of benefit to you. Your job is to find them. You will know them when you get a first treatment. Even if you experiment with a massage and feel it did not help, stay on the lookout for someone else to get a treatment from.

The bottom line is this: If the massage is intended to relax you – it will have benefits. If the massage is intended to release stress and trauma – it too will have benefits.

There is another benefit as well. Asking someone to help you is very therapeutic. I believe we can't heal ourselves from the traumas of life. We have to ask for help from others. Besides, it is a great gift to give yourself.

Research studies using subjects who have the symptoms of Parkinsons disease have found massage results in an improvement in daily functioning, better sleep and less stress. Progressive muscle relaxation has also been shown to produce higher dopamine levels.

You can find additional information on the effects of massage at the integrative healthcare website..

CAN EXPOSURE TO FLEA POWDER USED TO KILL FLEAS CAUSE PARKINSON'S SYMPTOMS? I WAS EXPOSED RECENTLY AND HAD AN IMMEDIATE REACTION.

Many people know that they were exposed to toxins but do not realize it is likely the factor causing their symptoms. There is a strong likelihood that the flea pesticide you were exposed to contained pyrethroid. Researchers have found that the symptoms of Parkinsons have been directly linked to exposure to this very specific pesticide.

Now the challenge for you is to identify a detox program that will succeed in releasing this toxin from your body. Although the toxin may have landed in your body in seconds, it will unfortunately take time, patience and dedication to eject it.

HOW DO YOU RECOMMEND WE DETOXIFY OUR BODIES?

Your question turns out to be huge indeed. I have used a naturopath doctor in Georgia (who I have actually never met in person), Ivy Faber. Ivy does Bioenergetic Testing to determine which toxins are problematic. She then recommends the detox protocol to use.

Naturopaths are great resources to help with detoxing. Herbalists have great resources, as are aroma therapists. Some medical doctors specialize in this area. Of course, exercise always helps the body to detox. Colon cleanses can be very useful as well.

In short, there are many, many possible approaches to consider. There are even detox programs that are designed to release specific toxins (like iron or other heavy metals).

I have actually tried different detoxes over the years which were purchased at food co-ops and health food stores. You can always tell if they are helpful because you begin to feel a lot better after several weeks.

Instead of doing a thorough review of alternatives, I ask my body through muscle testing which method I should use for now. The answer is often different depending on when I ask. Muscle testing is the "quick and clean" method. I do not have to think as hard. I am into making things happen now.

Perhaps my way stems from my impatience.   Perhaps I am just lazy. But, muscle testing works well for me and happens to be my way of making decisions about detoxes my body needs.

In the big picture, I think what matters is to acknowledge toxins to be a challenge for everyone. We all need to detox at least every year if not every six months.

I HAVE MASSIVE FAMILY ISSUES, STRESS ISSUES, PARKINSONS DISEASE AND AM 49. WHERE DO I START?

I have thought for some years now that everyone has huge family issues that come in one form or another. Many people deny them. Others gut their way through them. I have done both myself.

I think the key is just to start anywhere with doing something for yourself. Doing anything will get you started on the road to recovery. For example, I do the weekly Parkinsons Recovery Radio Program every Wednesday at 3:00 pm Pacific. You could listen in every week or listen to the replays. That is only one simple example you may not be able to do. Any act of commitment will get you off and running.

My feeling is – don't ponder over the right thing to do. Anything will do. Go to a funny movie perhaps, or a book, or exercise classes, or a new recipe or …

HAVE YOU HEARD OF LOW LEVEL LIGHT LASER THERAPY FOR PARKINSONS?

In a recent research article by Patricia A. Trimmer, Ph.D. from the University of Virginia and her coauthors reported promising results from using Laser Light Therapy to rejuvenate mitochondrial activity which is the source of energy in our cells for persons with Parkinsons.

The mitochondria in PD tissues are "metabolically and functionally compromised." Any treatment that nourishes the mitochondria will help with the symptoms of Parkinsons.

This study exposed neuronal cells to near-infrared laser light to determine whether the velocity of mitochondrial movement can be restored by low level light therapy (LLLT).

The results of their study supported their hypothesis. A single treatment with low level light therapy did restore axonal transport. The authors conclude that LLLT may be used as a novel treatment to improve neuronal function in patients with Parkinsons Disease. Of course, the exciting news is that laser light therapy is also safe and noninvasive.

HAVE YOU FOUND PAIN TO BE A SIGNIFICANT SYMPTOM IN PEOPLE WITH OTHER SYMPTOMS OF PARKINSONS DISEASE, AND IF SO, WHAT THEY DO TO FIND RELIEF?

Yes, I have received many reports from people who report pain is a very troubling symptom for them among others. First, from what I have learned, people get relief from pain by meditating. Meditation allows them to override all of the thinking that surrounds the "meaning" of the pain. We all put a head on top of our head, which makes the experience worse. That is one reason I have been motivated to record the weekly series of meditations.

Second, my observation is that there is typically a thought form that is buried beneath the pain. Once that is cleared and released, the pain resolves.

Third, a source of the pain is often unreleased trauma. Using one body therapy or another (we use craniosacral) helps with releasing trauma. Other therapies are helpful as well. Once the trauma is released, the pain resolves (if trauma is the primary causal factor)

Fourth, Lee Bender had a considerable challenge with pain over the years. You can listen to my interview with Lee on the August 13, 2009 to see what he does to get relief from his pain.

OUR BODIES GOT SICK BECAUSE OF SOME TYPE OF TOXICITY. AT LEAST THAT IS MY BELIEF. DO YOU AGREE?

It is certainly my belief too. Toxicity issues are not a primary issue for all individuals who have Parkinsons, but from my extensive work it is clearly a causal factor for a significant proportion of individuals. There is a large body of research that has unequivocally shown that toxins do contribute to the symptoms of Parkinsons.

HOW DO WE GET RID OF THE TOXICITY THAT IS MAKING US SICK?

There is no a simple answer to the question. In part it depends on the nature of the toxicity that is present in the body. When you know what toxin(s) are most troublesome, you will have a better idea of what detoxification protocols will be most effective. Once the toxins are eliminated, the neural pathways can be rejuvenated. Toxins do a good job of clogging them up.

Detoxing is not a one-day event. It is not a one-week event. I believe it needs to be a lifetime event. Eliminating toxins from our bodies is something we need to work on continuously. The good news is that there are many possibilities that can be very effective. Your body will thank you for detoxing and show its appreciation through a reduction in symptoms.

HOW CAN TOXINS OR STRESS BE REMOVED IF TRAPPED AT A CELLULAR LEVEL?

This is certainly an important question. There are a wide variety of detox methods that remove toxins and a wide selection of approaches that assist the body with releasing trauma. No gold standard exists for either because everyone's body is different.

Many people discover that one therapy will work for a while. Then, they have to switch off to another in order to continue the recovery process. Different methods are successful at different points in the recovery process.

© 2013 Parkinsons Recovery

One of the reasons I air the radio show every week is to offer a wide variety of choices you can consider. Whether my guest is a health care practitioner or a person who currently experiences the symptoms of Parkinson's, they usually tap into their approach for detoxing and de-stressing. People with the symptoms of Parkinson's talk about what therapies are working for them. It doesn't mean it will work for you - but it is a starting place.

I am guessing you were hoping for a much more simplistic answer -perhaps a few websites to visit. There are hundreds of resources out there for you to pick and choose from.

The most important step is to begin taking action now. Initiate your own exploration. Call or e-mail some of my radio show guests. Get more information. See what calls out to you.

You really can't go wrong. Most of the therapies people find are the most helpful are safe, non-intrusive and effective. The only side effect is improved health on some level.

CAN PARKINSON'S BE CAUSED BY PROBLEMS IN EITHER THE KIDNEY OR LIVER? IF SO, WOULD DETOXIFICATION OF THESE ORGANS HELP RELIEVE TREMORS?

Research has shown that many of the symptoms associated with a diagnosis of Parkinsons Disease - and there are many - can be caused by toxins. The kidneys and liver get clogged up with a residue of toxins that create a formidable bottleneck in the elimination system. New toxins that enter the body have nowhere to go other than hideaway inside the cells. Cells are a nice place to hang out.

My answer to your question is yes. Detoxes for everyone - those with a diagnosis of Parkinsons and those without - are a critical component of health and wellness. Think of detoxing your kidneys and liver to be the same chore as brushing your teeth. Both are necessary. Both need to be done on a regular basis.

Will a liver-kidney detox relieve tremors? The answer depends on whether you are also able to release the stress and trauma that may be trapped at the cellular level of your body. Toxins are impossible to release as long as trauma resides within the structural membrane of the cells.

I HAVE BEEN READING INFORMATION ON HOW TO RECOVER FROM PARKINSON'S DISEASE AND I CAME UPON AN ARTICLE THAT INDICATED ONCE YOU ARE ON THE PARKINSON'S MEDICATION YOU CANNOT RECOVER FROM THE DISEASE...THAT YOU CANNOT GO BACK SO TO SPEAK. DO YOU BELIEVE THIS TO BE TRUE?

No I do not believe this is true. What do I believe?

© **2013 Parkinsons Recovery**

Our thought forms determine our health and wellness. If you believe recovery is not possible for any reason - in your example because of the medications - recovery will not be possible. Period. End of story.

If on the other hand, you believe that recovery is possible, the magic begins. You will quickly begin to feel better. Transform your moment to moment thoughts and the miracle of life will unfold before your eyes.

I wrote Five Steps to Recovery to help people transform the thought forms that no longer serve their best and highest good. The steps help me moment to moment transform my own thoughts which do not serve my best and highest good. The challenge of transformation is tricky because we have as many as 50,000 to 70,000 thoughts each day!

I say to you today - believe in your heart, mind and soul that recovery will happen. Then sit back and enjoy the ride to recovery.

MY DENTIST DID HOURS OF RESEARCH & FOUND THE MOST HELPFUL THERAPY FOR PARKINSONS SYMPTOMS WAS USING MAGNETS & GOOD HYDRATION. REACTIONS?

First, I do hear over and over from people with Parkinson's symptoms that good hydration makes a big difference. Some people are getting good results from taking a homeopathic treatment that was designed to help their bodies become better hydrated called the Aquas.

Second, magnets alter the field which surrounds the human body. I do know there are companies which promote magnets as a device to clear blockages in the human energy field and thus help to restore energy and heal illness. I do not have any evidence from people with Parkinsons on the effectiveness of such devices.

I do know that the many forms of energy healing (Reiki, healing touch, energy healing, acupuncture, etc.) also help to clear blockages in the human energy field. Magnets are one approach to achieving this same goal.

The problem as I understand it is that if you get the poles reversed when you apply the treatment, the treatment can backfire. Instead of opening chakras and clearing the blockages, the chakras can shut down and blockages can be solidified. I have heard Barbara Brennan (a famous healer) warn against use of magnets because of the pole reversal problem. Apparently, use of magnets can either work big time or backfire big time.

I have an intuition that in the years ahead, such machines will be much more sophisticated. I can also add that of the many therapies that we now know help give symptom relief, I know of no therapy that helps everyone. Just because it might have helped someone else does not mean necessarily that it will help you out.

MY HUSBAND HAS BEEN DIAGNOSED WITH PARKINSONS DISEASE 7 YEARS AGO. HIS LATEST SYMPTOMS ARE: BURNING AND PAIN AROUND THE GROIN AREA, THIGHS AND SOMETIMES BACKSIDE. ANY SUGGESTIONS? I AM READY TO GIVE UP.

First, let me give my customary warning: I am not a medical doctor and am not qualified to diagnose and prescribe. My response is founded on my research findings and should be taken to a medical doctor for further discussion and evaluation.

My first reaction to the description of symptoms is that the pain may be caused by lymph that is backed up and clogged around the groin area. The only way to move lymph out of the body is through exercise.

Does your husband get exercise every day? I am guessing not.

What if exercising is too painful for him at this point? It may be painful at the beginning, but if my guess is on target, the pain will subside when he begins to move. A great technique for moving lymph is to jump on a trampoline. Everyone should do it. You can purchase small ones for home use for $30-$40 in the U.S.

Another possibility is for him to use a body inverter which he can use to shift the body so that his head is lower than the feet. There are little valves throughout the lymph system that prevent the lymph from slipping back down, so when you place the body upside down, the lymph moves up and out. There is no organ that pumps the lump as there is for blood (which of course is the heart).

A total inversion would probably be unwise, but positioning the body so that the head is lower than the feet can be helpful. Various health care practitioners might have such equipment you can experiment with. If he has other health problems, this idea might be unwise, so check it out with his doctor.

The challenge for him is likely that the lymph in his body is a thick mucus. Hydrating his body will be a great asset. John Coleman, ND, recommends that everyone with Parkinsons hydrate their body using a homeopath remedy called the Aquas (www.aquas.us). The thirst mechanism for all older persons shorts out, so the body needs a backup signaling system that will help the body tell him when to drink. At a minimum he should drink a lot of water.

My guess is that the more he can move his body, the more relief he will get from the pain. You of course might also want to examine very carefully the side effects of any medications he takes. This can also be a confounding factor which can directly contribute to the problem he is experiencing.

I must add, your last sentence jumps out at me

> *"Ready to give up."*

I note that you do not say whether you are ready to give up or he is ready to give up. If he is ready to throw in the towel, I would say to you – honor his wishes. A time comes for everyone when a decision is made to begin shutting down the body. Is this his time? If so, he will not move or exercise or do anything of the things necessary to relieve the pain.

Are you ready to give up? Believe me, this is totally understandable. It is so difficult to take care of someone you love who is ill. If you are ready to give up, it is time for you to take a break from care taking.

Take a short vacation with your friends. Get away. No one can take someone who is ill 100% of the time. Ill people take the energy away from healthy people. That is the natural process of what happens.

You need to get away to rejuvenate yourself. This sounds counterintuitive, but by taking care of yourself, you are actually able to do a much better job of taking care of him.

My guess about the cause of the pain may be wrong and you will have to move to another possibility, but I can virtually guarantee you that when he moves his body, he will feel better. It is the one sure fire suggestion I can offer that I know will yield relief.

I WOULD LOVE TO LISTEN TO YOUR STATION. HOW DO I GO ABOUT DOING THAT?

Parkinsons Recovery Radio Network is an internet radio program which means you can listen from anywhere in the world. There are two ways to listen.

You can call toll free 877-590-0733 (in the US) and listen in during the show. The call in number always stays the same and the program airs every Wednesday at 3:00 pm Pacific time (6 pm eastern time). If you do not live in the US and would like to ask a guest a question, connect to the radio show through your computer by visiting the following web address:

http://www.blogtalkradio.com/parkinsons-recovery

© 2013 Parkinsons Recovery

If you miss the live program you can always download any of the programs to your computer (the MP3 files) for listening at a later time. Or, you can download the MP3 file to your IPOD and listen while exercising (or doing other things).

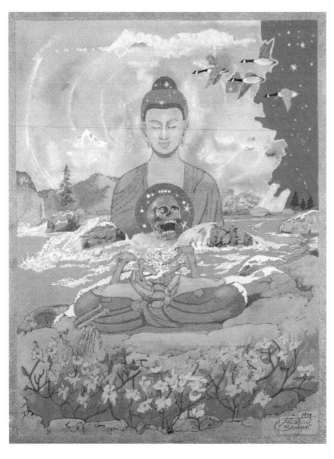

Buddha Nature (1999)
  Michael Sawyer

RESOURCES

PARKINSONS RECOVERY

The main website for Parkinsons Recovery contains links to all the other websites. If you can remember the words Parkinsons Recovery you can always link to all of the other websites that contain news, blogs, chat rooms, ways of tracking your symptoms, the Parkinsons Recovery radio program, links to books and other resources, and Parkinsons Recovery programs. Simply type in the two words into your browser "Parkinsons Recovery" and the top search result is the Parkinsons Recovery website.

http://www.parkinsonsrecovery.com

JUMP START TO WELLNESS

Parkinsons Recovery sponsors two day, hands on programs to provide the support and information that clear out and remove negative thought patterns that falsely convince you that recovery is hopeless. The focus of Jump Start programs is to help you release negative beliefs and thoughts that obstruct the recovery process and restore new thoughts that are conducive

© 2013 Parkinsons Recovery

to maintaining a state of balance and harmony. We also provide tools to jump start your recovery program.

www.jumpstart.parkinsonsrecovery.com

PARKINSONS RECOVERY BLOG

People have been submitting questions to me now for several years. I chew on them for a while, do research (usually that is, though sometimes I simply start writing when I am convinced I know the answer), incubate the answer, digest my analysis and post my thoughts on the Parkinsons Recovery Blog. On many of the postings you will see the question that was submitted and my response. You may also see comments from people regarding the question that was asked. Thankfully, people often post information I was totally unaware of which is particularly helpful (despite my valiant efforts at researching the answer).

http://www.blog.parkinsonsrecovery.com

Some of the postings are e-mails I have received on one aspect or another of recovery. People write their stories and talk about what has helped them. In addition to the question and answer postings, you will also find postings of stories that have been written by people with the symptoms of Parkinsons who have incredible insights on what has helped them feel better and what has obstructed their recovery. To visit the blog, click on the link above or enter the URL address above in your browser if clicking fizzles.

PARKINSONS RECOVERY CHAT ROOM

Everyone is invited to visit the Parkinsons Recovery Chat room which is open 24 hours a day. I visit the chat room from time to time with a smile on my face. We communicate through writing rather than talking here.

http://www.parkinsonsrecovery.net

To enter the chat room click on the link above or enter this URL address in your browser. Enter any name you wish others to see in the chat room. If you wish to be anonymous, enter the name of your dog or cat or pet squirrel. No password required. Everyone is invited. The chat room is open every day. All are welcome. Access to the chat room will always be free.

SYMPTOM TRACKER

We all have a tendency to focus on symptoms that are troubling. We all also tend not to celebrate improvement in symptoms that have resolved or vanished. Most people do not realize their symptoms are improving or that they are feeling better. If you do not acknowledge to yourself that you are feeling better, it will be difficult to maintain the commitment and focus that is necessary to heal.

Tracking symptoms with my Symptom Tracker is a great way to celebrate your progress and identify any areas that need extra attention. Symptom Tracker allows you to track your symptoms over time as often as you wish.

You can always find a link to Symptom Tracker on the Parkinsons Recovery main page at www.parkinsonsrecovery.com. Just click on the icon for Symptom Tracker and you will be taken to the log in page. This service is both anonymous and free. Or, to access Symptom Tracker directly, click on the link above or enter the following URL address in your browser:

http://www.symptomtracker.info/parkinsons/login.php

Start by logging onto the website and registering. To register, enter an email address and you create a password. That is it. Registration is entirely anonymous. The only "tricky" part of Symptom Tracker is that you have to remember the email address you used to register. If you forget your password it is no big deal. You can prompt the system to send you the password that you set up if you have forgotten it.

Once you log onto Symptom Tracker with your email address and the password you assigned yourself, you will answer a 39 item questionnaire known as the Parkinsons Disease Questionnaire 39. This survey instrument is widely used in the research literature. Once you answer all the questions you will receive a baseline snapshot of your current health situation.

You can then log on to symptom tracker and answer the same 39 questions every month or two. Each time you answer the questions you get a plot of your progress which shows areas of improvement and any areas you might want to discuss with your doctor. You of course are most welcome to print off the progress report and take it with you to your doctor's visits.

ON AND OFF TRACKING

Two sisters, one of whom has young onset Parkinson's, developed a program you can use to track on and off cycles if you are currently taking medications. This program helps you track the messages your body is sending on a day to day - hour to hour basis. They have generously made the program available for free. No personal information is collected. You don't even have to use your real name (but you have to remember the name you use so you can track your on and off periods over time).

http://www.datadrivenhealth.org

© 2013 Parkinsons Recovery

Fava Bean Blog

Interested in learning how you can grow your own fava beans, make a fava bean tincture and use it to get relief from your symptoms? Visit the fava bean blog to connect with a community of other people with Parkinson's who are growing their own fava beans and sharing their experiences.

http://www.favabeans.parkinsonsrecovery.com

Parkinsons Recovery Radio Network

I am a ham. I admit it. I have been acting since I was 1 hour old. What better outlet than my own internet radio program every Wednesday at 3 pm Pacific time (6 pm Eastern). I interview people with the symptoms of Parkinsons who tell their stories about what helps them get relief from their symptoms. I interview health care practitioners who tell us all what they have discovered helps people with the symptoms of Parkinsons feel significantly better.

I scan around the globe to interview anyone and everyone who has something to contribute. My idea is simple. The answers are hanging out in the ethers waiting to be documented. If I screen out any possibilities, I may miss finding therapies or treatments that have the potential to help a lot of people. I also love to interview people who discuss fresh ideas and offer new insights into healing.

You may find some of the people I interview a bit "out there." That doesn't bother me. I would much rather err on the side of being too inclusive than being too exclusive. Answers to pesky problems can be found in the most unexpected places. Working together and inclusively, we are unearthing some incredible answers to very difficult questions.

To listen to a live show, visit the Parkinsons Recovery Radio Network Page below:

http://www.blogtalkradio.com/parkinsons-recovery

If you do not have a computer, you can listen to the live show by calling the following toll free number if you live in the United States: (877) 590-0733. If you live outside the US, it is best to connect through your computer. You can talk with guests during the show using Skype. I have been hosting the weekly radio show since April, 2009. All shows are archived. You can download any radio show for free by visiting the radio show page above.

Explanations of Parkinson's Therapies

Some of my radio show guests are health care providers who discuss specific therapies in considerable detail. Below is a listing of shows that offer rich explanations of a therapy to treat the symptoms or a diagnostic approach to evaluate its cause.

© 2013 Parkinsons Recovery

All shows are archived and free to download. Visit the radio show page by clicking on the link below. Then scroll back in time to the date of the program you wish to hear.

http://www.blogtalkradio.com/parkinsons-recovery

Access Bars, Shereen Noon, October 10, 2012

Action Steps for Success, July 25, 2012

Amalgam and Crown Removal, Simon King, April 9, 2009

Anti-Aging Therapies, Mark Babizhayev, April 1, 2010

Arlon Bennett's Amazing Songs, Consider the Possibilities, December 5, 2012

BioAcoustics, Sharry Edwards, January 5, 2011

Bioenergetic Testing, Ivy Faber, August 5, 2010, August 31, 2011

Biophoton Therapy, Johan Boswinkel, September 26, 2012 and January 9, 2013

Chinese Scalp Acupuncture for Parkinsons, September 12, 2012

Color Therapy, Arlene Arnold, February 16, 2011

Dance, Pamela Quinn, September 30, 2010

Dance for PD, David Leventhal, October 19, 2011

Dehydration Remedies, Jaroslav Boublik, June 4, 2009

Depression Therapies, Roseanne Dobkin, August 19, 2010

Depression: A Natural Approach that Works, Kristen Allott, October 31, 2012

Detoxes and Parkinsons, Daniel Newman, December 10, 2009

Detoxes (Natural), Kristen Harper, January 2, 2013

Drumming, Heather MacTavish, April 22, 2010

Dynamic Energetic Healing, Steve Fenwick, January 21, 2010

Electromagnetic Pollution, Randy Mentzer, November 24, 2010

Electro-Stimulation, Donald Rhodes, July 20, 2011

Eliminate Harmful Toxins and Clean Green, December 12, 2012

The Emotion Code, John O'Dwyer, October 17, 2012

Emotional Freedom Technique, Bernadette Hunter, May 21, 2009

Essential Oils, Jean Oswald, September 17, 2009

Family Constellation Therapy, Dee Yoh, November 19, 2009

Fava Beans, Aunt Bean (Sandra), February 4, 2010

Feldenkrais, Irene Pasternack, December 8, 2010

Foot Whispering, Randy Eady, February 29, 2012

Forced Exercise, Jay Alberts, April 23, 2009

GigerMD Therapy, Jim Gray, October 3, 2012

Herbal Treatments for Parkinsons, December 19, 2012

Hypnotherapy, Steve Frison, February 9, 2011

Laughter Yoga, Gita Fendelman, April 8, 2010

© 2013 Parkinsons Recovery

Medicine Side Effects and Interactions, Randy Mentzer, November 25, 2009

Meditation, Norm Fischer, September 24, 2009

Music Medicine, Suzanne Jonas, January 14, 2010

Music Therapy, Matt Ford, January 26, 2011 & Wendy Magee, June 25, 3009

Multi-Dimensional Healing, Deborah Russell, November 5, 2009

Myofascial Release, David Howell, April 15, 2010

Natural Therapies, Laurie Mischley, June 24 and July 1, 2010

Neuro Feedback, Jacyln Gisburne, December 30, 2009, February 15, 2012 & July 18, 2012

Nutrition, Dorit, June 3, 2010

Pedaling for Parkinsons, Nan Little, November 10, 2010

QiGong for Parkinsons, Mington Gu, June 6, 2012

QiGong for Parkinsons, Bianca Molle, June 15, 2011

Physical Therapy, Kevin Lockette, June 10, 2010

Spiritual Integration, Michele Morgan, December 24, 2009

Stress Relief, Keith Zang, January 28, 2010

Swallow Safely, Joel Herskowitz and Roya Sayadi, July 22, 2010

Symptom Tracker, August 8, 2012

Tai Chi, Arieh Breslow, August 6, 2009 & Danny Loney, December 3, 2009

TMJ Disorder, Cheryl, October 21, 2010

Toxins and PD, Joe Hickey, August 10, 2011

Travel and Stay Healthy, November 7, 2012

Vibration Therapy, Lee Bender, August 13, 2009 and Holly Hughes March 4, 2010

Video Gaming (Wii) and Parkinsons, November 21, 2012

RADIO SHOW GUESTS ON THE ROAD TO RECOVERY

When you get discouraged about the prospects for recovery, I suggest you make it a habit to listen to one of my radio shows where my guest has Parkinsons Disease and has identified therapies that have made it possible for them to get sustained relief from their symptoms. Some of my guests are symptom free today. Others are doing significantly better today than when they were first diagnosed.

It has been inspiring for me to interview this impressive group who are pioneers of recovery. The shows will motivate anyone to take the actions needed to recover. Better yet, you will get unbelievable suggestions of what you can do for yourself to get relief from your symptoms.

Karl Robb March 20, 2012

Jim March 14, 2012

Judith Lynne March 28, 2012

Phyllis Rogers April 11, 2012

John Baumann May 23, 2012

Howard Shifke March 11, 2012

Tony February 15, 2012

Anne Atkin, January 11, 2012

Lexie October 5, 2011

Bianca Molle June 15, 2011

Lydia Epp March 23, 2011

Holly Hughes May 18, 2011

John Schappi May 4, 2011

Gord Summer December 29, 2010

Richard Secklin December 22, 2010

Richard London December 1, 2010

John Carlin November 17, 2010

Nan Little November 10, 2010

John Baumann November 3, 2010

Angela Wensley October 28, 2010

Cheryl October 21, 2010

Pamela Quinn September 30, 2010

Sue Richards September 16, 2010

John Coleman September 9, 2010

Elizabeth and Dave May 27, 2010

Paula and Jean May 20, 2010

Marilyn Murray and John Gold May 13, 2010

Heather MacTavish April 22, 1010

Gita Fendelman April 8, 2010

Lee Bender March 4, 2010

Holly Hughes February 18, 2010

Aunt Bean February 4, 2010

Karen January 7, 2010

Danny Loney December 3, 2009

Carol Meenan October 8, 2009

Mary Pauer July 30, 2009

John Ball July 23, 2009

Whit Deschner July 9, 2009

Leif Ogard June 18, 2009

Pioneers of Recovery May 28, 2009

PARKINSONS RECOVERY MINDFULNESS PROGRAM

© 2013 Parkinsons Recovery

One approach for reducing stress is to become mindful each and every moment of our waking lives. Mindfulness essentially means that we are present to what is happening now. When we focus our thoughts, feelings and sensations on present circumstances there is no opportunity to worry about the future or agonize over the past. Stress has little opportunity to rear its ugly head. When either fears about the future or worries about the past dominate, our life force is drained and enthusiasm for life is thrashed.

http://www.stress.parkinsonsrecovery.com

AQUAS HYDRATION FORMULA

The Aquas were designed as a homeopathic treatment to help the body hydrate. John Coleman, ND, says that the AQUAS played a significant role in his own recovery. Aquas were originally formulated and are now manufactured in Australia.

Because of the interest in the western hemisphere in the AQUAS, I set up a system for ordering them and answer questions about the Aquas. I learned all about the Aquas by taking them myself for several years and by interviewing the inventors. It really is a remarkable product. You can read up on the AQUAS by visiting the website below:

http://www.aquas4life.com

PARKINSONS RECOVERY MEMBERSHIP

After cutting away at the edges of learning what really helps people get better, it is now imminently clear to me that vigilance is required. It takes a commitment to eat nutritious food, to exercise, to find ways to relieve stress, to laugh yourself silly and to challenge your mind to create new neural networks.

A formidable challenge for most people is thus to maintain the motivation to do everything that is necessary to heal. It is so easy to become discouraged, to fall into the false belief template that you're a doomed to deteriorate.

All things considered I created a Parkinsons Recovery membership website that exposes you to all of the habits that are essential to a successful recovery program. I post fresh information on the member website every weekday that includes meditations and articles that contain the perspectives on healing Parkinsons that we have been developing through our work in Olympia, Washington. The meditations and visualizations offer novel ways to strengthen motor abilities, strengthen memory acuity and bring the body back into balance and harmony.

There is a ton of fun and interesting material that I post on the member website every day – jokes, healthy recipes, exercises, mind challenges - you name it. The membership costs $25 a month and requires access to a computer and interest in logging on regularly. To learn more, visit:

http://www.parkinsonsrecovery.org

PIONEERS OF RECOVERY

I receive many inquiries from people asking about the evidence I have gathered on people who are recovering and on therapies that have been proven to be useful. My information comes through interviews with people who are recovering. I also capture the wisdom of health care practitioners who have had great success in working with people with the symptoms of Parkinsons.

Interest in my research discoveries inspired me to create Pioneers of Recovery, a series of interview transcriptions with people who have been diagnosed with Parkinsons and who have found interesting ways to feel a lot better. The book and recordings also include interviews with health care practitioners who tell us their perspectives (and one comic!) on what helps people with Parkinsons. More information on *Pioneers of Recovery* is available by visiting:

http://www.pioneersofrecovery.com

Five Steps to Recovery

My research has clearly revealed there are many therapies, treatments and modalities that are helping people with the symptoms of Parkinsons feel better. I am personally curious about the underlying energy that feeds the symptoms and makes recovery challenging for some people. This debilitating energy comes in the forms of negative, low energy thoughts that obstruct the recovery process.

Thoughts are the most powerful force in the universe and will determine the final outcome of any healing process. I thus tackled the question – how can negative thought forms be transformed?

Pontificating on this question inspired me to write Five Steps to Recovery, a book and series of meditations which draw on the prevailing wisdom about how we manifest anything – health, wealth or happiness. I have translated all of the tried and true ideas of manifestation to the process of recovering from the symptoms of Parkinsons.

The work is available as a series of recorded meditations, a print book or a desktop book. For more information, visit

http://www.fivestepstorecovery.com

MEDITATIONS FOR PARKINSONS

I have recorded a series of meditations that were specifically created to help provide relief from stress and balance hormones naturally. Find more information on my meditation series at:

www.parkinsonsrecovery.info

Are you interested in learning how to meditate? Nancy Welch and I collaborated on a project to interview people who answered questions from persons who currently experience the symptoms of Parkinsons who were interested in learning how to meditate. Information about Nancy's book can be found by visiting:

http://www.medicinemeditation.com

TAI CHI

www.taichiwalking.com

www.taichifallsprevention.com

QiGong
http://www.chicenter.com

PHYSICAL THERAPY

www.parkinsonsmoveit.com

www.ohanapacificrehab.com

www.gigermdtherapy.com

DVDs
The When Less is More Health Video [VHS]

Move It: An Exercise and Movement Guide for Parkinson's Disease

Golden Motion - A Gentle Workout for the Young At Heart - Designed, Created, and Practiced on the Beautiful Island of Hawaii

NUTRITIONAL RESOURCES

Raw Food Diet - Dorit: www.serenityspaces.org

How to Reverse Depression and Anxiety - Kristen Allott, ND: www.dynamicpaths.com

© 2013 Parkinsons Recovery

Wahl's Diet: www.terrywahls.com

Nutritional Balancing - Larry Wilson: www.drlwilson.com

Connecting with Real Food: http://www.twotheroot.com

Coconut Recipes: The Coconut Lover's Cookbook

BOOKS
Laurie Mischley, Natural Therapies for Parkinson's

Donnie Yance, Parkinson's Disease and the Use of Botanical and Nutritional Compounds

Dorit, Celebrating Our Raw Nature: Plant Based Living Cuisine

Sandor Katz, Wild Fermentation

Roya Sayadi and Joel Herskowitz, Swallow Safely

Zhi Gang Sha, Soul, Mind Body Medicine

NATURAL MEDICINE
David Overton: www.natmeds.net/

Daniel Newman: www.rising-health.com

Dietrich K. Klinghardt: www.klinghardtacademy.com

Low Dose Naltrexone (LDN): www.ldnscience.org

DENTISTS
AMERICAN ACADEMY OF CRANIOFACIAL PAIN WWW.AACFP.ORG

Holistic Dental Association www.holisticdental.org

BOTANICAL FORMULATIONS AND MEDICINES

www.katesherbs.com

MUSIC THERAPY RESOURCES

www.innerharmonyhealthcenter.com

www.colostate.edu/depts/cbrm/

www.neurosong.com/index.php

THERAPY FOR EYE PROBLEMS AND CATARACTS

www.cataracts.parkinsonsrecovery.com

HYPNOTHERAPY

www.mindsighthypno.com

COLOR THERAPY

www.transformationaltools.com

ART THERAPY

www.jessielyle.com

HYDRATION THERAPY

www.aquas4life.com

VIBRATION THERAPY

www.vibrationtherapy.org

BIOACOUSTICS/VOCAL PROFILING

www.soundhealthoptions.com

CRANIOSACRAL THERAPISTS

www.IAHP.com/pages/search/index.php

BOWEN THERAPISTS

www.nsthealth.com

NEUROFEEDBACK

www.theconnectedself.com/index.php

COMPOUNDING PHARMACISTS

To locate a compounding pharmacist in your area, call 1-800-331-2498

COACHING

Bianca Molle: www.mettamorphix.com

© 2013 Parkinsons Recovery

Judith Lynne: www.partneringwithparkinsons.com

Holly Hughes: www.hollyhughes.info

Robert Rodgers: http://www.parkinsonsrecovery.us

Howard Shifke: www.fightingparkinsonsdrugfree.com

DANCE

www.pamelaquinn.net

www.brooklynparkinsongroup.com

www.danceforpd.org

www.salsaventura.nl

LAUGHTER YOGA

www.laughteryogawithgita.com

MEDITATION

Full Catastrophe Living

Every Day Zen: www.everydayzen.org

www.medicinemeditation.com

EMOTION CODE™

chichoices.com

ENERGY HEALERS

www.zeropointhealers.com

ESSENTIAL OILS

www.compassionateconsulting.net/

FELDENKRAIS™

www.feldenkrais.com/practitioners/find/

www.mindmoves.com

www.futurelifenow.com

Harmonic Healing

www.harmonichealing.com

DOCUMENTARIES ON PARKINSONS

Ride with Larry

BOOKS WRITTEN BY PEOPLE WITH PARKINSONS

John Bauman, Decide Success and Roadmap to Success

John Coleman, *Stop Parkin' and Start Livin'*

Whit Deschner, *Travels With A kayak*

Richard London, A Handbook for Life: A Practical Guide to Success and Happiness

Leif Ogard, *I Have Parkinsons but Parkinsons Does Not Have Me*

Phyllis Rogers, Over 40 and Gettin' Stronger

Karl Robb, A Soft Voice in a Noisy World

Anne Atkin, Living and Laughing with Parkinsons

BLOGS BY PERSONS DIAGNOSED WITH PARKINSON'S DISEASE

www.fightingparkinsonsdrugfree.blogspot.com

www.asoftvoice.com

www.biancaschichat.com

www.partneringwithparkinsons.blogspot.com

parkinsonsand5htp.blogspot.com

www.parkinsonstampabay.org

WEBSITES OF ARTISTS FEATURED IN ROAD TO RECOVERY

Alan Babbitt   http://www.abproductions.com

The photographic image on the book cover is by Alan Babbitt who was diagnosed with Parkinson¹s Disease in 2003. Alan's tremor is a unique and I might add essential asset to his "Tremor Enhanced" photographic work. Alan explains that his work has "broad appeal among movers and shakers of any kind - runners, dancers, nervous people, heavy coffee drinkers - really, anyone who moves or wants to be moved." Alan's images are a guiding inspiration to the spirit and intent of Road to Recovery.

Anne Davis   annepaints.shutterfly.com

Cindy Deluz   www.cindydeluz.com

Edwin Ferran   www.hap46st.com

                  www.facebook.com/video/video.php?v=102703349748869

Judith Giddings   www.edgeoftheforest.com/judith.htm

Carol McLeod   pwnkle.com

Mary Pauer   www.marypauer.com/MarysART.html

Michael Sawyer   www.michaelsawyerart.com

Peter Thompson   www.peterthompson.ca

INDEX

© 2013 Parkinsons Recovery

© 2013 **Parkinsons Recovery**

testosterone, **74**, **318**

tetrachloride, 98

the poor man's hula, **262**

Therapeutic Goods Administration, **235**

Therapeutic Touch, **245**

therapies, **18**, **19**, **22**, **25**, **34**, **42**, **55**, **57**, **58**, **59**, **60**, **72**, **74**, **81**, **84**, **94**, **135**, **136**, **137**, **138**, **140**, **141**, **149**, **155**, **172**, **189**, **245**, **246**, **248**, **253**, **287**, **317**, **325**, **328**, **331**, **337**, **342**

Thieves, **233**

thought forms, 19, 70, 129, 316, 342

thoughts, **19**, **38**, **39**, **52**, **63**, **64**, **65**, **66**, **68**, **69**, **70**, **71**, **82**, **83**, **84**, **85**, **129**, **130**, **137**, **141**, **142**, **149**, **150**, **162**, **189**, **209**, **210**, **292**, **315**, **316**, **334**, **335**, **342**

Thyromin, **232**

TMJ Disorder, 117, 339

Toby Christiansen, **137**

toxicity, **102**, **250**, **328**

toxin cleanses, **189**

toxins, **19**, **37**, **54**, **74**, **75**, **80**, **81**, **83**, **84**, **85**, **88**, **89**, **90**, **91**, **93**, **94**, **95**, **97**, **98**, **99**, **100**, **101**, **102**, **103**, **104**, **105**, **106**, **117**, **120**, **128**, **135**, **136**, **144**, **154**, **155**, **156**, **164**, **235**, **236**, **250**, **280**, **281**, **315**, **316**, **318**, **326**, **328**

Toxins, **81**, **89**, **91**, **93**, **94**, **97**, **98**, **100**, **105**, **140**, **154**, **189**, **237**, **328**

Training the Brain, 240

trampoline, **280**, **331**

trauma, **23**, **25**, **38**, **54**, **71**, **72**, **74**, **80**, **81**, **83**, **84**, **86**, **87**, **88**, **89**, **103**, **104**, **106**, **117**, **136**, **144**, **146**, **147**, **153**, **154**, **189**, **216**, **245**, **308**, **316**, **317**, **320**, **325**, **328**

Trauma, **81**, **83**, **86**, **103**, **144**, **146**, **189**

treatment, **20**, **21**, **35**, **53**, **56**, **57**, **58**, **74**, **137**, **139**, **145**, **154**, **163**, **191**, **203**, **214**, **224**, **225**, **235**, **249**, **256**, **280**, **283**, **284**, **287**, **325**, **327**, **330**, **341**

tremor, **72**, **80**, **173**, **201**, **203**, **282**, **283**, **284**, **285**, **313**, **314**, **316**, **348**

tremors, **45**, **71**, **72**, **224**, **233**, **283**, **284**, **285**, **305**, **316**, **318**

trichloroethylene, 93, 98

tripeptide, **174**

UDPRS, **202**

unconscious processes, **160**

Unified Disease Parkinson's Disease Rating Scale, **202**

University of Kentucky, **250**

University of Pittsburgh, **198**

unwinding, 23, 146, 152

Unwinding, **23**

urine, **102**, **129**, **167**, **273**

urine sample, 91

© 2013 Parkinsons Recovery

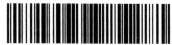

39199785R00205

Made in the USA
Middletown, DE
08 January 2017